Learning Redefined

Changing the Images that Guide the Process

Dennis R. Rader

Building Democracy

Press

Democracy has to be born anew in each generation
—and education is its midwife.

John Dewey

410 Conway Street—Suite 4
Frankfort, Kentucky 40601
606-627-2855
Hogsonice@yahoo.com
www.Learning-Redefined.com

Front Cover: "Sisyphus," by Titian

Back Cover: "Rainbow Way," by Judy Hart

Cover Design by Gumption

ISBN 978-0-578-03176-7

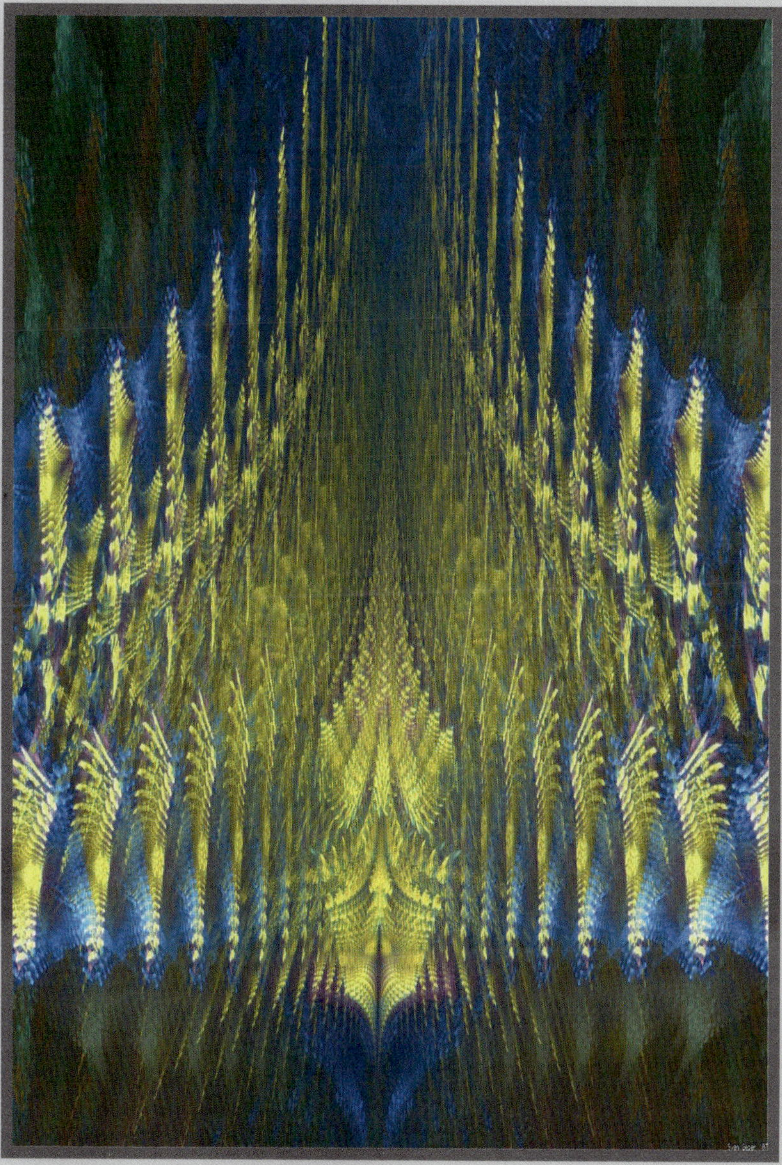

"The Road Ahead" by Sven Geier

When old words die out on the tongue, new melodies break forth from the heart; and where the old tracks are lost, new country is revealed with its wonders.

Rabindranath Tagore

Introduction

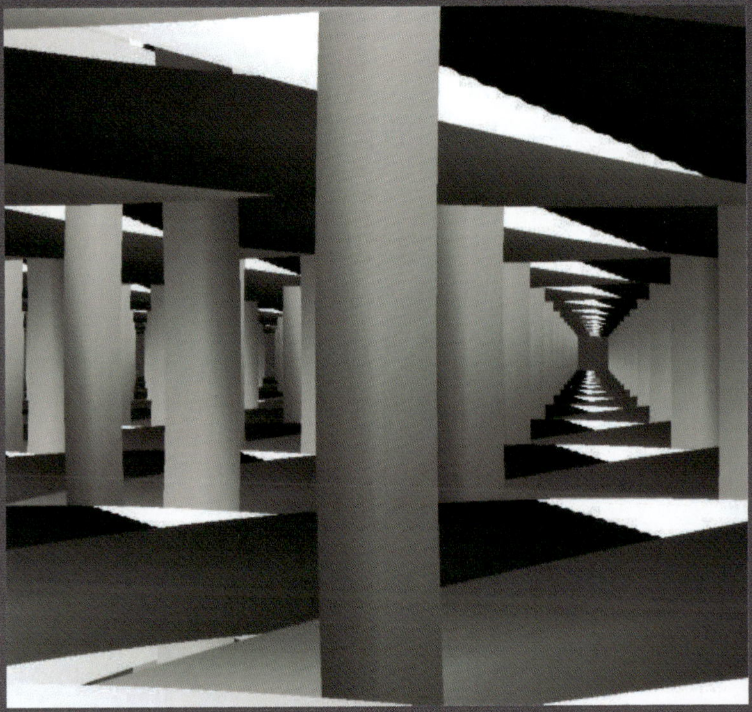

"Gallery of the Mind" by Ken Keller

If I were asked what has been the most powerful force in the making of history, you would probably adjudge me of unbalanced mind were I to answer, as I should have to answer, metaphor, figurative expression. It is by imagination that men have lived; imagination rules all of our lives. The human mind is not, as philosophers would have you think, a debating hall, but a picture gallery. Around it hang our similes, our concepts.

W. MacNeile Dixon

Image is everything; until we change our vision of a stimulus, to revision, which means to look at with "fresh eyes," our responding will not change. Worthwhile reform is not possible without revision. The metaphors harbored within our minds determine our methods and even our materials. The central picture—the **operating metaphor**—generates a constellation of supporting pictures. Until we change the operating metaphors guiding our behavior, we cannot reform (which, after all, means reshape) our methods.

The pictures in our mental galleries can free us—or they can trap us. Wisdom, in essence, is the capacity to perceive—and therefore escape—whatever entraps us. Do we have, or can we develop, the wisdom necessary for escaping our predicaments? The task is much harder when the problems are the systemic results of our own pictures, when they reside within our own beliefs and assumptions.

A helpful way to image the needed redefinition of learning is moving the educational process from a fixation on exercising and measuring the left-side of the human brain to more inclusion of practices that excite and inform the right brain. The left brain, however, is easier to feed since it deals with easy-to-measure things such as facts, sequences, and cause-to-effect connections. The right brain is harder to educate because it deals with hard-to-measure factors such as inspiration and pattern-recognition. The left brain loves text, the stringing together of words, or facts, or formulas; the right brain loves context, the big picture, the metaphors, the insights, and the understandings. (This is, of course, a simplification, but you get the picture.)

Daniel H. Pink, in his book, *A Whole New Mind: Why Right-Brainers will Rule the Future,* believes that the new economy of the Conceptual Age will call for increased capacity for right-brain thinking. He elaborates on the distinction between the two sides of the brain:

> The left converges on a single answer; the right diverges into a Gestalt. The left focuses on categories, the right on relationships. The left can grasp the details. But only the right hemisphere can see the big picture.

Pink's work is a call for a redefinition of learning, and thus teaching as well as schooling. It is also a call for a redefinition of how we put together books. This book incorporates pictures with words to help the left and right brains communicate with each other as the mind strives to construct a perspective, a comprehension, a wider image of the reality.

The challenges and opportunities of the emerging new economy demand a redefinition of learning. Otherwise, the educational process will be analogous to "fighting the last war." That would be particularly ironic, since the future is the business of education. We need a new Gestalt, one that pulls us out of our habitual convergence upon single answers, such as the current fixation on the easily measured exemplified by systemic stupidities such as No Child Left Behind. It is not just the categories—it is also the relationships.

The Newtonian Metaphor helps us see causalities while the Quantum Metaphor helps us see contingencies. The left brain resonates with the Newtonian Metaphor: There is a casual chain. We only have to ascertain the categories. The right brain prefers the Quantum World; it says that the Newtonian image may be true, but it is incomplete. It does not provide the prediction and control heretofore assumed. The Newtonian image is an inadequate explanation. We also have to comprehend the relationships, and that makes the world complicated indeed.

The left brain likes Newton and says, "If this—then that."

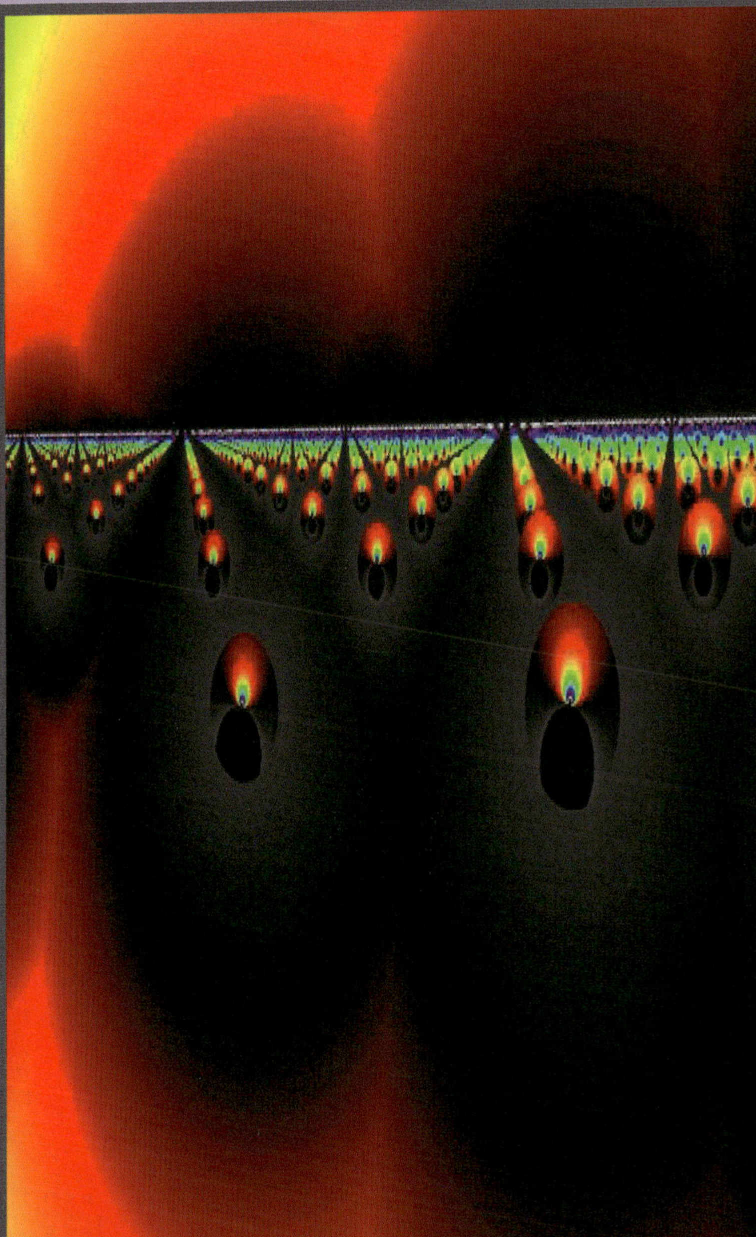

"Cue Ball Array" by Lynda Sweetman

The Quantum right brain loves the words of the poet Charles Olson:
"It's not either . . .or, but not only, but also . . . and also."

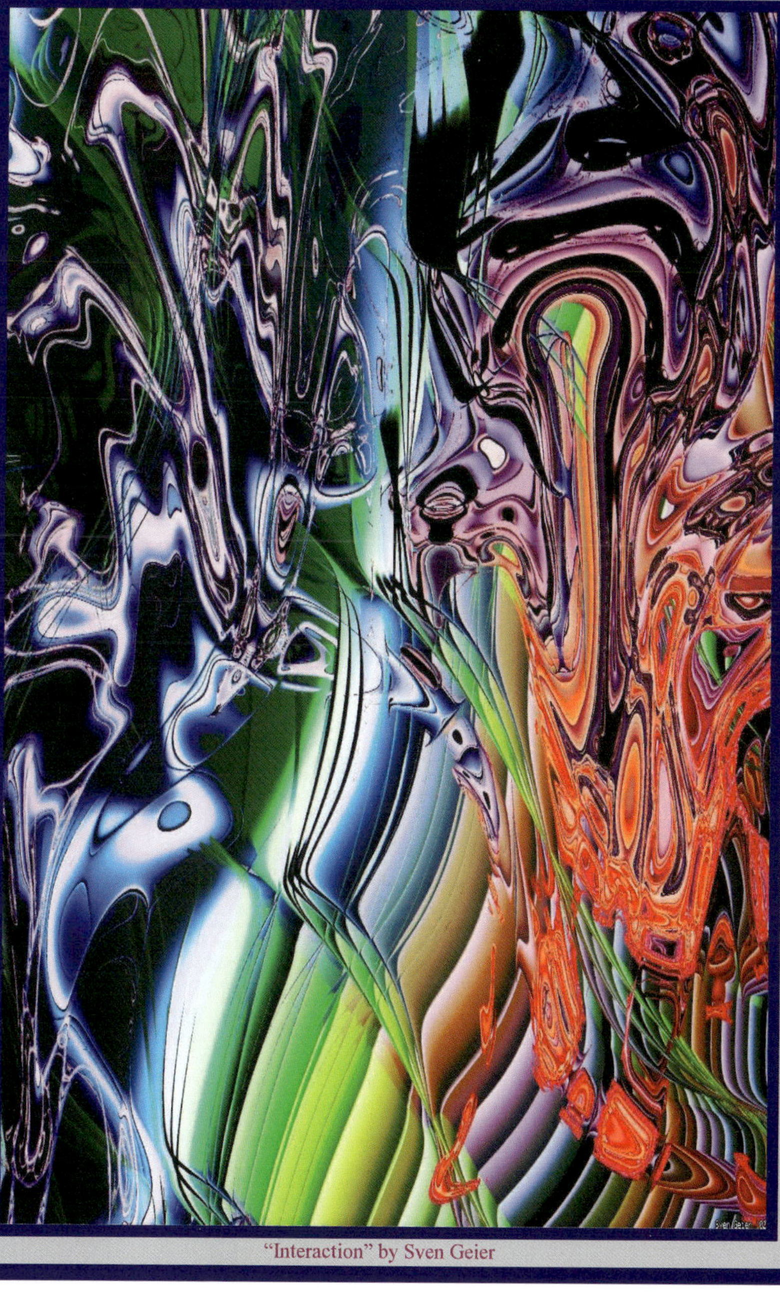

"Interaction" by Sven Geier

Both the Newtonian and Quantum images have something to say—but the complete picture lies in the application of both metaphors. There is causality, but there is also, always, contingency. The context of reality is forever unfolding. The world is dynamically complex. Causalities and contingencies continuously interact; they twirl and dance, submerge and emerge, and ebb and flow. Prediction and control is conditional, ephemeral, and often illusory.

We cannot throw out the word "learning." It is too big, too embedded in our language and culture. But we can redefine it. We can change the meanings of our words, their interpretations, their connotations, in order to reveal a new country with its wonders. The new sciences will help us in this endeavor, especially neuroscience and its insights into how the brain likes to learn.

This book attempts, through essay vignettes, pithy quotes, and brief stories, to inspire and inform conversation about how we define learning. The way we presently learn is challenged by the increasing dynamic complexity of the times. The image that worked in past decades, to some degree at least, will not suffice for tomorrow's predicaments and opportunities. Unless we redefine it, we will continue teaching in the same ways and learning the same lessons. We will therefore continue getting the same results.

Learning is who we are: we specialize in learning. Other animals can learn, but like the giraffe that has specialized in eating leaves high in the trees, we stand head and shoulders above all other learners. We have even evolved art, language, and culture to help us learn. How we define learning, then, is integral to the definition of ourselves. If our focus is the learning of duties, then we become duty-bound. If society has corralled our learning into the pursuit of fashion, then we become fashion-plates. If our focus is learning tribal connections, then we become parochial in our mindsets. Gossip, sports trivia, and worship of the famous can likewise fence-in the desire to learn. Learning is so much a part of our environment that, just as water is to fish, it is hard for us to envision it and realize its impacts upon our perception and thinking.

A worrisome concern for me as a college professor is the present definition of learning in the majority of my students. So many come to me with the attitude of "Just tell me what you want me to know." And they think they are being good students with that approach. After all, they have good grades to show for it. They have been taught by our educational system to be the passive recipients of transmitted knowledge. They don't understand that the democratic spirit within them has been crippled by their own schooling.

I fear this attitude of passive learning more than ordinary ignorance or incapability. Those can be dealt with much more easily. But the harbored image of learning as the passive reception of transferred information is scary. The image guides students to not think about what they are learning. Thinking, by the light of that guiding image, is not only unnecessary but disruptive. A nation of citizens who believe that learning is a passive activity, something akin to watching television, will not have a future as a democracy. Citizens who have the habit and capability of thinking for themselves are a necessary condition for the maintenance and development of democracy.

The teacher/author/scholar bell hooks, in her book, *Teaching to Transgress: Education as the Practice of Freedom,* writes:

> When I was a [college] student, I embraced any professor who wanted to create more progressive teaching practices. I still remember the excitement I felt when I took my first class where the teacher wanted to change how we sat, where we moved from sitting in rows to a circle where we could look at one another. That change forced us to recognize one another's presence. We couldn't sleepwalk our way to knowledge. Nowadays, there are times when students resist sitting in a circle. They devalue that shift, because fundamentally, they don't want to be participants.

By the time professor hooks gets her students, they have undergone at least twelve years of schooling dominated by a definition of learning that engrains passivity and irresponsibility. They don't want to participate because they have been taught by the system that participation is not only unnecessary, it is a bother. Participation—true engagement—disrupts curriculum design.

A fundamental reason for this book is that I have grown to dislike an increasing percentage of my college students. Don't get me wrong. I like them as people, and some I have grown to treasure, even love. But I don't like them as students. Only a few have impressed, excited, and inspired me. There have been moments of real learning and instances of individual successes—and semesters where classes jelled as learning communities. But on the whole, my students lack pizzazz, interestingness, and potential as learners. Where are the students fired with intrinsic motivation, with questions, not just about the syllabus, homework, and the damned tests, but about the subject? Where are the students imbued with dreams and therefore charged with the responsibilities to make them real? Not just students driven with desire to get a degree in order to get more status and make more money and therefore buy more stuff—but students who dream of learning, growing, and contributing. Where are the students who wish for understanding, who yearn for meaningful lives and wisdom? Why so many disinterested and disengaged students—present but not really involved? Where are the self-directed learners everyone seems to desire? The vast majority of students come to me dominated with one of two attitudes about learning: either resistance or compliance. Neither attitude is good.

What have we done? What will be the systemic results of the operating metaphors currently dominating educational practice in this country? What happens when people don't strive to reveal truths for themselves, who do not construct their own revelations—who wish to sleepwalk their way to knowledge? Many educators have noticed that our students lack critical thinking skills, so curriculum has been designed to remedy the problem. But the curriculum is itself handicapped by the present dominating definition of learning. How can a system that generates passive learning educate for critical thinking? The short answer is: it can't, because thinking is based on initiative; it is active, not passive.

All thinking can be considered critical, in that it perceives the significant in situations and makes adjustments accordingly. It is certainly not a mere collection of skills. It is both a habit and an emergent, holistic capability. Thinking is, most importantly, an action, a construction, a statement of interest, concern, and assertion on the part of the learner. It is the personal contribution of the learner to the learning. Passive learning therefore suppresses thinking, by systemically saying that thinking is both unnecessary and disruptive to the curriculum as designed and implemented. Our correct-answer schooling constantly says, "This is significant, so learn (memorize) it. There is no need to construct your own understanding, for that won't be tested, anyway." That is why our students lack critical thinking skills.

My syllabi point out that the only way a student can get an A in one of my courses is by creating a project germane to the subject that expresses and informs their initiative. They can attend every class, do all the homework, and ace every test, but without that project the highest grade they can get is a B. For me, the grade of A denotes excellence—which can only be achieved through personal interest and initiative, through individual contribution. Creativity is integral to excellence, especially in these dynamically complex times.

But our students have been taught otherwise. They have been taught a simplistic, passive definition of learning. They have been taught that simply studying is learning—though it is not. Learning, in the best sense of the word, occurs only through the engagement of interest, imagination, and initiative. Learning is a creative action on the part of the learner. It is not a reaction to the demands of either teachers or curricula. Students have been taught that memorizing is learning. It is not. Until an interpretation is developed and meaning constructed within the learner, learning has not occurred. The passive reception of transmitted data is not learning, though that is the prevailing image.

Information, the product of learning, is a personal action, a construction. Real learning is always a response—not a reaction—to the knowledge presented. It is a complicated, emergent phenomenon we can call response-ability, which is entwined with imagination, interest, and initiative. It is certainly not passive. But response-ability has been systematically ignored and discounted. Imagination, interest, and initiative have been systemically suppressed by a congested curriculum, incessantly lecturing teachers, and pervasive tests.

John Holt said, "The biggest enemy to learning is the constantly talking teacher." This is true, but teachers are compelled to lecture by the impacted curriculum and the almighty tests—by the present definition of learning. Acquiescence, not response-ability, is also desired in our teachers.

Passive learning is the prevailing image of the process in American society today. That image has systemic and pernicious effects that, left to molder and fester, will rot away our substance and potential. We have the task to redefine learning, to give it a more robust, individualistic, and, most importantly, active image. Learning is a personal construction or it is a hand-me-down. And people who become addicted to hand-outs will not have the initiative and integrity to fend for themselves. They will not be the citizens necessary for a democracy.

We need a serious and intense conversation in this country about our definition of learning. How does our schooling promote or degrade that definition? What are the systemic effects of that definition? Are those the results we truly want?

The nature of the process determines, to a great degree, the nature of the product. That product is nothing less than ourselves, our habits and capabilities, and, most importantly, our responsibilities. Students who do not perceive and understand the responsibility for their own learning will have that responsibility assumed by others. The students who come to me harboring the image of learning as the passive reception of teaching scare me because they are too easy to teach what some authority wants them to learn. But the democratic spirit is still alive and well within them. Most come around to the challenge to find and define themselves and what they care enough about to contribute, to themselves, to the subject, and to the rest of us. They want to engage their initiative and, ultimately, their responsibility—because they still believe in their uniqueness and that they have something special to contribute.

> Our socialistic philosophy of schooling—founded on the image of "scientific" prediction and control—hasn't killed our democratic spirit yet, but it has been working at it, daily, hundreds of days a year, in hundreds of thousands of classrooms across the land for many decades now.

Real learning is too fierce, too robust, too intense, too idiosyncratic, too passionate, too individualistic, and at the same time too dependent upon the synergistic effects of the learning community to be scientifically managed. (That is why we have fixated on educating for the left side of the brain and neglected the right side: to avoid the messiness and impose "scientific management" on the process, a problem we will return to). There are simply too many relevant conditions and contingencies in real learning. Real learning combines training, via the left brain, with initiative, the synergizing impacts of the right brain. Prediction and control machinations can only interfere with real learning—which they have systematically done.

Educating the right brain calls for more conversation, reflection, and projects in our schooling, for they weave learning into evolving intellects. Without them, imagination, interest, and initiative are neither respected nor informed, resulting in resistance or, worse, acceptance on the part of the learner. But those processes play havoc with the present design of schooling, which is fixated on the forced ingestion and assessment of easily-measured knowledge bits.

Imagination, interest, and initiative are generated by the right-brain. They are therefore too emotional and unpredictable—and too hard to measure—for the present definition of learning. That is why they have been ignored. But we should educate for the right-brain along with the left-brain. We need the synergistic impacts of imagination, interest, and initiative. Those factors increase our intelligence, capability, and wisdom. More importantly, they—because they tap into the power of the democratic spirit—excite and encourage personal ownership and responsibility.

If nothing else, such thinking will open up and enliven the debate about who we are, what we are doing, and what we will become. We are talking about nothing less than the mind's definition of itself and how that definition will evolve. Jonah Lehrer writes, in *Proust was a Neuroscientist:*

> The head holds a raucous parliament of cells that endlessly debate what sensations and feelings should *become* conscious. These neurons are distributed all across the brain, and their firing unfolds over time. This means that the mind is not a place: it is a process. As the influential philosopher Daniel Dennett wrote, our mind is made up "of multiple channels in which specialist circuits try, in parallel pandemoniums, to do their various things, creating Multiple Drafts as they go." What we call reality is merely the final draft. (Of course, the very next moment requires a whole new manuscript.) [Or picture.]

Our mind is indeed a debating hall, a head full of raucously-firing neurons—but the most important component of that debating hall is its picture gallery. Which images will we hang up and discuss and learn from? Which ones will we assign to the basement, and, eventually, the dustbin? Which ones do not even exist yet? Which ones can never exist, because the cultural conditions suppress them? What will be the images, the operating metaphors, we will choose to guide our perceptions and inform our actions?

The task to redefine learning, and through that process redefine teaching and schooling as well, will determine who we will become. Hopefully, the following quotes, stories, and essay vignettes will help us investigate the present image of learning. We need to take that picture down off the wall and look at it more carefully, to turn it this way and that in order to better understand its positive and negative effects. Then we can develop a more powerful definition of learning—one aligned with our democratic principles.

NOTE—The question arises: "How does one write a book with the right brain in mind?" That is why the design of this book incorporates features that require explanation: picture, color, rhythm, story, and conversation. The next five vignettes explain their contribution.

Picture

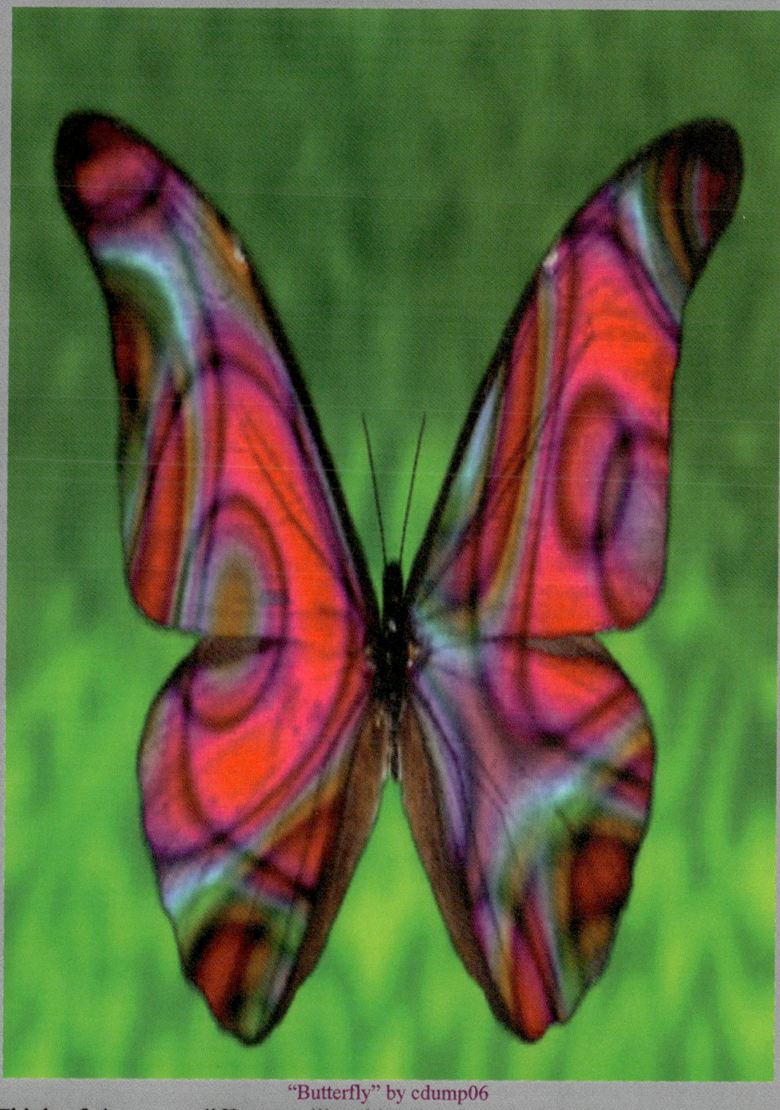

"Butterfly" by cdump06

Think of the . . . . difference like this: the right hemisphere is the picture; the left hemisphere is the thousand words.

Daniel H. Pink

Pictures add perspective as well as color to the work. They also change the rhythm; they lift the eyes, and thus the mind, from the march of the words, thus moving the brain from left to right. This affects the rhythm as the mind then flows back toward the left as it leaves the interpretation, appreciation, and/or puzzle of the picture. Pictures also prepare the mind for story as it strives to ascertain their meaning. They contribute to the conversation, if, for no other reason, by exciting the question, "Why did the author incorporate this image?"

I chose Titian's Sisyphus for the cover of this book because the educational process, as presently defined, is so often Sisyphean, the endless drudgery of pointless tasks. The picture is a clear and vivid statement of the problem. Every endeavor to fix a problem, as Einstein pointed out, ends up Sisyphean when approached by the same consciousness that created it. Granted, the boulder of ignorance, weakness, and incapability will always burden us, but must it be the same old boulder? Do we not progress onto the lifting of other, different boulders? Bottom line, the educated person should be more response-able. If not, all the effort, of both teachers and students, is Sisyphean. The front cover is a warning, a statement about the present situation, meant to bother the reader, at least on a subconscious level.

I chose the fractal "Rainbow Way" by Judy Hart for the back cover because rainbows are not only colorful but hopeful, for they indicate the coming of sunny skies. They also cover the whole spectrum of light, just as, hopefully, *Learning Redefined* will help open the whole spectrum of human capability. Hart's fractal intimates an explosion of potential. Also, Iris, the Rainbow Goddess, frequently carried messages to humans of her own initiative, in itself a great message. (We will return to Sisyphus and Iris.)

The image of the butterfly on the previous page prepares the mind for words about transformation, for it is a well-understood metaphor of moving from a cocoon (with all the connotations inherent within the context of that word/image) to a seemingly unpredictable change—a complete metamorphosis. The caterpillar in the cocoon cannot imagine its future, of course, but can we imagine ours? We think we can, or we can certainly try, but can we? Much can be said, implied, intimated, suggested, alluded to, and illustrated with a picture. The image of the butterfly says a lot to the attentive brain; it prepares us for better comprehension of the accompanying words. The butterfly says beauty, flightiness, transformation, and chaos—and it, like the rainbow, embodies hope. (We will return to the power of the butterfly.)

The butterfly is also an important image in chaos theory, for it represents the power of resonance (a positive feedback loop) within a dynamic system. In theory, a butterfly, despite its fragility, weakness, and flittiness, could cause, with one flap of a puny wing in Brazil, a hurricane in Texas.

James Gleick, in *Chaos: Making a New Science,* writes:

> The Butterfly Effect acquired a technical name: sensitive dependence on initial conditions. And sensitive dependence on initial conditions was not an altogether new notion. It had a place in folklore:
>
> ***For want of a nail, the shoe was lost;***
> ***For want of a shoe, the horse was lost;***
> ***For want of a horse, the rider was lost;***
> ***For want of a rider, a battle was lost;***
> ***For want of a battle, the kingdom was lost!***
>
> In science as in life, it is well known that a chain of events can have a point of crisis that could magnify small changes. But chaos meant that such points were everywhere. They were pervasive.

We don't like to image the world so contingent upon swirling, bubbling points of chaos; that reality disrupts our desire for prediction and order. But the reality of every moment rests upon the fragile substance of wind from distantly flapping butterfly wings. A metaphorical butterfly flapping a flimsy wing may have changed the history of the world. The ironically named "butterfly ballot" story is elaborated on by Daniel H. Pink in his book, *A Whole New Mind*:

> The nonpartisan investigation found that what decided the outcome in Palm Beach County—and therefore determined who would become leader of the free world—wasn't an evil Supreme Court or recalcitrant chads. It was bad design. The bewildering butterfly ballot confused thousands [out of millions} of voters and cost Gore the presidency, according to the professor who headed the project. "Voters' confusion with ballot instruction and design and voting machines appears to have changed the course of U.S. history."

Pictures also prepare the mind for the comprehension of metaphors, a right-brain capability. It can be argued that metaphorical perception is essential to intelligence, that, in fact, lack of metaphorical perception is blindness to those complexities beyond literal perception. A metaphor is a picture that illustrates the reality of something else entirely: knowledge that an iceberg is 90% underwater helped Freud perceive the subconscious mind. The physicist Robert Stetson Shaw says,

You don't see something until you have the right metaphor to let you perceive it.

This book depends upon metaphorical perception—for the real power of language is ultimately metaphorical. Language provides us with images, whether we realize them or not, for we are perceptual specialists. We have expanded the capabilities of our eyes with the power of our imagination to bring unseen realities "into sight," solidified but continuously developed over eons through ever-evolving language. The book utilizes logical arguments and stories, but the key concept is the operating metaphors that govern not only how we see ourselves but our world and our endeavors within it. What is our insight horizon, bearing in mind that "horizon" means the limit of what one can see?

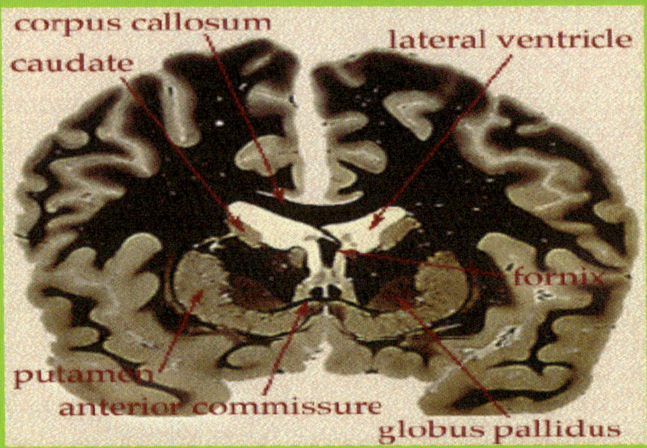

A key focus of Learning Redefined will be the *corpus callosum*, the thin bridge of nerve tissue that connects the brain's left and right hemispheres. It is where the words and the pictures interweave to evolve our perspectives and capabilities. Shouldn't education focus on thickening this thin bridge, certainly metaphorically, and perhaps even literally? It certainly should not be ignored. It should be an integral part of the educational picture.

Many of the images in this book are fractal art, for several reasons other than they are attractive, colorful, and intriguing: They challenge us to interpret them holistically. They exercise the right side of the brain as the mind strives to impose meaning on the image. Fractal art is also borne of complexity science and chaos theory, the new sciences that have contributed much to better understanding of how the brain operates.

Quantum physics teaches us that reality is not as stable and solid as we have presumed. The world is relational, emergent, and interactive, even at subatomic levels. Reality is not as easily knowable as we would like. It is not as predictable and controllable as we have assumed. Newtonian physics is not mistaken, but it is inadequate for comprehending and explaining interactive complexities. The physical world is dynamically complex all the way down to its simplest constituents. The social world is even more relational and interactive, resting on a rubble of unpredictable contingencies and emergent realities—chaos points.

That is why the philosopher Hubert Dreyfus says,

It is interpretation all the way down.

Science once considered the right brain stupid, mute, agraphic, dyslexic, word-deaf, and apraxic, incapable of higher cognitive function. This was the prevailing image only forty years ago. Psychologists and educators went along with this metaphor, of course, which accounts, to some degree, for why the right brain has been ignored in our schooling. The problem is that the action of interpreting depends upon the interaction of both sides of our brain. The right brain, it turns out, is not stupid at all; its functions were only beyond the measurement capability of science at that time. The left brain provides the necessary details but the right brain puts those details into perspective, giving us the whole picture.

Jonah Lehrer, in *Proust was a Neuroscientist,* writes:

> The most direct evidence of our diffuseness comes from the shape of the brain itself. Though the brain is enclosed by a single skull, it is actually made of two separate lumps (the left and right hemispheres), which are designed to disagree with each other.

In other words, not only outer realities but our inner realities, our identities, are subject to interpretation all the way down. W. MacNeile Dixon is correct—the mind is less of a debating hall than it is a picture gallery. We are governed more by the metaphors we can grasp and choose to harbor than we are by the logic of particular situations. The picture comes first; debate only fills in the details. What we see is dictated from the top down. The mind governs what the brain and the eyes see. Interpretation determines perception more than the other way around. That is why our operating metaphors are so powerful; they determine what we see and thus do. Interpretations transcend perceptions. Experience, after all, is our interpretations of events. We can return to the importance of philosophy here, in its purest meaning, the love of wisdom. True wisdom has more to do with our metaphors than our logical conclusions, than even our supposed experiments, since they were predominantly mere debating points mustered to support a hidden metaphor. The metaphors beget the methods which in turn beget the materials. Since this is the case, the wise thing to do is watch our metaphors with an imaginative and critical eye, for they are us.

We are blind to our operating metaphors because they are so essential to us. We recognize and question them at the peril of confusion, befuddlement, and inability to act. We ignore and do not question them at the peril of fundamentalist certainties, unearned clarities, and inability to consider. But, since the mind is more of a picture gallery than a debating hall, we must accept that, if we are to control our actions, to author ourselves, then we must be aware of and comprehend how our metaphors guide our methods of perception and action.

The new cosmic reality portrayed by quantum physics informs us that the world is full of relationships. And the meaning of those relationships has to be interpreted. Simplistic cause-to-effect connections do not exist in reality, only in theory. The world, both physically and socially, is dynamically complex. The left brain is Newtonian—the right brain is Quantum. We need both working in tandem in order to grasp, analyze, synthesize, and interpret the world—and ourselves. We need the words, and we need the pictures.

> The imagination is a necessary ingredient of perception itself.
>
> Immanuel Kant

Color

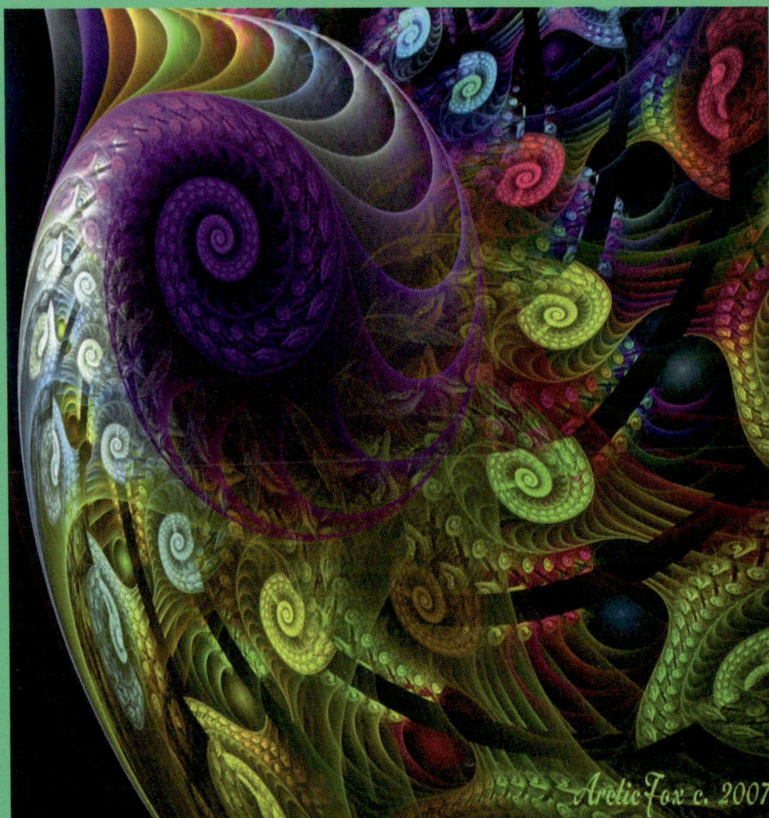

"Peacock" by Artic Fox

Neuroscientists are now confirming in the laboratory what the Egyptian, Buddhist, Mayan, Chinese, and medieval European illuminators knew all along: **Colorful visuals are a powerful stimulus to learning.** Neuroscientists have found that when we read in black and white, many regions of our brains—such as those that process color, form, motion, orientation, and position—are effectively shut down, put in sleep mode (Zeki, 1999). The most effective learning strategies motivate readers by **activating** their emotions (LeDoux, 2003). Adding color and design to our literature is a way of activating these emotions in different areas of the brain (Zeki, 1999).

Valerie Ruth Kirschenbaum

Few animals have color perception. The vast majority see only grays or limp sepia-like tones. Color perception is important to us for evolutionary reasons: they alerted us to dangers and opportunities, for they helped us spot predators and find fruits. Perhaps that is why they came to have emotional impact.

We have ignored this truth for the simple reason that we had no choice; the printing world could only work, feasibly, in black and white. Recent technical advancements help us escape that impediment. Learning Redefined heeds the advice of neuroscientists that the most effective learning strategies motivate by **activating** the emotions. Emotions, such as interest, are essential to the emergence of imagination and initiative—to constructive, worthwhile learning. That is why I have incorporated color—as well as design—whenever possible.

A Cautionary Thought

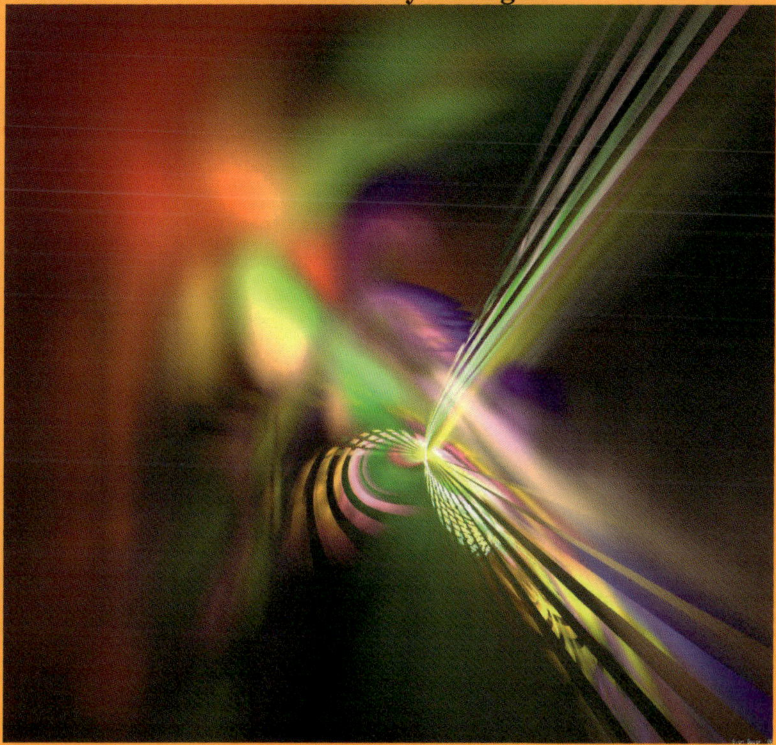

"Prismatic" by Sven Geier

Our schools, I believe, are not ineffective because they do not know what happens at synapses or the chemistry of neurotransmitters, but rather they have yet to address the brain as the organ for learning, and to fit instruction and environment to the "shape" of the brain as it is now increasingly understood.

Leslie A. Hart

Rhythm

The Rhythm Method

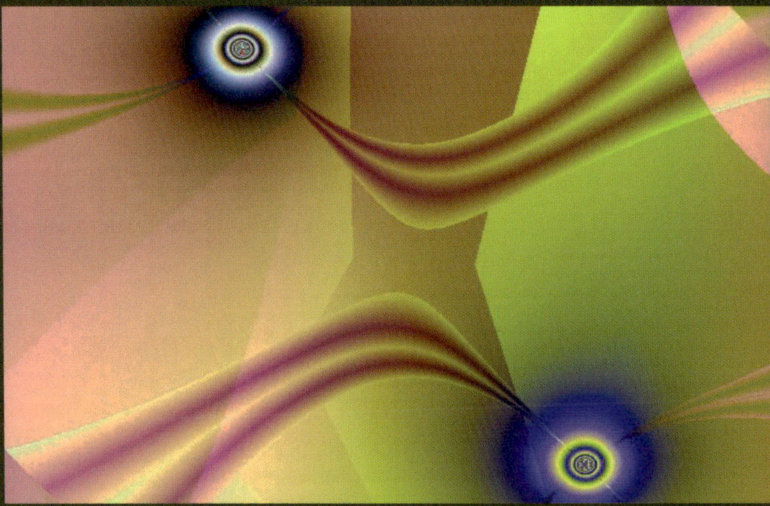

"YinYang" by Alex Thomas

Studies on how the brain best likes to learn validates the philosopher Suzanne Langer's understanding of rhythm, which is, in essence: "Rhythm is not the regular occurrence of an event [like the steady beat of a hammer on a nail]—but a period of tension begetting a period of resolution which in turn begets another period of tension, and so on." This book therefore moves from pithy quotes to essay vignettes to the occasional story. It utilizes short sections instead of chapters. It is not an exhaustive investigation but a let's turn it this way and that approach: diverging facets in search of a converging perspective.

Successful teachers understand that human learning is rhythmic. Ignoring or fighting that rhythm is counterproductive: the students disengage from the process. Once the brain disengages, either in boredom or resistance, inertia carries it further away from the hopes and designs of the teacher. Learning occurs in an interactive, dynamic balance between attention and relaxation. Rhythm also affects writing: novels are getting shorter; the graphic novel is exploding in popularity; and the long; thoughtful letters of yesteryear are replaced by short, succinct, grammatically unkempt emails. The attention span of young people in particular, but readers in general, continually shrinks. Movies and TV are getting "jumpier." The temporal distance between tension and resolution and tension again is getting shorter and shorter.

Who knows whether this shrinking of the attention span is good or bad? It just is. Perhaps this is natural in an increasingly dynamically complex world. We can only hope that sustained focus is possible whenever necessary. Years ago my father taught me how to be a good hunter. Don't go through the woods focused on looking for deer. Be quiet, be attentive, but enjoy the walk while attuned to anomalies, the sudden quiet of birds, the flicker of an ear, the snap of a twig, the color out of place. The best hunters are right brain thinkers. Their attention span skips from here to there, looking for the unusual, for the interesting, for the hint of something important. The farmer cannot allow his attention to wander, for suddenly he is plowing his wife's flower bed. He must stay within the furrows of his plan. But the good hunter has ADD, with a heightened sensitivity to the interesting, the better to find the out-of-the-box significant.

A consistent theme in this book is the tension between initiative and training. Training is less mindful of rhythm than initiative. Training likes to push while initiative thrives in a different environment. Learning redefined will incorporate the wisdom of neuroscientists in the use of rhythm. It is more research-driven than the present definition of learning, which harbors a paradigm [of prediction and control] that resists scientific findings questioning that image. Programmed instruction perceives learning to be a continuous process. It is assumed that, with the right techniques of manipulation and instruction, the learning process can be made constant. That is why educationists with programmed instruction mindsets do not hesitate to eradicate "unnecessary peripherals" such as art, music, and physical education, and even recess periods.

Richard Saul Wurman, in his book, *Information Anxiety*, comments:

> A widely held myth, fostered by the regimen of school, is that people should learn continuously. But when do people really learn? We learn at moments rather than continuously, and it's the acceptance of moments of learning that allows you to make full use of them. If you believe you're supposed to learn continuously and you don't continuously learn, then you'll be full of anxiety and guilt. You'll be distracted from learning because you're too busy worrying about *not* learning.

Learning—that has lasting nutritional value—occurs during moments of conversation and reflection. It is not continual but rhythmic. The present definition of learning wrongly pictures learning as a steady, continuous process. Students, sitting in their classrooms listening to the drone of teachers imparting the curriculum know they are rarely if ever learning anything worthwhile. They then either feel anxious about not doing what it seems they are supposed to be doing or they resent the environment of pernicious and constant invalidation.

I once observed a teacher of the year in her large, metropolitan district hammer instructively at her fourth-grade students for three straight days. She did it nicely, with hugs and candy and well-articulated lesson plans. She obviously cared for her children; they loved her and worked hard. The present definition of learning considered her the best teacher practitioner out of many thousands. But what were the systemic effects of her constant though velvet hammering? Where were the opportunities for initiative instead of more training, for intrinsic rather than extrinsic motivation? After three days I had to leave to attend to other projects. And to be honest, I wanted to leave; three days was enough for me. Where were the opportunities for either reflection or conversation? The curriculum called for discussions—but they were nothing more than periods of knowledge-bit regurgitation. There was no rhythm to her teaching, and I wonder and worry about the long-time ramifications. How much anxiety and guilt swirled around in the minds of those little children? There was joy in pleasing the teacher—but what was happening to the joy of learning? Can there be the sheer joy of learning for its own sake without personal initiative and intrinsic motivation?

An ecological perspective of the learning process recognizes rhythm. Learning is not constant. Conditions can be established and maintained that increase occasions of learning. But an instance of learning is something that periodically emerges from the interaction of such variables as knowing, thinking, interest, and initiative. Constant pushing only invites resistance and resentment, or worse, passivity.

The future asks an important question: which party really has Attention Deficit Disorder, individual students with over-stimulated minds or schooling with its under-stimulating addiction to the uninteresting? I suspect social evolution will find the latter guilty of ADD—with its fixation on decontextualized but easily transmitted and assessed data bits. Future historians will wonder how we could categorize so many of our students unable to adjust to the "assumed to be natural" rhythm of learning dictated by the present-day definition. The real attention deficiency is within the system itself. We have failed to pay attention to what really matters and how the brain really learns.

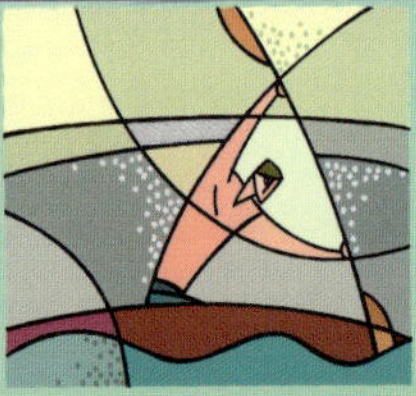

We operate in our schools as if teaching and learning should occur continuously. We should know better. We should understand that there is a rhythm to learning, just like any human endeavor. Real learning, common sense and personal experience tell us, depends upon periods of "mull and muck." We mull over an idea with reflection; we muck around with it through conversation. The presentation of an idea provides the tension; mulling and mucking provide the resolution. When we remove opportunities for conversation/reflection-driven as well as project-based learning, such as the arts, from our schooling, we prevent the necessary mulling and mucking. Room must be provided for interest and understanding to flower, and for comprehension and initiative to find avenues for expression. Otherwise, the learning is without rhythm—or life.

Story

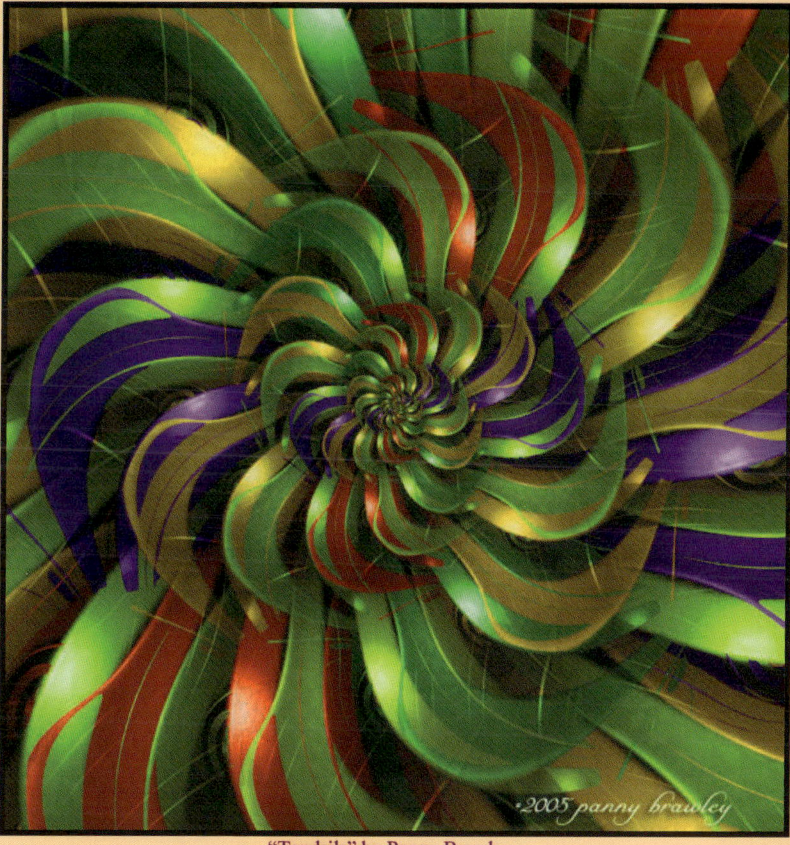

"Tendrils" by Panny Brawley

Stories are "more true" than facts because stories are multidimensional. Truth with a capital "T" has many layers. Truths like justice or integrity are too complex to be expressed in a law, a statistic, or a fact. Facts need the context of when, who, and where to become Truths. A story incorporates when and who—lasting minutes or generations and narrating an event or series of events with character(s), actions, and consequences. It occurs in a place or places that give us a where.

Annette Simmons

Stories can investigate realities that are far more complex and dynamic than simplistic knowing can handle. Their multidimensionality helps us perceive contingency and context. They are at the heart of true literacy regarding any subject. The ability to read fully, with in-depth interpretation and comprehension, depends upon awareness of story. With story, we can move toward the capacity for critical thinking, the capacity to perceive the significant in situations. Annette Simmons, in *The Story Factor: Inspiration, Influence, and Persuasion through the Art of Storytelling,* writes:

> Even if a story is not literally true, it is a very good representation of what is True because it can weave the relational aspects of facts with space, time, and values. Story can hold the complexities of conflict and paradox.

Story provides the framework for contextual awareness, for perception and understanding of relational factors. When we know the story, we see and comprehend the previously hidden or misinterpreted. Story carries us on the magic carpet of metaphor to new perspectives about our problems and new possibilities for products to fashion. Story awareness expands emotional intelligence, sometimes exponentially. Story is at the heart of emotional intelligence because unless we know the story, "we don't get it." Without story awareness, we are "clueless." We are therefore blind to the situational realities. Without story, we can neither find nor forge the pattern of situations. We cannot construct meaning. Without knowing the story, we cannot author ourselves, or our circumstances.

Stories can excite, inform, expand, and parameter conversation. They indicate the movement of a dynamically complex process, the exploration of understandings and meanings in an ongoing dialogue. Stories provide a sense of community, a cohering feeling of shared concerns, values, and investigations. Stories give listeners opportunities for understanding and resonance—and for clarification and dissonance. Stories develop the emotional intelligence of organizations, whether they are sports teams, corporations, political entities, or classrooms and schools: What are the stories that resonate enough to become part of history, or serve as indicators of the envisioned future?

Stories indicate the life—its health or lack thereof—of organizations. Are the stories told and retold negative or positive? (How many teachers have been made—or undone—by even one story?) Do the stories encourage exploration and conversation, or suppress them? Are they inclusive or exclusive? Do they nourish community, or fracture cohesion? Stories always indicate the truth of often immeasurable realities, the history, vitality, and potential of relationships.

As learning is redefined, the importance of emotional intelligence will be increasingly stressed. The work of Daniel Goleman and others has pointed out that the capacity to solve problems and fashion products has much to do with the emotional factors of intelligence. Intelligence is a lot more complicated than our curriculum and our tests have heretofore perceived. An effective approach to increasing emotional intelligence is *hearing and telling stories* that are rich in examples, symbolism, metaphors, and inspiration. Stories are not as concise and direct as abstract principles or fact statements, but they are richer in content and, most importantly, context. They are important for dealing with ambiguities, which is especially relevant in turbulent times.

Stories also speak to the "heart" in a way that nothing else can. They invite participation in thinking and understanding whereas abstract principles and fact statements frequently condone passive knowing at best. Stories invite feelings, for they have less fear of their murkiness. They are more likely to inspire learners through the provision of insights and understandings.

People ignorant of the story are, in effect, illiterate in the situation. Facts cannot be accumulated to the point where they indicate either the content or the context of the whole. They can help but cannot provide interpretation. Literacy in any endeavor means to be able "to read the situation." Story is the best way to excite, inform, and encourage literacy of any kind. Story is at the core of interpretation. Stories, like analogies, help us see the hidden, the hidden beneath the delusion of denial and the confusion of context and complexity. Their power is metaphorical: stories carry our imaginations into different realities, frequently forging pathways of understanding in the process. They are often closer to the truth than any single fact or strand of facts.

A Key Concern: Initiative, the contribution of self, is at the heart of active learning, for it comprises the wings of imagination, the shape and substance of personal responsibility, and the bricks of integrity. Without initiative, we are passive learners. We will acquiesce rather than imagine, copy rather than invent, deflect rather than assume responsibility, and slide into sleaze and weakness rather than forge integrity and strength.

But initiative is a puzzle. Where does it come from? What are the sources of gumption, resourcefulness, uniqueness, pluck, enterprise, self-reliance, and individuality—the desire to self define and author oneself? Why do some people have it in spades, and others retreat into passivity and victimhood? Why does initiative sometimes contribute to society, and at other times is self-centered, only concerned with self contributing to self? Can we educate for initiative? Can we help people express and establish their best selves through the exercise of their initiative? Stories help us figure out the puzzle of initiative and its ecological relevance to the educational process. Literature has never forgotten the importance of initiative. Every novel, and most short stories and movie scripts, is a study of initiative and, ultimately, integrity. What is the self and what does it have to offer, and will it manage to make that offer, are the recurring themes of literature. In the final analysis, literature consistently says to the reader, "You only have it in you if you have it within you to get it out."

This is the interface between literature and initiative, and why I have mixed short scenarios with educational considerations. Stories synergize reflection—and conversation.

Conversation

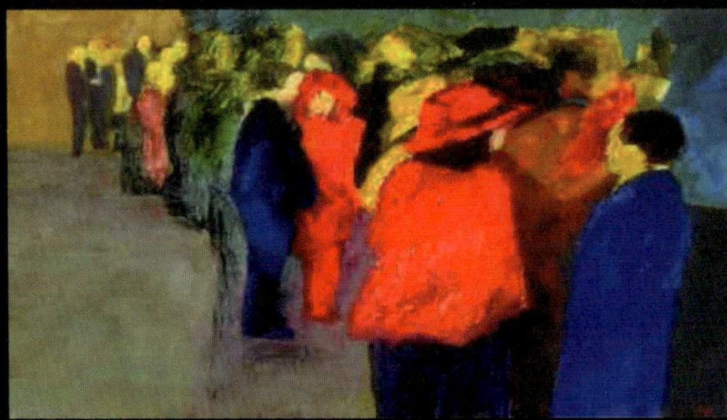

"Conversation" by Piet Noest. Visit www.galeriaaniela.com.au

The success of conversation consists less in being witty than in bringing out wit in others; the man who leaves after talking with you, pleased with himself and his own wit, is perfectly pleased with you.

La Bruyere

Formal education, up to this point, has been dominated by the image of presentation. Teachers present the material, hopefully with some wit, and students take notes and regurgitate the "acquired" information at test time. Discipline, of course, consists of paying sufficient attention to the presenter in order to get the information. Teachers, in turn, attend college classrooms and in-service workshops dominated by presenters doing the same thing to them. The result of all this presentation is, in theory, education.

Research into how the brain learns says for us to rethink the image of presentation. Presentation is, of course, necessary in some cases. But it is not how the brain likes to learn. It prefers projects, stories, reflections, and conversations. We need to replace the image of presentation with that of conversation, within which stories are an integral part, and that hopefully occur in the process of working on projects.

What does conversation do?

A conversation must carry either the actuality or the potential of growth. Otherwise, the interaction is merely discussion at best, or worse, noise. Conversation contains dialogue, the exchange of understandings and meanings in the endeavor to construct better information. Conversation is inclusive, for it encourages and nourishes individual voice as it develops a community of vision. Conversation helps us find the "turning points" necessary for the life of the mind.

Conversations encourage, carry, and increase truth. Truth improves personal and organizational capability, especially in dynamically complex situations. Truth constructs meanings that are strongly (though flexibly) moored to reality. The flexibility is necessary because situations constantly change. Conversation increases personal and organizational intelligence.

Conversations can be intrapersonal as well as interpersonal. Reflection is an internal conversation about a concern, problem, or project.

A conversation is a kind of project, sometimes without a given agenda, or at least without stultifying guidelines. It is a project dedicated, perhaps subconsciously, to building awareness, comprehension, understanding, and capability, characterized by mutual trust, lack of fear, and engaged desire for contribution.

Conversations excite and inform. They generate reflection and inspiration. Most importantly, they exist within an environment characterized by trust and respect, where learners are encouraged to participate in their own learning. Ownership, community, and self-directed, life-long learners will emerge when the image of conversation controls the process rather than the image of presentation.

Conversations turn the ongoing dialogue this way and that. There may be a theme, and in the case of schooling and writing, there must be a theme. But there are also opportunities for rhythm and diversion, for breaks in the routine, for lifting of noses off the grindstone, for the humorous refreshments. The turning can come from either teachers or students—depending on their imagination, interest, and initiative. The turning is fundamental to the nature of true conversation, which is etymologically based on the concept of turn, as in convert, conversely, or convertible.

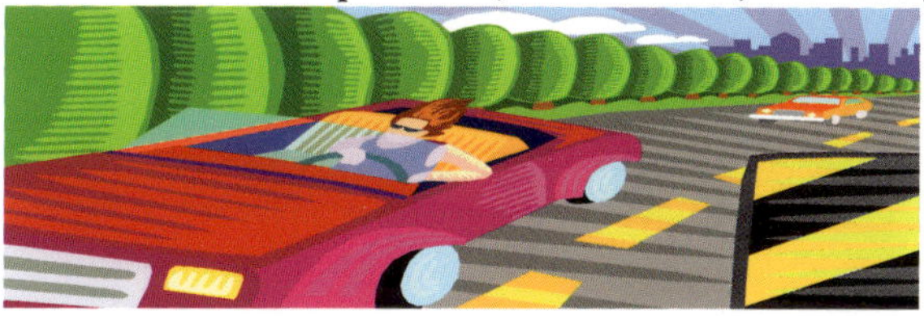

Conversation is integral to the construction of information—the New Productivity. An educational process that fails to prepare students for conversation is failing to prepare them for productive employment. Conversation requires emotional intelligence, and capacities such as the ability to think reflectively, spontaneously, and predictively. Schooling that neglects empathetic and creative imagination, vigorous and responsible initiative, and the give and take of conversation is failing to prepare students for the New Productivity.

Conversation is brain-based learning. The brain dislikes lecture and deals with it through resistance, resentment, subterfuge, and passive

> learning. The human brain prefers projects, where learners construct something perceived by them as meaningful. This includes conversation—the place where awareness and understanding are constructed. Conversation is necessary for worthwhile learning.
>
> Conversation is, by definition, an antidote to in-the-box thinking for it frees imagination, interest, initiative, and, we should add, integrity, to "turn" the flow of attention and interpretation wherever challenges and possibilities dictate.
>
> Conversation is therefore a self-correcting process promoting systemic change—for it revises the images guiding interpretation and direction and reshapes the conditions affecting development and productivity.
>
> Conversations bring out the wit in others while presentations merely display the wit—or lack—of the presenters. Leaders help others develop their wits.* (Remember: teaching is a leadership position.)
>
> Conversation is what we have evolved to blend and synergize the capabilities of the left and right brains. It strengthens the corpus callosum. It is where logic and intuition interweave, where facts and imagination dance.
>
> Most importantly, the habit of and capability for conversation is essential for the transmission and nourishment of the democratic spirit.

The image of conversation has guided, to the degree possible, the design of this book. Each vignette says, in effect, let's turn the investigation and look at it this way for a moment. Readers are encouraged to turn the pages this way and that until something engages their imagination, interest, or initiative. The value underlying this approach is that it is more important to think than it is to know. Both are necessary, but presentation is all about knowing while conversation is all about thinking. The image of a linear presentation, through the advance of some logical argument, is a secondary concern. The hope is to excite thoughtful engagement rather than provide training—to provide opportunities for resonance or dissonance, reflection or deflection, consideration or rejection.

*According to *Brewer's Dictionary of Phrase and Fable*, edited by Ivor H. Evans, there are only five wits: the first of which is common sense; the others are imagination, fantasy, estimation, and memory. Wit means understanding—from the old English *witan*, to know. So, the expression, "to keep your wits about you," means to maintain a firm grasp of your common sense, imagination, fantasy, estimation (or judgment), and memory. If you can manage that, then you can maintain self-possession despite the attempts of any situation to disconcert you. **Only five to keep track of?—should be easy.** Present schooling is fixated on the wit of memory, however, distilling it to a lethal dose. Schooling that had increased concern for common sense, imagination, fantasy, and judgment would generate an explosion of excitement and potential.

Learning Redefined

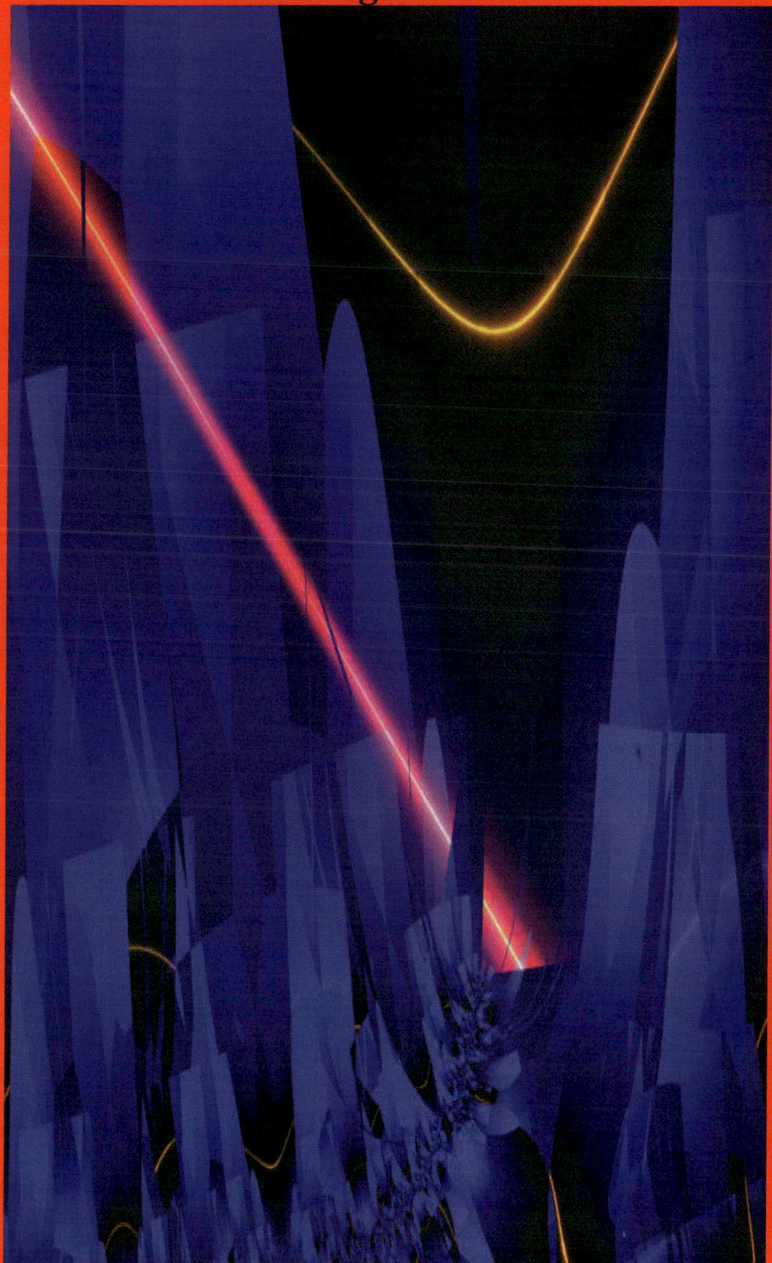

"Searchlight" by Vicky Brago-Mitchell

—1—

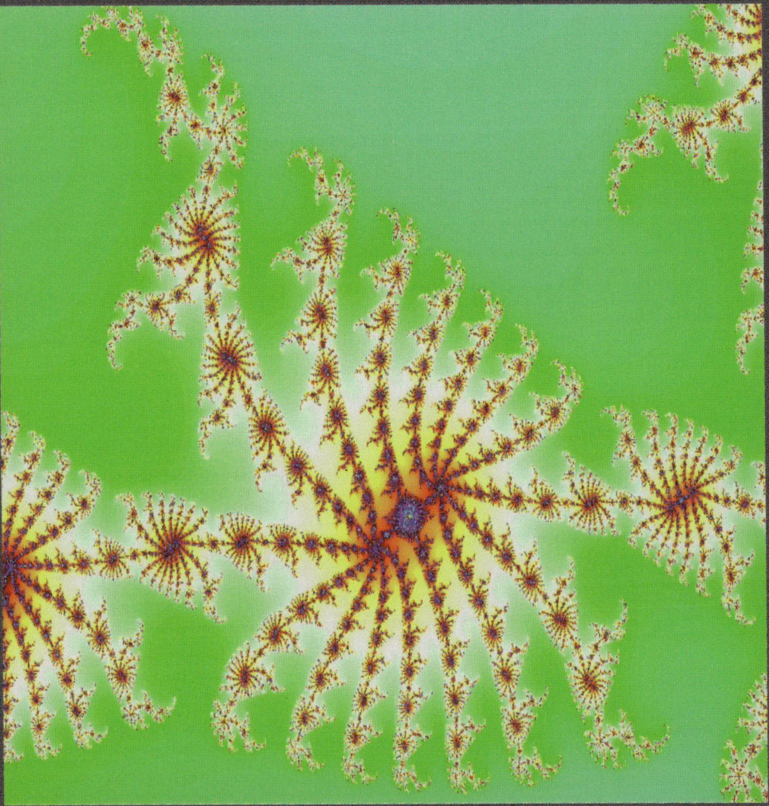

"Dancers" by Kevin Atkinson

Uncovering strongly held assumptions, beliefs, and values that shape action may be difficult and painful, but also powerfully catalytic. People able to see how their actions are shaped by their views—leading often to unwanted results, often wholly contradictory to their intentions—learn from that experience. While it is not always easy for people to change their beliefs or actions, the first step is to recognize their existence.

Victoria J. Marsick

Language, which not only houses our thoughts but even the potential of our thoughts, in essence consists of dead and living metaphors. Metaphorical perception allows us to understand the nature of one reality by using the perception of a dissimilar reality to provide the necessary light. As mentioned earlier, a condition for Freud's theory of the subconscious was the personally and culturally held realization that ninety percent of an iceberg was submerged. George Lakoff and Mark Johnson, in *Metaphors We Live By*, comment:

> The concepts that govern our thought are not just matters of the intellect. They also govern our everyday functioning, down to the most mundane details. Our concepts structure what we perceive, how we get around in the world, and how we relate to other people. Our conceptual system thus plays a central role in defining our everyday realities. . . But our conceptual system is not something we are normally aware of. In most of the little things we do every day, we simply think and act more or less automatically along certain lines. Just what these lines are is by no means obvious.

Everyday practice depends upon the prevailing philosophical perspective; a truth that most people rarely consider. Value-decisions therefore permeate our behavior, whether we are aware of them or not. Values affect our assumptions about how we deal with the world, whether we had any part in their construction or not. This is necessary; we can't invest the consideration required to place value on everything. But our approval is nonetheless placed, even if it is tacit or ignorant. As the economist Lord Keynes pointed out, underneath whatever dominant theory governs our present economic behavior lie the value-decisions of dead economists. Beneath those value-decisions rests a centralizing vision, one that coheres the threads of the theory into a meaningful pattern. Sometimes we stand on the shoulders of giants, but other times we depend upon intellectual midgets or emotional misanthropes, and sometimes even ghosts. The validity of that central vision may have been inaccurate to begin with or it may have outlived its usefulness. But it nonetheless governs everyday practice until the costs of its guidance generate either enough aggravation for fundamental change or result in an economic collapse.

Victoria J. Marsick, in her article, "Transformative Learning," discusses the work of Jack Mezirow on how we change our fundamental perspectives:

> Mezirow's theory revolves around the realization that adults filter all of their experience through "frames of reference that define their life world." These structures of assumptions . . . selectively shape and delimit expectations, perceptions, cognition, and feelings . . . (and) set our "line of action." Frames of reference are broad, comprehensive "habits of mind: that show up in different situations as specific "points of view" that shape interpretation of a specific event. Habits of mind and points of view can be psychological, political, social, cultural, economic, or epistemological.

Our interpretations guide our perceptions more than vice-versa. Debates rarely change the images the guide our behavior. Reflections and conversations are better at changing the operating metaphors guiding our methods and materials. Debates are effective only to the degree that they excite and inform conversation, remembering that reflection is a conversation with oneself. Without conversation and/or reflection, the operating metaphors are hidden and thus unchangeable.

A Cautionary Exchange

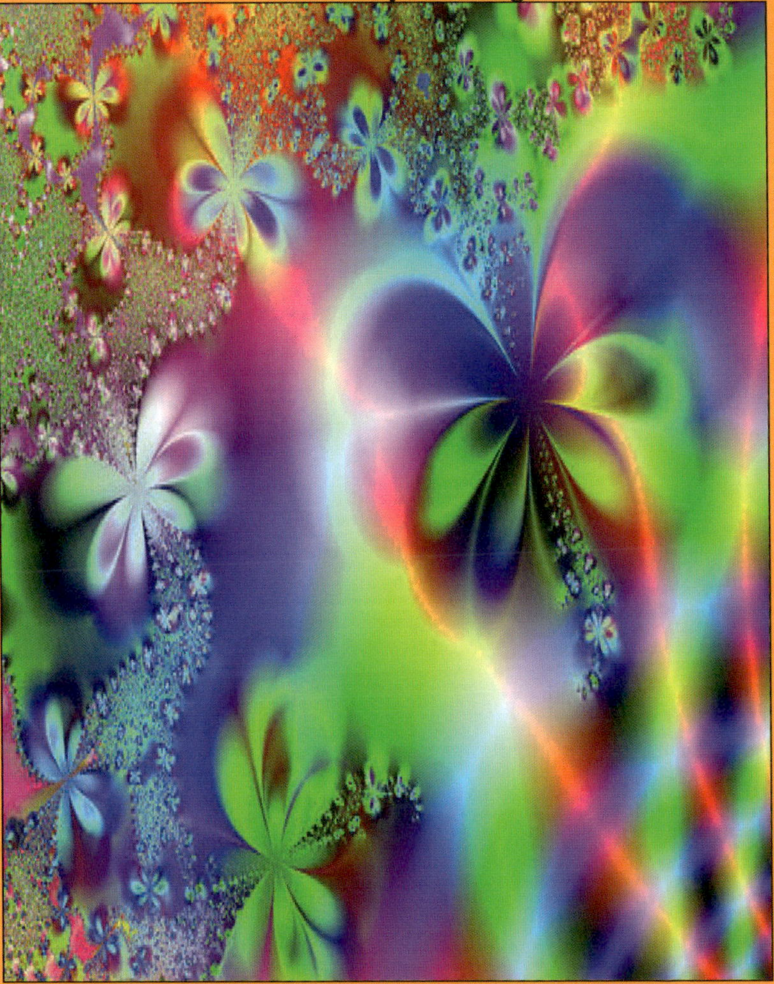

"Fractal Flies" from flickr.com/photos/18602777@N00/917312501/

"Oh, they're there, all right," Orr had assured him about the flies in Appleby's eyes after Yossarian's fist fight with Appleby in the officers' club, "although he probably doesn't even know it. That's why he can't see things as they really are."

"How come he doesn't know it?' inquired Yossarian.

"Because he's got flies in his eyes," Orr explained with exaggerated patience. "How can he see he's got flies in his eyes if he's got flies in his eyes?"

Joseph Heller, in *Catch 22*

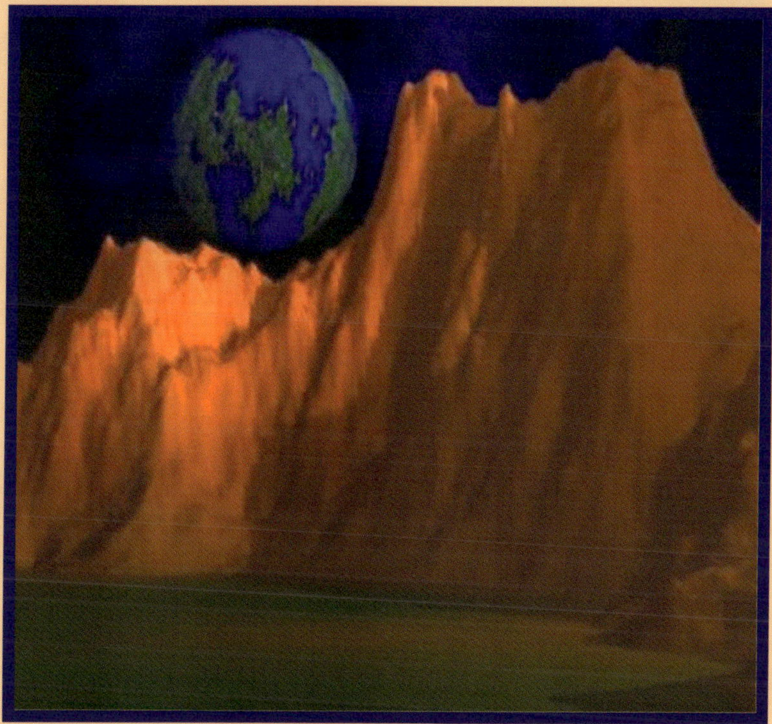

Art by Merlin Hughes

Our mental models determine not only how we make sense of the world, but how we take action.

Peter Senge

Sometimes an act of learning accomplishes little; the news that the shoe store has a sale causes us to run out and get a new pair of sneakers but that's no big deal. Sometimes it can change everything, the insight that completely changes one's perspective. The most important learning occurs when visions change, when we "revision," when we see with fresh eyes.

One revision can be worth a thousand minor adjustments. However, while minor adjustments are easily measured, revisions are not. But if we are to succeed at redefining learning, it will be through insights that give us new understandings that eventually accumulate into a new comprehension. Our mental models, our operating metaphors, govern how we perceive and deal with the world. They are analogous to fields: in some fields some things will simply not grow, regardless of the efforts of farmers and the desire of plants to sprout, blossom, and flourish. The conditions are just not favorable to growth, or, at least, growth for that particular kind of plant. As mental models and operating metaphors change, different kinds of ideas can grow.

Ignorance of our operating metaphors makes us not only susceptible to stupidities like hypocrisy but failures to be successful. We cannot really be successful unless we know who we are. It has to do with "locus of control." If we are not aware of the images that push and pull us, then we are not in control. Susan J. Bethanis, in her article, "Language as Action: Linking Metaphors with Organizational Transformation," writes about the power of metaphor:

> The concept of metaphor will be explored here as the energy source of language. Metaphors make language come alive: language becomes action because metaphors can spark people to different actions. Metaphors are more than the clever, figurative nouns that we first learned about in elementary school (e.g., that person is a rock: this relationship is a peak and valley). Metaphors are not merely figures of speech—they are figures of thought. G.B. Madison suggests that a "metaphor is more than just an odd way of saying things with words, it is a superbly effective way of doing things with words, of altering our way of being-in-the-world."

Metaphors such as "teachers as the sage on stage" have been under assault for decades now. That image of teaching, nonetheless, still governs much of the educational process. Constellating pictures emanate from that operating metaphor: students as "empty vessels to be filled," "good schools as filled with quiet and pacific students," "and effective schooling as indicated on simplistic memory tests." Pictures have enormous power: the domino theory was an integral cause of the Vietnam War; our national leaders at the time envisioned that, if Vietnam became communist, all the surrounding countries would topple into the evil empire (another image).

Families can be twisted by their operating metaphors. "Don't hang your dirty laundry out in public" often covers up abuse. Bullies are governed by the image of "if bigger than you then I can push you around." The list of harmful mental models is long. Mental models can also do a lot of good. Some positive examples are the minister who takes the image of shepherd seriously; the leader as servant, the politician as change agent.

The issue is: operating metaphors are hard to recognize and change. But to the degree they blind us to relevant realities, they weaken and endanger us. Learning redefined will increasingly incorporate the importance of recognizing operating metaphors and learning how to discard negative ones and create new ones. Otherwise, we will lose that locus of control referred to earlier. Regardless of how much you know, if unaware of your operating metaphors, then you can only behave from an ignorant perspective. If you allow some other force to impose images of how you should behave, then that force has control over you. Such ignorance can also make us unwittingly hypocritical, in that we fail to act in accordance with what we espouse.

The following story illustrates a person ignorant of her operating metaphor:

> Leaving a faculty meeting, I walked down the hall of a major university. Passing by a classroom full of graduate students, I saw and heard a colleague holding forth about a subject. Behind the lectern, the professor commanded the attention of about thirty-five students. I moved just beyond the door to where I was out of sight, and stopped and listened. For the next thirty minutes I heard no noise from the students, all practicing, experienced teachers, except a few coughs, chairs being moved, and note scribbling. Finally, bored, exasperated, but also amused, I left the scene. The class had been going for about forty-five minutes before I got there, and I could stand the monotony for another thirty, so for at least an hour and fifteen minutes the professor had lectured authoritatively, citing considerable research, about the evils of "teacher talk."

Ignorance of our operating metaphors makes us stupid; we behave without intelligence, neither solving our real problems nor fashioning desired products. The professor was ineffective in her teaching—though we should consider the possibility that maybe she served, paradoxically, as a cautionary example. Ignorance of our operating metaphors frequently compels us to be self-defeating without even realizing it. Metaphors are the peaks of our learning. They carry us into otherwise unseeable worlds. And, sometimes, we cannot truthfully see what we do because we don't harbor the proper metaphors. We are blind to our own efforts. As we redefine learning, we will increasingly focus on the power of metaphor—especially those that govern our behavior.

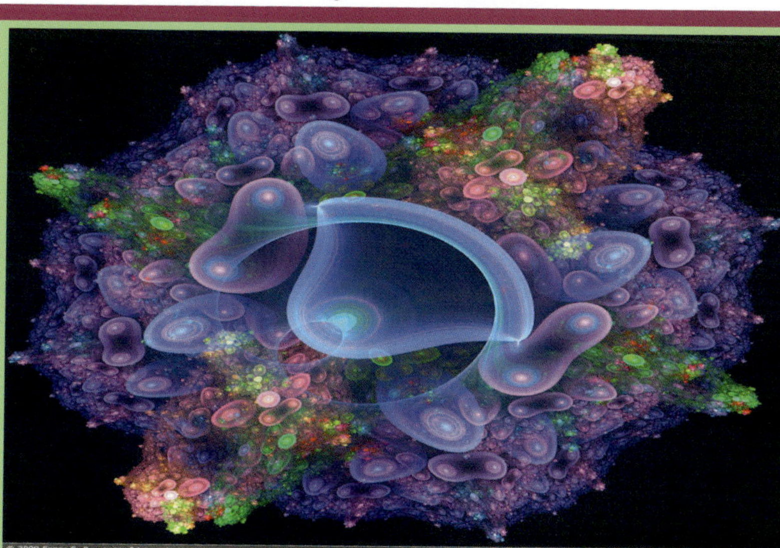

"A Flock of Blobs" by Exper Giovanni Rubaltelli

Getting rid of a delusion makes us wiser than getting hold of a truth.

Ludwig Borne

—2—

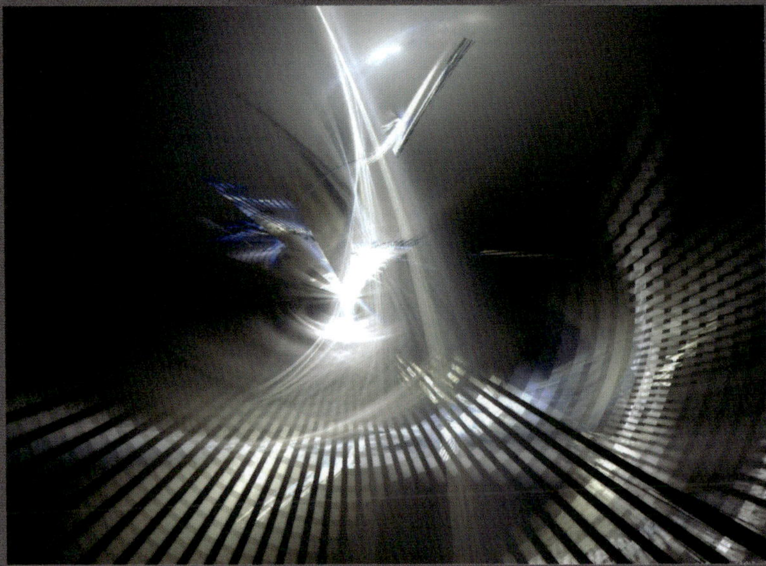

"Breakthrough" by Sven Geier

That is what learning is. You suddenly understand something you've understood all your life, but in a new way.

Doris Lessing

Words are often surrounded by a galaxy of beliefs and assumptions. A word like "love" is thick with hidden meanings and changing connotations. Our understanding of love changes as it responds to individual and cultural experience. In important ways, we love differently today than we did yesterday, though the word itself has not changed in appearance or denotation.

The word "learning" projects various pictures: the child playing a game, the adult working a cross-word puzzle, the teacher in front of a class, students in a classroom, or the scientist at work in a laboratory. But these are just quick snapshots of a very complicated animal, the learning that is going on. Most of what is happening, or not happening, we cannot see. None of those preceding images guarantee that learning is taking place. Or at least learning that is constructive, beneficial, and contributing.

Students can be adept at appearing to learn. Teachers can be snookered, and they can be mistaken about what is going on:

> One student consistently came to my class late, then sat at the back of the classroom and stared out the window. He never contributed to the

> subject, human development. He had a perpetual scowl on his face, and given that he was a huge lineman for the football team, his attitude intimidated everyone, including me. Nonetheless, one day I decided that the problem had to be addressed, so I informed him that we would have a private conference after class in my office. This huge, seemingly angry young man followed me down the hall. When I turned to close the door I found a sad young man with tears in his eyes. The stories that I frequently used to illustrate the subject under study reminded him of his mother, who had died the previous semester. She also told stories to get her points across. He was perpetually late because he hated the sadness it made him feel; though he always forced himself to attend. He stared out the window because the stories and discussions gave him so much to think about. He apologized and promised to change his attitude and behavior. I told him that, because of his explanation, he could continue his present course, even arriving late if he felt the need. He was learning from me and the subject. But what if he had encountered a teacher with a traditional image of learning?

Some years ago I worked on a team to redesign a middle school in San Diego. The district wanted us to turn it into a learning academy. It was our job to redefine the place, to align it with its new name. The team, which consisted not only of educators but anthropologists, businesspeople, and politicians, ran into one problem that turned out to be a tough nut to crack. The principal's definition of a good school, a good classroom, and a good teacher was wrapped around several pictures: quiet, empty hallways during class time, teachers standing in front of classrooms talking, students sitting in their seats, focused on the teachers, and taking notes. We had an intense, ongoing debate striving to educate those pictures out of his and several other heads. But we succeeded. The principal, and others, began to see that learning did not have to take place within the framework of those pictures. That, in fact, those pictures guaranteed that the place would not be a learning academy but a regular, traditional middle school.

With that new philosophy—with that new picture gallery—the school had a chance at becoming a true learning academy. Sad to say, other interests, in particular the need to teach to the tests, soon reasserted the dominance of the previous pictures. I doubt if the school is still, in a true sense, a learning academy. The dominate paradigm, the curator of the pictures that guide our behavior, soon straightened out the gallery, removing the pictures that did not fit the program. The embedded definition of learning demanded quiet hallways, teachers in front of class, and students dutifully sitting in their seats. That was the picture, and there was no changing it at that time. I wonder how the principal—now educated about the nature of learning—dealt with the pressures to disregard his new understanding.

Metaphors govern our perception; they either constrain or expand our understanding. They limit our horizons, and when they change, increase them, though we should harbor the caution that they can change for the worse and also decrease the limit of what we can see. Sometimes, we cannot truthfully see the reasons for our actions, and their consequences, because we don't harbor the proper metaphors. We are therefore blind to our own efforts. We have not answered the old admonition to "know thyself" until we are aware of our operating metaphors.

Lasting, worthwhile change must be cultural and philosophical, for it is our operating metaphors, our mental models that guide our methodologies. Practice is ultimately derived from image. The only change that is really worthwhile is systemic change. Anything else is just tinkering; the real work doesn't get done. Real learning, as the author Doris Lessing points out, is when we construct a breakthrough into a new understanding—in this case, of learning itself.

Cautionary Thoughts: While we frequently trot out concern for self-directed learning, we unconsciously establish and maintain conditions for passive learning. The pervasive "hidden curriculum" weighs down occasional words to the contrary. Even passionate teachers fall into the trap of herding students down the programmed track with canned discussions and prescribed group work. The ethos of schooling does not reward right-brain activities such as initiative, imagination, or even—or perhaps, especially—personal interest. So many so-called "discussions" simply reinforce the lesson plan. True exploration of a subject, led by initiative, imagination, and interest, always threatens to jump off the curriculum track. It takes real leadership/teaching for genuine exploration.

Neil Postman provides other negative factors within the hidden curriculum that emanate from the present definition of learning:

—Passive acceptance is a more desirable response to ideas than active criticism.
—Discovering knowledge is beyond the power of students and is, in any case, none of their business.
—Recall is the highest form of intellectual achievement, and the collection of unrelated "facts" is the goal of education.
—The voice of authority is to be trusted and valued more than independent judgment.
—One's own ideas and those of one's classmates are inconsequential.
—Feelings are irrelevant in education.
—There is always a single, unambiguous Right Answer to a question.
—English is not history and History is not Science and Science is not Art and Art is not Music, and Art and Music are minor subjects and English, History, and Science are major subjects, and a subject is something you "take" and, when you have taken it, you have "had" it, and if you have "had" it, you are immune and need not take it again. (The Vaccination Theory of Education?)

—3—

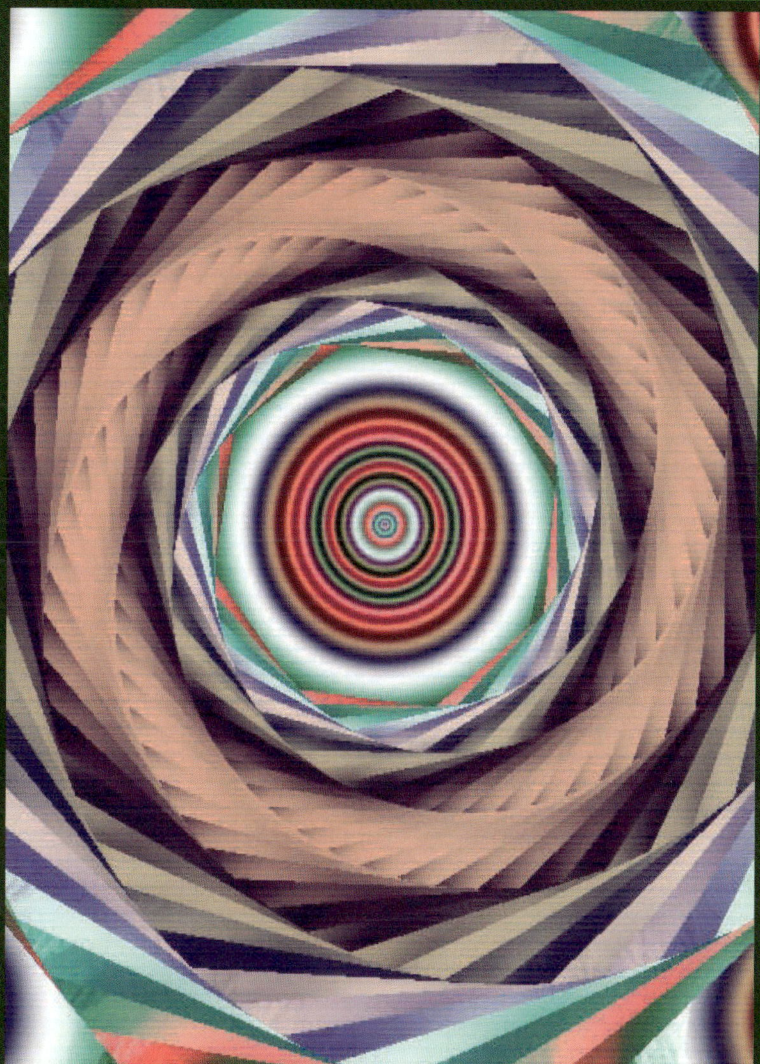

"Iris of Contemplation" by Ken Keller

"Put that in your pipe and smoke it" is an assertive, perhaps even arrogant, way of punctuating a conversation, which basically means "Please contemplate my arguments against your delusions."

So what is the mental model governing the American educational process? It is a centralized-controlled, top-down perspective driven by faith in the "scientific management" of a dynamic, holistic process. It is a lock-step process addicted to allegiance to the directive of "being on the same page." The one word that sums up this operating metaphor and its constellating methods and materials is **Socialism.** The American educational system, including the persistent and pervasive calls for a standards-based and data-driven process, is socialistic in its very foundation—its philosophy.

Democratic principles rarely find their way into the educational process. While Marx and Engels were the fathers of communism, the metaphorical father of the socialistic process was an American economist by the name of Frederick Winslow Taylor. Lenin loved him: "We should try out every scientific and progressive suggestion of the Taylor system." And Soviet Russia did so, with the eventual result of its collapse.

> America will lose [the economic competition] because its people are infected with a disease of the brain, called Taylorism.
>
> Konosuke Matsushita

Regrettably, the American educational system, from its early philosophy and design to this day, also loves Taylorism. The present definition of learning fits hand-in-glove with the socialistic metaphor. It pushes for a standardized process producing standardized products. The result is training which crowds out initiative in both teachers and students. Our system of schooling has not yet collapsed, but the conditions for the collapse are building. The present American educational system as it is now designed should collapse, since it is based on a socialistic metaphor—at odds with our most cherished principles and values. But the system has been in operation for over a hundred years. It has its proponents, the vast majority of whom do not realize the socialistic roots of their perspective.

We often fail to understand how philosophy (the constellation of our mental models) governs behavior, how metaphors beget methods and materials. Every day in hundreds of thousands of schools, administrators and teachers—who believe in the democratic spirit—school in ways founded on Taylorism, an essentially socialistic perspective.

The operating metaphor of Taylorism and the constellating methods and materials resulting from that perspective so loved by Lenin found a home in the heart of American educators because they envied the credibility and capability of scientists. They wanted the prediction and control of science, and Taylorism promised that. Taylorism is especially seductive to educators, who tire of explaining their endeavor to those who consider it an easy though amorphous profession. It is also stressful to labor diligently at a task so hard to measure, so the profession loved the Tayloristic methods of assessing the easily measured. The supposed clarity of scientific management was too attractive.

We desired the prediction and control promised by Taylorism so much that we forgot about the importance of interaction and the emergent natures of learning and maturation. We systematically grasped at those powers—even if it meant ignoring how the resulting methods suppressed intrinsic motivation—even if it meant neglecting our democratic principles.

In the early part of the twentieth century, an education administration professor by the name of Franklin Bobbitt, of the University of Chicago, took on the role of transferring Taylor's economic principles into the business of education. He was too successful. Ray Marshall and Marc Tucker, in their book, *Thinking for a Living: Education and the Wealth of Nations*, elaborate:

> Bobbitt believed with Taylor that efficiency depended on the centralization of authority and definite direction by the supervisors of all processes performed . . . The worker (that is, the teacher) . . . must be kept supplied with the detailed instructions as to the work to be done, the standards to be reached, the methods to be employed, and the appliances to be used . . . The results of the planning department had to be transmitted to the teachers so that there can never be any misunderstanding as to what is expected of a teacher in the way of results or in the matter of method. This means that instruction must be given as to everything that is to be done. Thus were the principles of scientific management used to elevate the authority of the supervisors and limit the freedom of the teacher.

There is nothing wrong with either standards or data, per se. It is when they are used to "scientifically manage" what is in essence an interactive, holistic, and emergent process that we run into trouble. When standards and data are used to suppress both teacher and student initiative, we should worry. When standards and data are used to centralize a perspective that suppresses individual judgment and decision-making, we should worry. When standards and data are used to crowd imagination and individuality out of our curriculum and schools, we should worry. Most of us harbor and treasure the spirit of democracy in our hearts. We believe in the Democratic Promise. So why do we school our children with a socialistic operating metaphor and the resulting top-down driven methods and materials?

Put that in your pipe and smoke it—I chose this assertive, even arrogant, directive because it puzzles me how we have lost touch with our democratic values. Why don't we understand the damages caused by our methods and materials? Are we willing to pay the costs of redefining learning, and in so doing change the way we teach and assess? Or shall we continue on the present path, even though it erodes the imagination, initiative, individuality, integrity, and intellectual capability necessary for a democratic citizenry? How can we educate for a democracy through socialistic metaphors, methods, and materials? Why don't we see the absurdity of our schooling?

—4—

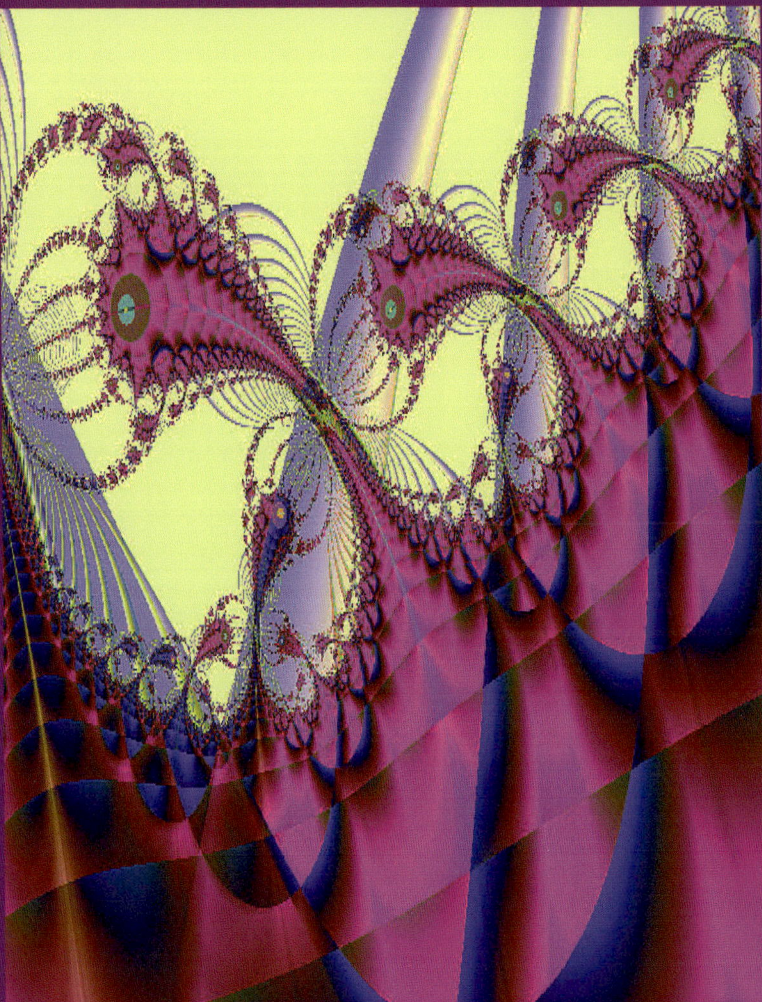

"Rolling Void" by Ken Keller

The problem of American secondary education resides in its mediocre sameness rather than in fragmentation. Today we need no new consensus, but, rather, an agreement to help our adolescents break out of our existing mediocre harmonies.

Theodore R. Sizer

S.O.S.—Same Old Schools

A reasonable assumption is that schools in a democracy would be characterized by individuality and distinctiveness—but that is not the case. The synergistic effects of initiative are smothered by a culture of socialistic metaphors, methods, and materials. The idiosyncratic energy of democracy is constrained by the standardization needs of an authoritarian bureaucracy. Individual and institutional identities that are characterized by eccentricity, or, at least, distinctiveness are a natural corollary of self-formation, a truth that is unacceptable to a socialistic perspective—which desires to "scientifically manage" the process. The Tayloristic operating metaphor hammers down innovation, individuality, and uniqueness in its desire for standards and the status quo.

Theodore R. Sizer, in his book, *Horace's Compromise: The Dilemma of the American High School,* points out:

> This big country contains numerous educational jurisdictions, with authority decentralized [politically not culturally]. Nonetheless, as one visits communities one is gradually struck by how similar the structure and articulated purpose of American high schools are. Rural schools, city schools; rich schools, poor schools; public schools, private schools; big schools, little schools; the framework of grades, schedules, calendar, courses of study, even rituals, is astonishingly uniform and has been so for at least forty years.
>
> In most schools, I visited biology and social studies classes, and I could soon predict the particular topics under study during a given month in Bio 1 or U.S. History, whatever the school. While the texts had different covers and authors, their commonness was stunning.

No matter what the community, no matter what the student body, no matter what the situation, we respond with the same old schools. A socialistic, bureaucratic culture cannot respond to individual circumstances. A governing template, the mediocre harmonies referred to by Sizer, must be followed. Standardization is demanded, not a standard of excellence, but a standard of sameness. We want everyone to be on the same page. Ray Marshall and Marc Tucker, in *Thinking for a Living: Education and the Wealth of Nations,* comment:

> American schools operate on design standards set by legislators, state school boards, chief state school officers, local school boards, superintendents of schools, and central office staffs. The standards are remarkably uniform, they stifle innovation, and because so many individuals and bodies set them, no one can be held responsible for the failure to provide results.

Sameness provides bureaucratic protection: "This is the industry standard; this is how everyone perceives and approaches the tasks." The degree of sameness in our schools despite the diversity of supposedly responsible individuals and institutions indicates that the socialistic, bureaucratic culture controls our profession.

Bureaucrats like autopilots; they do not like reflective practitioners who wrest initiative and take responsibility from the system.

Bill Creech, in *The Five Pillars of TQM: How to Make Total Quality Management Work for You*, sums up the socialistic mindset and bureaucratic approach:

> When problems arose, those on high would initiate a predictable flurry to reprogram the central autopilot: Change the rules. Write tighter regulations. Idiot-proof the procedures. Reprogram all the mindsets. That response nearly always lagged far behind the need and rarely reached the actual cause of the trouble. As a result, today's solutions became tomorrow's problems. Those closest to the problem, who understood it best, were not empowered to fix it before it grew—so it did.

The suppression of individuality in our educational institutions has far-reaching negative ramifications upon the individuality of our students, and thus their integrity, character, and responsibleness. What this means to the fundamental conditions of a democracy will be deciphered by future historians—but it is safe to suppose that individuality is integral to the foundation of a democratic citizenry. The very spirit of democracy is antithetical to any form of monoculture. A homogeneous ecosystem, of either theory or practice, is, like a genetic one, highly susceptible to disease-carrying viruses. Why do we allow the socialistic metaphors, methods, and materials of our very own educational process to suppress the health and vitality of our natural diversity?

A Cautionary Story

I once applied for a position at a university that will go unnamed. The interview went well until the administrator spelled out the goals of the institution. It was a selling point, he was proud to claim, that, if a student had to drop out of a class at any time, program design guaranteed that there would be no problem. The student could return, even a year later, even with a different instructor, and pick up the class exactly where he or she had left off. In other words, class meeting number ten in Educational Psychology 601 always covered the same material, regardless of students, instructors, and, presumably, world events or natural disasters. Interaction was absolutely not at the heart of their educational approach. It would have been hard to squeeze any in at the fringes. We did not form a professional relationship. However, that university system has done well, with a history of expanding its campuses into numerous states. Unique schools, especially at the college level, still exist, but the pressure for sameness is strong and growing.

Have we made a culture-wide decision to no longer value individuality? Have we decided that training is so much more important than initiative that it should be suppressed? Have we decided that uniqueness, of either perspective or response, is no longer a desirable value?

Our educational system says that we have.

—5—

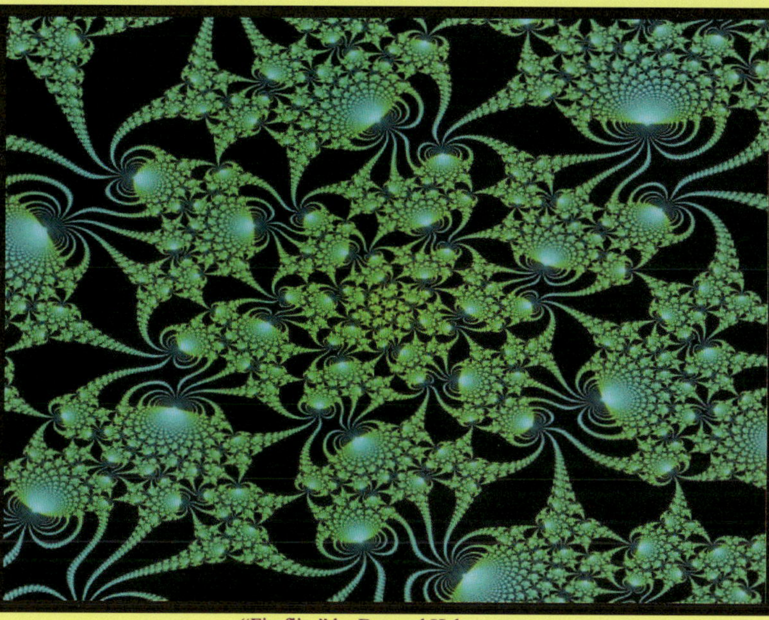

"Fireflies" by Bernard Helmstetter

There are only little daily miracles, illuminations, matches struck unexpectedly in the dark.

The character Lily, in Virginia Woolf's *To the Lighthouse*

I image the life of the mind, whether individual or social, as a huge dark field at night sporadically lit by the haphazard dance of fireflies. Genuine reflections and conversations are rare and seemingly happenstantial. Little daily miracles of insight and connection exist, matches struck unexpectedly in the dark. But the field is not only huge but forever expanding; and along with the unexpected flowers and hidden beauties are noxious weeds and unknown beasties.

We need a new understanding of human development, one that supports and correlates with a redefinition of learning. The present theories are too Newtonian in metaphor; they fail to incorporate the quantum reality. Human development is messier than we wish to believe, less often caused by the logical sequences that make us comfortable. Human development is more often an unpredictable emergence—emanating from the boil and toil of underlying conditions, bearing in mind that one of the most important underlying conditions is the mind itself. We are more capable of self-genesis than present theories assume; our thinking has more to do with who we are and will become than we presently think. We have more mystery in us than our present understanding of human development.

The firefly image illuminates the happenstantial and flitting (because of those wonderful butterflies) process of mental life. It may seem ephemeral, but we do nonetheless somehow acquire relatively stable structures such as perspective, intellect, judgment, capability, and, even, experience. Insights do build into understandings which do construct comprehensions which do inform and guide our capacity for decision and action. Even wisdom occasionally occurs. Butterflies do emerge from their cocoons. The illuminating reflections and conversations, no matter how sporadic and brief their life sometimes, leave a product we can call education.

We have history, science, philosophy, religion, art, and, perhaps most importantly, literature, to help us gather the flickering insights into steady beacons of illumination. However, we are occasionally blinded by the rays of yesterday's light. Much of our trouble in the educational world is the product of the scientific management philosophy, one that had co-evolved with a theory of human development wrapped around deterministic notions—such as behavioralism. The resulting operating metaphors are counterproductive when applied to a holistic endeavor such as schooling, and stultifying when used to envision the puzzle of human development. The metaphors, capabilities, and credibility of science have been used systematically in the perpetuation of this woodenheadedness in the educational endeavor, often over the strenuous objections of real scientists. But now the science has changed, particularly in the form of neuroscience, which is changing our understanding of how the brain learns and thus the nature of human development.

Just as the world used to rest on the back of a giant turtle, the brain used to be perceived as fixed at birth. New neurons could not be added. This was the commonly held belief as recently as the 1980's. Neurogenesis did not exist; the brain was a set-in-stone computer-like program—not malleable, not capable of regeneration. It could respond to stimuli; it could construct experience, but its potential was set at birth. The ramifications of this image fit in with the desires of the positivist philosophy: all we had to do was learn the intricasies of the program, and we would be able to predict and control student behavior and learning. (The mind itself had to be ignored, for it was way too messy.) But the notion of the fixed brain ran into trouble, the self-correcting process of science.

As Jonah Lehrer writes, in *Proust was a Neuroscientist*:

> The genius of the scientific method, however, is that it accepts no permanent solution. Skepticism is its solvent, for every theory is imperfect. Scientific facts are meaningful precisely because they are ephemeral, because a new observation, a more honest [or capable] observation, can always alter them.

The image of neurons as fixed at birth had served to exclude any evidence to the contrary. It had guided the perceptions and behavior of scientists, psychologists, and educators for more than a century. But all that was about to change, as Lehrer points out:

> In 1989, Elizabeth Gould, a young postdoc working in the lab of Bruce McEwen at Rockeller University, in New York City, was investigating the effect of stress hormones on rat brains. Chronic stress is devastating to neurons, and Gould's research focused on the death of cells in the hippocampus. But while Gould was documenting the brain's degeneration, she happened upon something miraculous: the brain also healed itself.
>
> Confused by this anomaly, Gould went to the library. She assumed she was making some simple experimental mistake, because *neurons don't divide.* Everybody knew that. But then, looking through a dusty twenty-seven-year-old science journal, Gould found a tantalizing clue. Beginning in 1962, a researcher at MIT, Joseph Altman, published several papers claiming that adult rats, cats, and guinea pigs all formed new neurons. [But] . . . his results were ridiculed, and then ignored.
>
> As a result, the brand-new field of neurogenesis vanished before it began. It would take another decade before Michael Kaplan, at the University of New Mexico, would use an electron microscope to image neurons giving birth to new neurons. Kaplan discovered these fresh cells everywhere in the mammalian brain, including the cortex. Yet even with this visual evidence, science remained stubbornly devoted to its doctrine. After enduring years of scorn and skepticism, Kaplan, like Altman before him, abandoned the field of neurogenesis.
>
> Reading Altman's and Kaplan's papers, Gould realized that her mistake was not a mistake: it was an ignored fact. The anomaly had been suppressed.. . . Gould spent the next eight years quantifying endless numbers of radioactive rat brains. But the tedious manual labor paid off. Gould's data shifted the paradigm. More than thirty years had passed since Altman first glimpsed new neurons, but neurogenesis had finally become a scientific fact.

The science of neurogenesis is barely a decade old. But it is the lever with which we can bring the necessary change in our definition of learning. Lehrer points out that "the brain, far from being fixed, is actually in a constant state of cellular upheaval." What current theory of learning incorporates this reality? We assume that neurogenesis should be a goal of the educational process. This is an arguable position, for neurogenesis is neither predictable nor controllable. That reality wreaks havoc with the operating metaphors of the present definition of learning. But disorder, not order, is at the core of our individuality and our freedom. Lehrer writes:

> This is the triumph of our DNA: it makes us without determining us. The invention of neural plasticity, which is encoded by the genome, lets each of us transcend our genome. We *emerge*, characterlike, from the vague alphabet of our text. Of course, to accept the freedom inherent in the human brain—to know that the individual is *not* genetically predestined—is to accept the fact that we have no single solutions.

> Every day each one of us is given the gift of new neurons and plastic cortical cells; only we can decide what our brains will become.
>
> . . . In order to create the wiggle room necessary for individual freedom, natural selection came up with an ingenious, if unnerving, solution. Although we like to imagine life as a perfectly engineered creation (our cells like little Swiss clocks), the truth is that our parts aren't predictable. . . Molecular biology, confronted with the unruliness of life, is also forced to accept chaos. Just as physics discovered the indeterminate quantum world—a discovery that erased classical notions about the fixed reality of time and space—so biology is uncovering the unknowable mess at its core. Life is built on an edifice of randomness.

We need a new understanding of human development as we redefine learning in order to stop designing and imposing curriculum predicated on Newtonian-guided assumptions? How can we instead create and maintain learning environments guided by operating metaphors emanating from a new theory of human development—one enlightened by the findings of neuroscience?

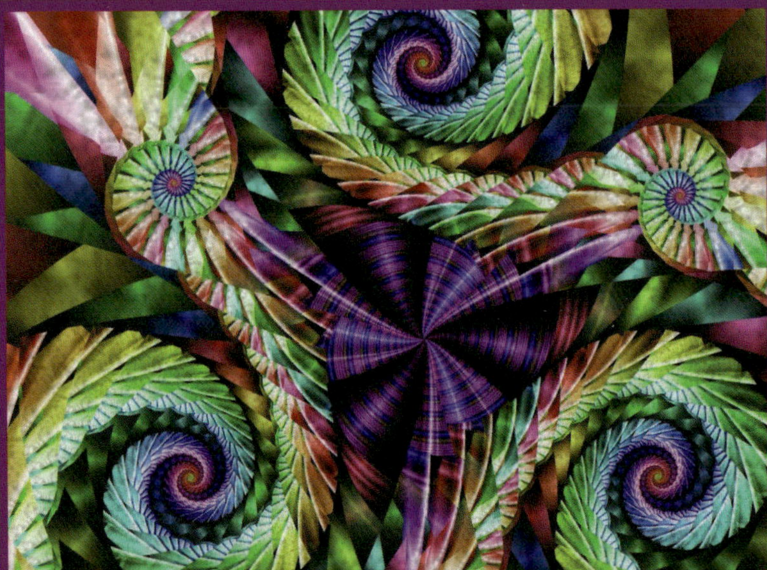

"Twist" by Sven Geier

The human mind is the largest, thickest, and toughest knot in the known universe. Neuroscience suspects that, since it is a process and not a thing, we can never find a Gordian perspective with which to address the mind. It is too dynamically complex, individual, idiosyncratic, ever-changing, and ever-evolving. There is too much magic in us to ever be fully nailed down.

A Cautionary and Ironic Truth

Hans Christian Andersen recognized (in 1835!) the stultifying potential of the mechanistic image, as opposed to the organic image, when he wrote "The Nightingale." The organic nightingale was banned from the castle because it would not always sing on command. The mechanical one, however, was more predictable, for it always did as it was told. But the mechanical bird eventually broke down and poisons accumulated—until the organic nightingale returned to save the kingdom. Andersens's intuition over a century and a half ago is now supported by neuroscience. We have hurt the song of ourselves by suppressing the image of the organic nightingale in fixation on the mechanical one.

Lehrer discusses the work of Fernando Nottebohm, who proved neurogenesis necessary for bird song:

> To sing their complex melodies, male birds needed new brain cells. In fact, up to 1 percent of the neurons in the bird's song center were made fresh every day. "At the time, this was a radical idea," Nottebohm says. "The brain was thought to be a very fixed organ. Once development was over, scientists assumed that the mind was cast in a crystalline structure. That was it; you were done."
>
> Nottebohm disproved this dogma by studying birds in their actual habitat. If he had kept his birds in metal cages, depriving them of their natural social context, he would never have observed the abundance of new cells that he did. The birds would have been too stressed to sing, and fewer neurons would have been created. As Nottebohm has said, "Take nature away and all your insight is in a biological vacuum." It was only because he looked at birds *outside* of the laboratory's vacuum that he was able to show that neurogenesis, at least in finches and canaries, had a real evolutionary purpose.

We need to ask some important questions:

—What are the environmental conditions best suited for encouraging and informing neurogenesis?

—Can they exist in the traditional classroom?

—Does the constant testing generate the birth of new neurons—or is it neurotoxic?

—Which classrooms consistently succeed—or fail—at generating neurogenesis?

—What does a neurogenic classroom or school look like?

—What is the relationship between the image of the organic nightingale in our schools and the growth of integrity in our students and citizens?

—Can we not equate the "aliveness" of our schooling with the expression of our democratic faith?

—Is that relationship not worth assessment?

—How can we redesign our schools of education and professional development to where teachers are helped bring life back into the educational process?

—What can we do to escape the contraints of the mechanical images and replace them with organic ones?

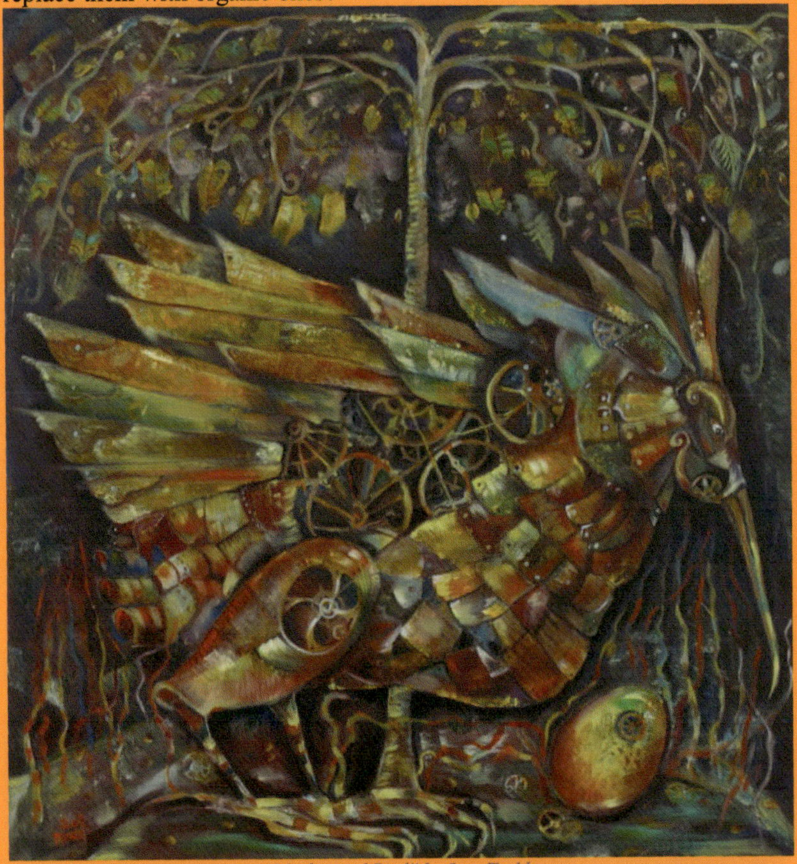

"Mechanical Bird" by Igor Tyshler

For you see, ladies and gentlemen, and, above all, your Imperial Majesty, with a real nightingale one can never calculate what is coming, but in this artificial bird, everything is settled. Everything is fixed before-hand. It is this way, and no other! We can take him to pieces, we can open him up and understand with our human mind, how the mechanism works, how his wheels are put together, how they move, and how one thing follows another.

Hans Christian Andersen

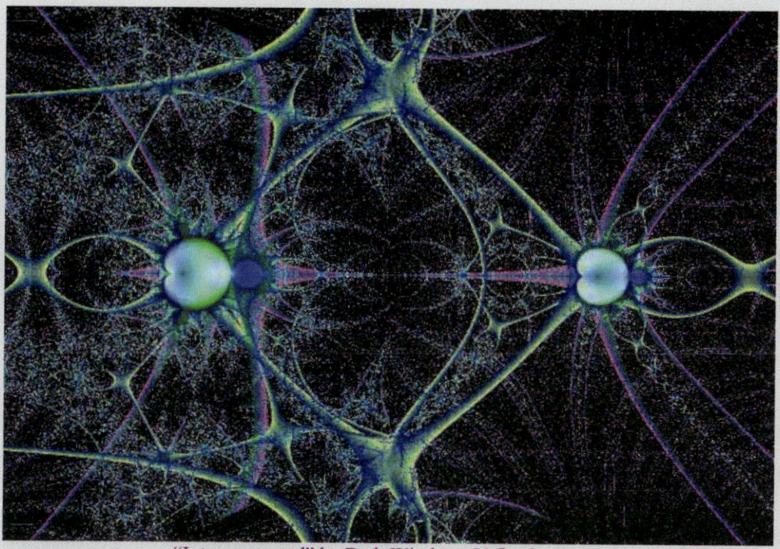

"Interconnected" by Beth Windozer50@yahoo.com

Imagine the brain, that shiny mound of being, that mouse-gray parliament of cells, that dream factory, that petit tyrant inside a ball of bone, that huddle of neurons calling all the plays, that little everywhere, that fickle pleasuredrome, that wrinkled wardrobe of selves stuffed into the skull like too many clothes into a gym bag. The neocortex has ridges, valleys, and folds because the brain kept remodeling itself though space was tight. We take for granted the ridiculous-sounding yet undeniable fact that each person carries around atop the body a complete universe in which trillions of sensations, thoughts, and desires stream. They mix privately, silently, while agitating on many levels, some of which we're not aware of, thank heavens. If we needed to remember how to work the bellows of the lungs or the writhing python of digestion, we'd be swamped by formed and forming memories, and there'd be no time left for buying cute socks. My brain likes cute socks, But it also likes kisses. And asparagus. And watching boat-tailed grackles. And biking. And drinking Japanese green tea in a rose garden. There's the nub of it—the brain is personality's whereabouts. It's also a stern warden, and, at times, a self-tormentor. It's where catchy tunes snag, and cravings keep tugging. Shaped a little like a loaf of French country bread, our brain is a crowded chemistry lab, bustling with nonstop neural conversations. It's also an impersonal landscape where minute bolts of lightening prowl and strike. A hall of mirrors, it can contemplate existentialism, the delicate hooves of a goat, and its own birth and death in a matter of seconds. It's blunt as a skunk, and a real gossip hound, but also voluptuous, clever, playful, and forgiving.

Diane Ackerman

—6—

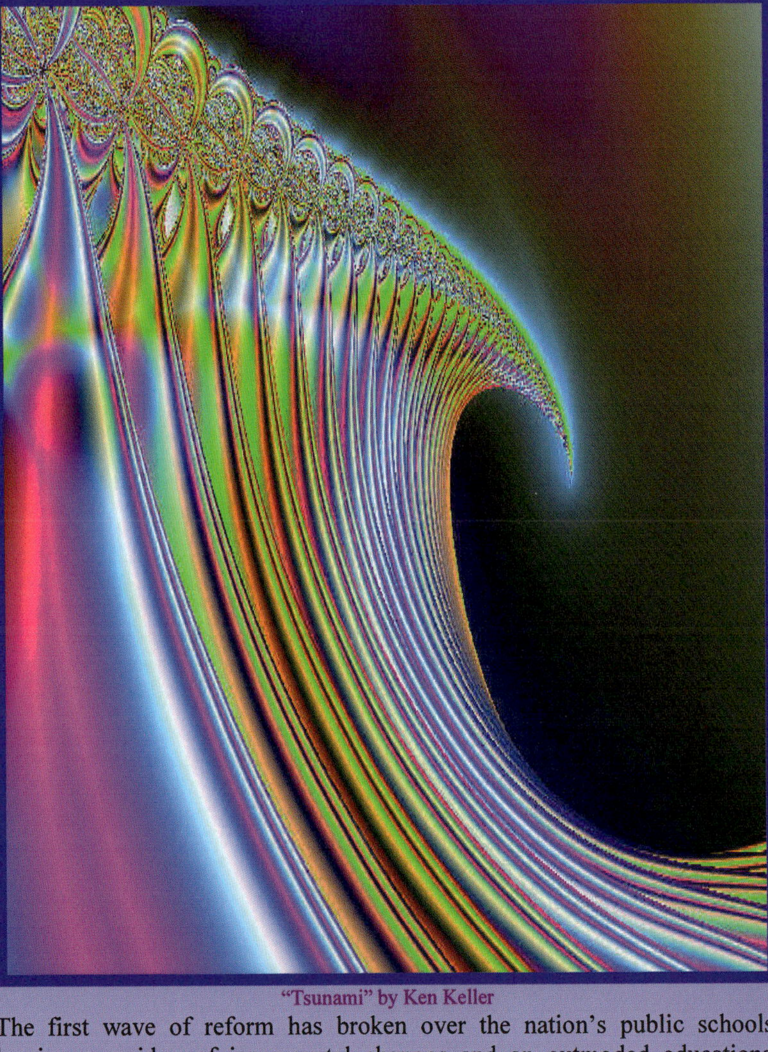

"Tsunami" by Ken Keller

The first wave of reform has broken over the nation's public schools, leaving a residue of incremental changes and an outmoded educational structure still firmly in place. The second wave must produce strategic change that restructures the way our schools are organized and operate. We've been tinkering at the margins of the education problem for too long. It's time now to get to the heart of the matter.

David Kearns

Learning—and teaching—redefined goes to the heart of the matter. Waves of reform that do not originate from revision, or manage to generate revision, will fail. However, each wave pressures people to rethink their operating metaphors as evidence accumulates that there are poisons within the system.

Robert. J. Marzano, in his book, *A Different Kind of Classroom,* advocates learning-centered instruction:

> I believe that the "heart of the matter" of any educational reform or restructuring is the relationship between the teaching and learning processes. We know that effective teaching mirrors effective learning, yet as educators we have not mounted a serious effort to organize teaching around the learning process. Instead, we have viewed education as an institution or an administrative system or a set of instructional techniques (Banathy 1980). We have not examined the learning process and then built instructional systems, administrative systems, indeed, entire educational systems that support what we know about the learning process. We have not built education from the bottom up, so to speak.

It may seem absurd that we have not centered our schooling on the learning process, but we have not. We have instead centered the process on easily measured and supervised methodology and assessment. That way we can claim effectiveness despite the mounting evidence to the contrary.

Another systemic culprit for failure to base our schooling on the learning process is scientism. William E. Doll, in his book, *A Post-modern Perspective on Curriculum,* writes:

> The social sciences, including education, in trying to "scientize" their disciplines have adopted a shallow and mistaken view of what constitutes science. The point is that in using [Newtonian] physics as a model the social sciences have excluded the concept of interaction. This has had devastating effects on curriculum, for, as both Dewey and Piaget have pointed out, it is interaction that forms the heart of growth.

Interaction, the messy, often unpredictable matrix of intermingling initiatives coming from students as well as teachers, is at the heart of worthwhile, effective learning. Its very messiness and complexity compelled the education world to ignore interaction, even if it is at the heart of intellectual, emotional, and spiritual growth. Learning redefined will bring our attention back to the importance of interaction through changing the operating metaphors that guide the process. Only then will we stop tinkering and get the necessary work done.

> When a practitioner becomes aware of his frames [of perception], he also becomes aware of the possibility of alternative ways of framing.
>
> Donald Schon

—7—

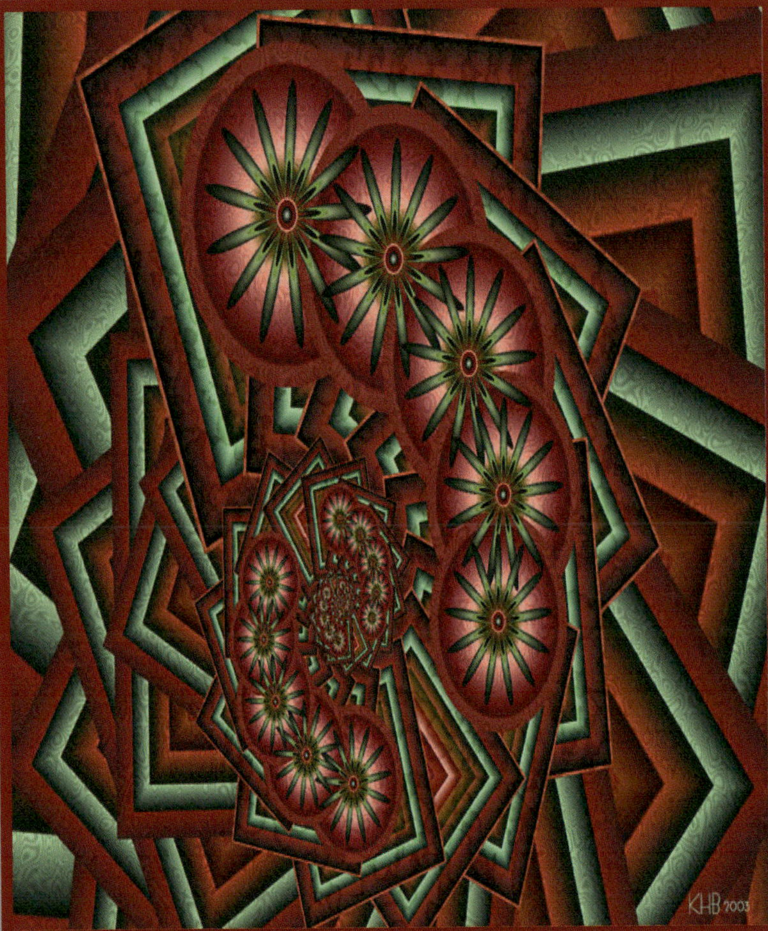

"Windowboxed" by Panny Brawley

It is the unfortunate dilemma that initiative and training are both necessary [for the healthy educational process] and that training is apt to kill initiative.

Alfred North Whitehead

The primary focus of *Learning Redefined* is bringing a balance between training and initiative into the educational process. Initiative is a cardinal concern because without it much of what we desire is not possible, such as life-long, self-directed learners, such as critical thinking, such as individual character and personal responsibility. Initiative—within both our teachers and our students—is essential to the necessary redefinition of learning. Initiative is at the heart of active learning—and it nourishes the right-brain while training exercises the left-brain. Initiative is what prevents boxed-in windows. Through initiative we construct our own horizons, our own limits of what we can see. We forge our own interpretations and meanings.

> Initiative is a cardinal capability. It lies at the heart of understanding, creativity, response-ability, and integrity. Initiative occurs when learners contribute to the learning, when they think about it, constructing their own interpretations, meanings, and uses. Most importantly, initiative is at the core of the democratic spirit.

The image of training, however, has crowded out the importance of initiative in our schooling—just as Alfred North Whitehead feared way back in 1916. Training, because it is more easily measured and supervised, has pushed initiative out of the educational dynamic. Training fits in with the socialistic design of our schools. Initiative is disruptive and derailing to the prediction and control machinations of our educational system. Training is, as Whitehead understood, necessary. However, if distilled to a lethal dose, training will suppress imagination and responsibility. It will generate passive learners. It will also wear and tear against our potential as individuals, and as a society.

Carol Caughey, in "Becoming the Child's Ally—Observations in a Classroom for Children Who Have Been Abused," writes:

> Since initiative is required for the evolution of self, children may act in apparently destructive ways in order to maintain this sense of initiative. Of apparent maladaptive behaviors, Virginia M. Axline says, "It could be that it is the most effective way that he has discovered to control the situation and is therefore a satisfaction to him, because it is an expression of his power to direct and individualize himself."

The energy of initiative is intimately bound up with identity development. It is how we explore, express, and define ourselves. Initiative emerges from intrinsic motivation, the desire to author ourselves, which, as Axline points out, can be for either good or bad, for contribution or disruption. Through initiative we construct associations between what we are learning and who we want to become. We think—which is how identities establish ownership of themselves. Initiative is not only entwined with both critical and creative thinking, it is bound up with the development of personal integrity and responsibility. Is it any wonder that its suppression is a condition for the emergence of disruptive and destructive behavior? Initiative is also integral to the functioning of the right-side of the brain; its suppression should be resisted, especially in a democracy.

Two negatives result from the suppression of initiative:

- Both society and individuals lose potential. This is especially true of creative potential.

- Students resent and resist a process that suppresses their initiative—or worse, they capitulate to it.

Initiative is how we get a sense of movement and momentum in our lives. It is how we feel like we have traction, that we are getting somewhere. Initiative is the constructive energy that expresses who we are and what we want to become. It also establishes the parameters of our responsibility. As Adolph Eichmann maintained, people who are not allowed to have initiative in certain areas cannot be held responsible for those areas. We hanged him anyway, though he had an argument. The ultimate pragmatist, Eichmann claimed that the metaphors guiding his methods and materials were the responsibility of those in charge. Nose to the grindstone, it turns out, is not an acceptable excuse for ignorance. We are responsible for the whole of what we do. We hold people responsible (and therefore response-able) for their initiative, or lack of it, even if it has been trained out of them. Pragmatism is no refuge for faulty or evil ideals or moral laziness; we cannot escape the weight of our metaphors. Free will is always there, within us, whether we cherish it or not.

We hold dearly the cultural value of freedom and responsibility. But we can't logically, or fairly, call for them at the same time we crowd initiative out of our schooling through an excessive focus on training. Our democratic spirit demands that we provide an educational system that encourages initiative in both teachers and students.

A Cautionary Story

I asked a group of college students sitting at the same table in the cafeteria what they were reading for an English course:

"Big Blonde," one answered.

"A short story by Dorothy Parker," added another.

"What's it about?" I asked. One of my favorite stories, I wanted to know what they thought, what was their interpretation. They gave me a good summary of the characters and the story line.

"That's good. So what does the story mean to you?" I asked.

"I don't know," a student answered. "The professor hasn't told us yet."

"He's supposed to talk about it in the next class," contributed another.

"But what is your interpretation of it?" I pressured.

"What do you think?" the pressured student directed her question to a fellow teacher sitting at the table.

"She won't tell you," I intervened. "What do you think it means?"

But neither she nor the others could answer. They were waiting for the "right answer" from an authority.

—8—

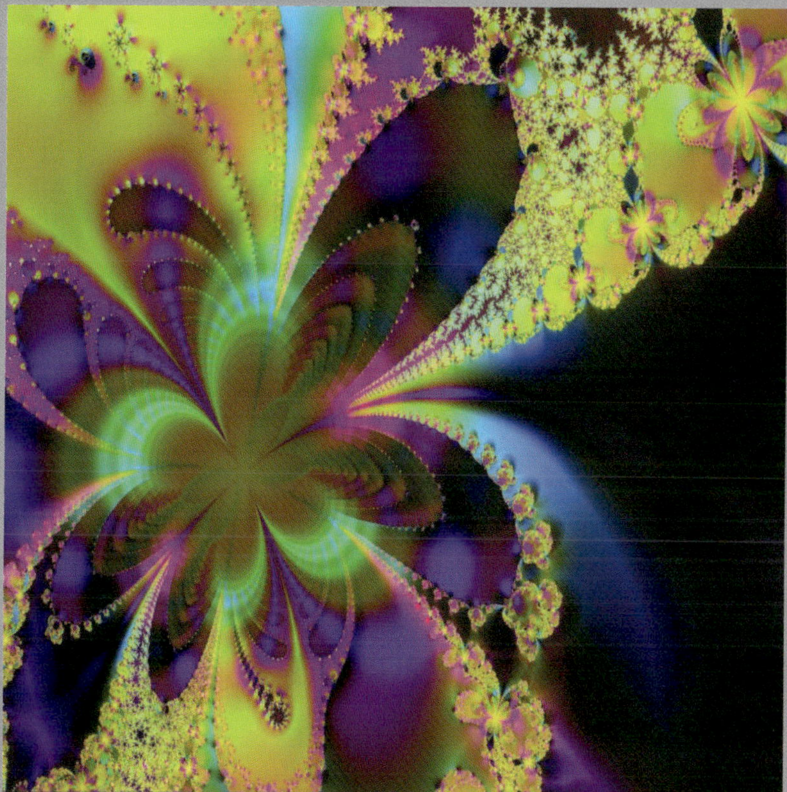

"Butterfly Echoes" by Lauren Zorn

We need a new educational paradigm which looks to the nature of learning rather than methods of instruction. Learning, after all, is the process by which we have moved every step of the way since we first breathed; the transformation that occurs in the brain whenever new information is integrated, whenever a new skill is mastered. Learning is kindled in the mind of the individual. Anything else is mere schooling.

Marilyn Ferguson

As we increasingly recognize how expert-driven practices have disrupted our capabilities and sense of purpose, we will develop the new educational paradigm Marilyn Ferguson called for, one "which looks to the nature of learning rather than methods of instruction." Learning is kindled through initiative. Anything else is just schooling. Theodore Roszak, in *The Cult of Information: the Folklore of Computers and the True Art of Thinking,* writes:

> Too much apparatus, like too much bureaucracy, only inhibits the natural flow. Free human dialogue, wandering wherever the agility of the mind allows, lies at the heart of education. If teachers do not have the time, the incentive, or the wit to provide that; if students are too demoralized, bored or distracted to muster the attention their teachers need of them, then that is the educational problem which has to be solved—and solved from inside the experience of the teachers and the students.

When we understand that teacher intellect is more important than teacher training, we will be well on the way to recovering our educational strength and vitality. It is intellectual activity, the gathering of insights and understandings, not training, the gathering of instructional apparatus, which is best able to perceive and deal with the dynamic, interactive nature of learning. Training is too formulaic, too locked-in to habits of manipulation, too blinkered by simplistic "pedagogical agendas." It is the intellect of teachers which enables them to perceive and deal with the roller-coaster of predicaments which characterizes classroom life. Intellect, after all, is the capacity to understand the dynamic complexity of emergent realities. Teachers with developed intellects and accrued experience are increasingly able to meld unpredictable developments into the fabric of their classrooms. Teachers with intellect more often manage, somehow, to dissolve student resistance and establish learning communities. They become artists at making possible futures more real for others, which necessitates a tremendous breadth and depth of understanding about the hesitations and barriers that interfere with actualization of potential.

However, intellect and experience can only go so far without systemic support. Therefore, the following is an integral component of the necessary paradigm shift:

To transform educational practice from an expert/bureaucrat driven endeavor to one that is teacher/community/student driven.

The reason educational practice needs to become more teacher-driven is that the process should be more learner-focused. The practitioner on the scene of the interaction, with the most elaborate understanding of the student's resistance, desires, and capabilities, should be the one determining the methods and materials at any given time. The professional involved in the situation is the one who can best design and maintain the conditions for learning, who has forged the working relationship with the individual students.

Ferguson's call for us to look to the nature of learning rather than methods of instruction fits in with our concern for bringing initiative back into the educational mix. Training prefers methods of instruction, for they can be more easily supervised and evaluated. But understanding the nature of learning and the idiosyncratic expression of it in individual learners is produced by the initiative of teachers. Here we are talking about teacher intellect, teacher judgment, and teacher responsibility. This is messy territory, one avoided by perspectives addicted to prediction and control machinations. Learning Redefined, as well as Teaching

Redefined, and, ultimately, Schooling Redefined, will not be afraid of that messiness, for it is the by-product of minds at work, of hearts engaged.

Teachers can only nudge—not control—human development. The teacher's intellect is attuned to the indicators of possible resonance. We look for moments where we can play the butterfly. One of the most important conditions within any learning environment is the presence of butterflies. They flit about, fluttering this way and that, appearing here, now there. Carried by interest, sometimes by enthusiasm, even by focus, the butterflies can, at any moment, dramatically change what had been perceived as a complete comprehension into a different definition entirely, with the merest flutter of one wing. Learning is synergistic; it is not bound by linear rules of development. It is emergent; it is, in many ways, an instance of unpredictable development. Learning rarely proceeds, as the old definition would have it, in a step-by-step sequence. As Deborah Walker and Linda Lambert write, "Learning is not uniform and cannot be specified in advance; it is not assembled like parts of a machine, but rather evolves in nonlinear ways from the experiences and attitudes of the learners."

The Butterfly Effect is an integral part of learning redefined. This Quantum reality is defined as:

A special sensitivity to initial conditions.

One thought, either internally created or carried by conversation can change the entire picture. It all depends on the initial conditions within the learner or group of learners, because there are resonant and even contagion factors in learning. Other conditions are: the nature and intensity of the curiosity, the presence of mutual trust and credibility, the comprehension already in place, the level of excitement, the relevance factor, and even such variables as fear and courage.

A Cautionary Example: The state of New York once specified over 1,800 discrete learning skills in reading that progressed in a neat, orderly fashion from the first to the twelfth grade. The state had a curricular map that produced people who could fill out all the workbooks and even pass all of the skills tests, but still not know how to read. Reading, after all, is a holistic capability, a reality easily neglected by the old definition of learning. The necessary synergy never developed because the instructional conditions suppressed it. The linear fixation killed the butterflies essential to the emergence of reading capability. The emergence of reading does not hinge upon the accumulation of discrete learning skills—no matter how numerous or insistently stamped into the learner. Reading emerges from a critical mass of factors such as modeling, curiosity, interest, initiative, imagination, and self-directed learning. It is a relational capability with a complicated ecology of interacting energies, many of them right-brain in genesis.

—9—

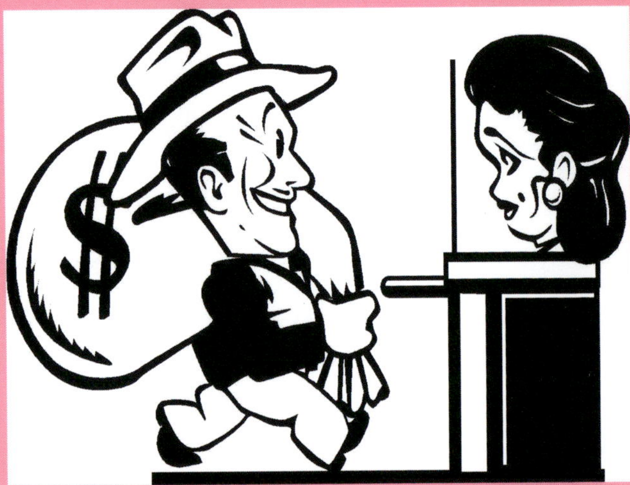

The banking [image] is Paulo Friere's metaphor for pedagogy, in which the transmission of knowledge from teacher to student is likened to the depositing of money in a bank. The student's knowledge and breadth of schooling is wholly dependent on what teachers place in their accounts. By this Friere underscores that students are indoctrinated and are without the critical thinking skills to free themselves from educational tyranny.

George David Miller and Conrad P. Pritscher

Students who do wish to succeed academically too often approach learning with a passive attitude. They have been taught by their schooling that education is an information-injection process where ownership and intrinsic motivation are neither expected nor rewarded. They have been infantilized by what the Brazilian educator Paulo Friere warned us about, the banking concept of education.

Democracy, in its purest sense, should be a raucous activity, but we strive to indoctrinate our students into complacent acceptance of predigested information. We pressure our students to become knowers of inherited knowledge bits rather than creators of understanding, the constructors of their own intellects and judgments. This does not bode well for a vital and vigorous democratic citizenry in the future.

In most classrooms, in most textbooks, and in most curricula, the banking image morphs into that of making foie gras, where geese or ducks are force-fed. In short, our students are gavaged. Wikipedia elaborates:

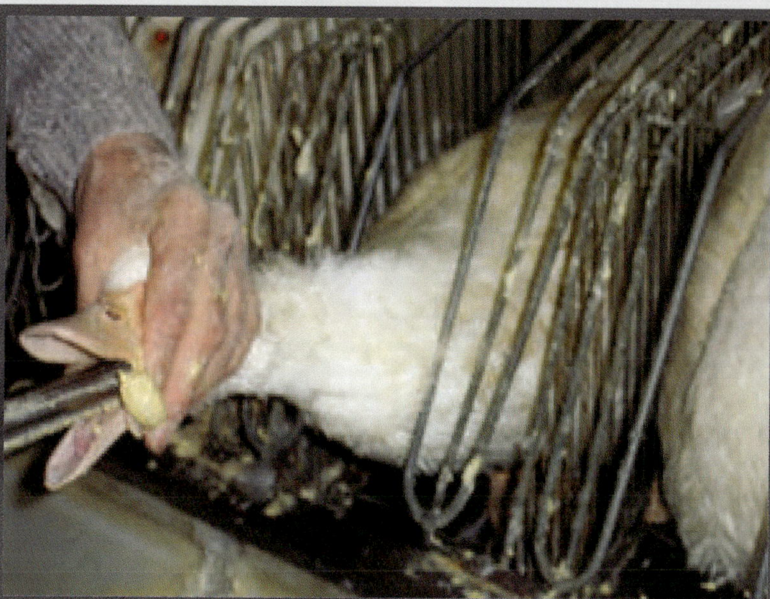

Force-feeding is also known as **gavage**, from a French word meaning "to gorge." This term specifically refers to force feeding of ducks or geese in order to fatten their livers in the production of foie gras. Gavage can also refer to the practice of administering liquids (such as medicine) to laboratory animals via a tube or syringe.

The toxic practice of gavaging is the banking metaphor pushed to an extreme. Gavage works with geese and ducks because they lack a gag reflex. However, our students do have a gag reflex, which is resentment and resistance of different forms. But the constant and pernicious gavaging forces them to draw shallow, tortured breaths as they strive to deal with an educational system governed by an operating metaphor fixated on easily transmitted and measured knowledge bits.

As Marion Brady writes in his book, *What's Worth Teaching?*

> Knowledge is an entity that can be "divided" into "bits" to be "passed on," "taken in," "absorbed," "stored." Teachers "cover the material." We "cram" to prepare for an examination. Familiar metaphors for educating tend to be some version of spoon-feeding—an adult selecting food, preparing it, bringing it to the child, cutting it into pieces, determining the sequence of presentation, picking up the individual pieces, and putting them into the child's mouth. All the child has to do is swallow and keep it down.

How much damage is done in the systemically ordained gavaging attempts? How much effort is wasted? How much imagination is suppressed? How much initiative is lost? How much intellectual growth is stunted? How much counter-productive resentment and resistance is generated? How much are the souls of the assaulted students diminished? How much capability and potential are lost?

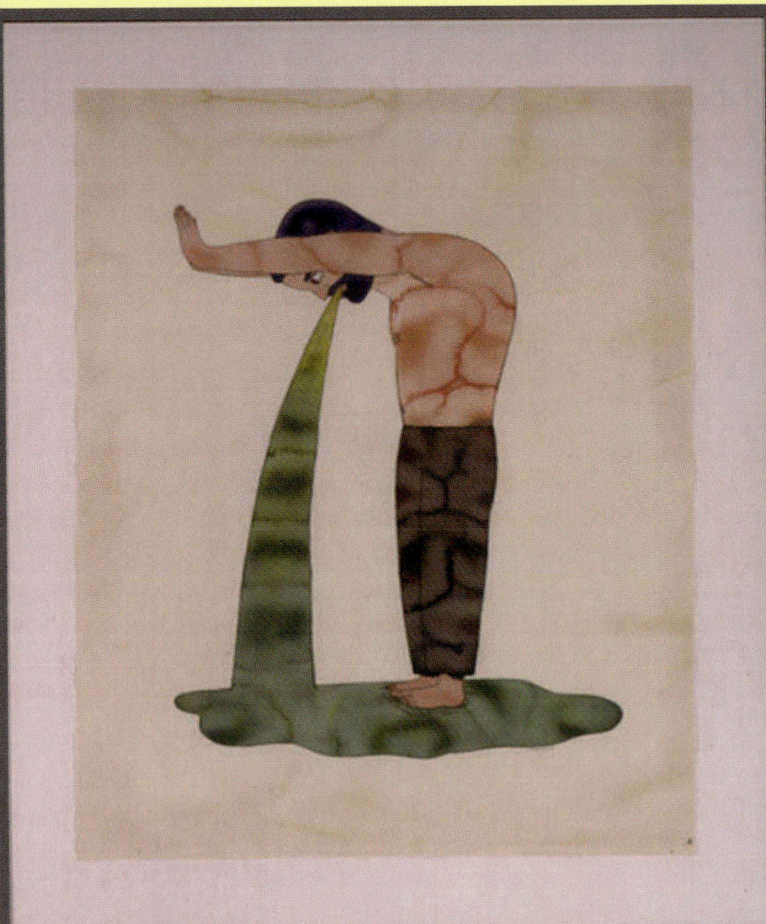

Art by Antonio Eligio Fernandez

In addition to banking, another metaphor we can use for education is bulimia. Students binge on facts until their bellies are full and then expel them on exams. Input then output, and what is the state of a student's body of knowledge? Skeletal and enervated. They learn nothing that will stick with them. What they learned did not remain in their systems long enough to give them nutrients necessary to become insightful and live happy and meaningful lives.

George David Miller and Conrad P. Pritscher

The banking metaphor underlying educational practice is bankrupt because it neither stimulates nor nourishes student growth. The systemic response (one form of resistance) to this bankruptcy is often bulimic learning. Intellectual nutrition is not a focus in an educational culture dedicated to instructional prediction and control. What matters most is knowledge acquisition that is easily measurable. Significant learning is crowded out by surface learning; contextual understanding is neglected in pursuit of congelated knowing. (Congelated knowing is the accumulating of knowledge bits separated from their contextual flow.) The result is schooling that fails to develop intellects in an excessive focus on temporary knowledge exchanges between teachers and students.

Most teachers have heard this sentiment from their anxious, clamoring students:

> "Hurry up and give us the test before we forget everything."

The students are ready at that moment to jump through the necessary hoop. They realize that whatever they have learned is of no nutritional value to them, that its presence within their minds is both disconnected and temporary. Their teachers also recognize this lack of contribution to growing intellects and souls. The culture of their profession, however, compels the absurdity of bulimic learning.

The cultural conditions that generate bulimic learning also pressure for anorexic teaching. Interpretation and utilization of acquired knowledge, the stuff of critical thinking, is not expected and often not allowed of either our students or teachers. Substantial learning is crowded out by conveniently measurable learning. Substantial teaching is crowded out by curricular packages and instructional procedures that are amenable to administrative prediction and control.

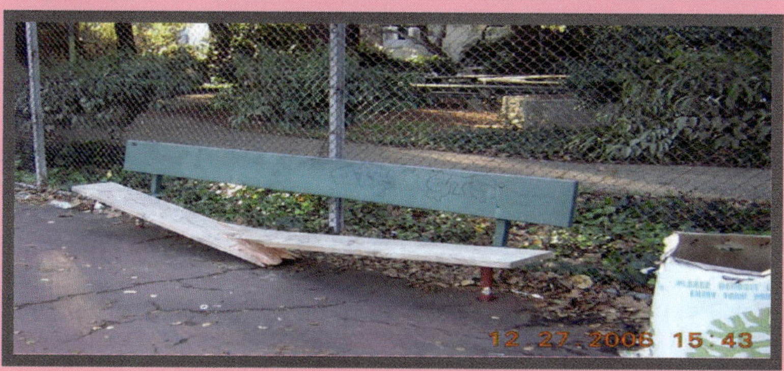

It is not what you say—It is what they hear.
Red Auerbach, Legendary Coach of the Boston Celtics

The banking metaphor has been "bankrupt" for a long time. The supposition is that it was ever helpful to the human need and desire to learn. There is good reason to suspect that most worthwhile learning has occurred despite the suppressive effects of schooling as transmission and regurgitation of decontextualized knowledge bits. Bankrupt means, by the way, "broken bench." Banking began in Italy with moneylenders sitting on special benches. When a lender lent beyond his resources, the other bankers would break his bench. The meaning is clear in the image, the broken bench cannot support the assumption or belief.

Students are the victims of a coverage/measurement fixated curriculum. They have been compelled, day in and day out, for years, to listen to constant lecturing, fill out endless worksheets, and take the increasingly ubiquitous tests. As a result of our educational system, they have learned to resent and resist the educational process. They have become adept at <u>not hearing</u> what teachers say, because they have been systematically taught in ways the human brain hates to learn. Linda Hargan, the founder and CEO of the Collaborative for Teaching and Learning in Louisville, Kentucky, boils the bankrupt dogma down to a saying,

I don't know why they didn't learn it—because I taught it.

We need to get off of that broken bench and change the perspective completely around. In other words, we need to redefine learning. We need a new perspective on the process, one the reverse of the present approach, one where, as Hargan says, "The focus isn't on 'I taught it,' but on 'they learn it.'" Teacher or curriculum-centered instruction in essence claims "I said it," while student-centered instruction is focused on "what did the students hear?"

Lecture can be effective, but it has to be done well, and it can't be constant. In a coverage-fixated culture of education, lecture becomes the only possible way of teaching. Another dynamic, of course, is the increasing student to faculty ratios. Beyond a certain number, lecture is necessary, as is a simplified grading strategy. (Although I know of and in two cases have seen teachers standing behind lecterns propounding at classrooms of only a few students; in one class in California, a solitary student.)

The culture of lecturing has by now been distilled to a lethal dose; the students we receive these days are the result of an educational environment toxic to the engagement of learners. Their initiative in the construction of their own learning has been systemically ignored and suppressed; the result being the collateral suppression of ownership and responsibility. Engagement, after all, is disruptive to coverage—it leads students away from the mandated material. In reaction, students have learned not to hear whatever teachers say, at worst, or, at best, listen to only whatever is necessary in order to slide through the system. They have learned resistance—not engagement—to the learning process. They withhold reflection and conversation, the only ways lecture can be turned into intellectual, emotional, or spiritual nourishment.

Dewey offered the analogy of the car salesman who had a fantastic sales pitch, but the question remained, "Was he a good salesman if the customer left without buying a car?" We need to listen to the wisdom of Coach Auerbach, who never had a losing season and won nine championships in his eighteen years as head coach of the Boston Celtics. "It is not what you say—it is what they hear."

—10—

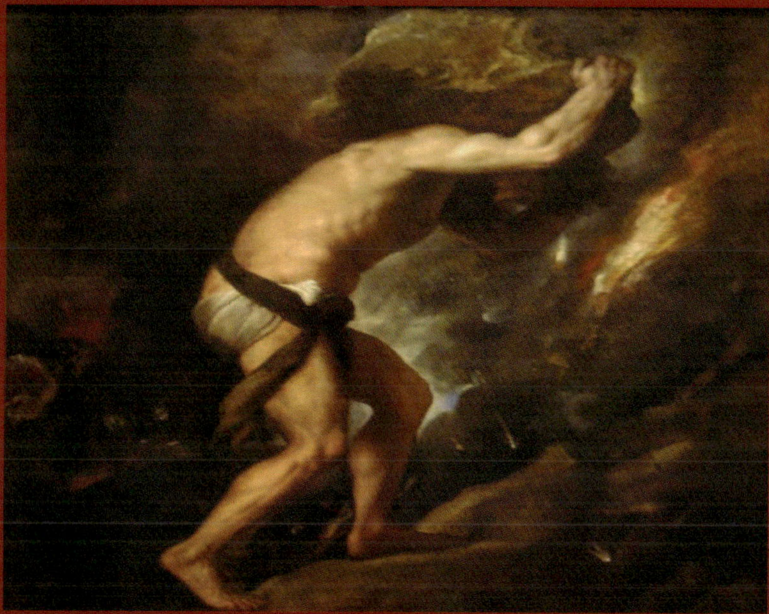

"Sisyphus" by Titian

Sisyphus, because of his audacity, was punished by the gods to roll a huge boulder up a hill, only to watch it roll down again, and to repeat this fruitless endeavor throughout eternity. Sisyphean can be used as an adjective meaning that an activity is unending and/or repetitive. It also refers to tasks that are pointless and unrewarding.

Why is our schooling so often Sisyphean? Why are so many math and English college professors teaching lessons that were taught years before—though not learned? I frequently find myself puzzled and frustrated because a high school graduate cannot write a complete sentence or interpret a simple text. Remedial education is a hot field in universities these days—and getting hotter. Increasing numbers of students arrive from our public schools not prepared for college level work. Why?

Many of my colleagues blame the students. They are so far behind because they are too lazy, spoiled, or simply too dumb. I think all those factors exist to some degree—but they are rare. Lack of intelligence is especially rare. What are not rare are curriculum-damaged students. They have undergone over a decade of a system of stultifying experiences in the forced-ingestion of knowledge bits. They have been gavaged into a lack of curiosity and initiative resulting in malnourished intellects. They think learning is the successful regurgitation of temporarily memorized knowledge bits, and they have either bought into that definition or spent time and energy resisting and resenting it. They have learned to play the game (going along to get along) or play the system (finding ways of not doing the work). They have either accepted or rejected the present definition of learning, and neither path prepares them for tomorrow's world.

Our students lack a developed intellect, the capacity to understand a subject or endeavor, and that makes them unable to do things, like write a persuasive, thoughtful, complete sentence or construct a personal interpretation. Worse, they often think they know, because they have the grades to prove it; they don't have the understanding to understand that they lack understanding. They don't know that they don't understand—and that is not their fault!

A colleague told me of a situation with a freshman advisee who wanted to become a physical therapist, a degree program that requires a good "working knowledge" of math:

> She flunked the math portion of the entrance exam. Placed into a remedial math course, which does not contribute to the requirements for graduation, she complained, and so did her parents. After all, she had a solid B+ in math on her high school transcript. I checked when she said that, and it was true. I urged her to take the test that would place her out of the remedial requirement. She did—and flunked it as well. She was angry, complaining that she had had all that stuff over a year ago and she had forgotten it. When challenged that she should have reviewed her math knowledge, she responded that she should not have to review. She knew the math and she had the grades to prove it.

What she didn't realize is that though she "knew" the math, at least well enough to pass the ubiquitous tests, she didn't understand it. Understanding is what prevents the educational process from being Sisyphean. When we reach an understanding, a residual picture of the process remains to guide future efforts in similar situations. If she had understood the math, a quick review would have sufficed or it would have come back to her during the challenge exam. (Howard Gardner has been urging us to educate for understanding for decades, but assessing the temporary ingestion of knowledge-bits is easy; understanding is difficult to measure.)

Education should not be such a Sisyphean endeavor. Sure, we forget things, and sometimes we simply fail to "get" things, but, overall, capability should be built by the process. It may not be a rigid sequence of ever upward-flowing constructed abilities. It may be gradual, sporadic, episodic, explosive, or transformative. We can even apply negatives to the process: "He was educated into an ivory tower from which he cannot escape, or, she suddenly found herself knowing more than she could handle." We more or less cycle ourselves upward in regard to capability, in awareness, in perspective, in ability for understanding and developing interpretation. Isn't the ideal that we shoulder the boulder up the mountain in order to qualify for a bigger, different boulder? Must it be the same damned old boulder?

What does the educational process accomplish if not the growth of our **intellectual capital**, a curious term indicating the collection of intangible abilities (such as creativity, emotional intelligence, accrued affinities and goodwill, cooperativeness, developed capacities, ability to think individually and socially, imagination, and historical knowledge of the organization, its stories) that can create **intellectual property**? Intellectual property is produced by intellectual capital coupled with intellectual effort. Intellectual capital, however, as opposed to physical capital, such as machines, buildings, and cash reserves, is ineffable and intangible. Perhaps the term intellectual capital is a little too mercantile for our purposes, but it is at least an attempt by economists to somehow measure the intangibles that are really the best products of the educational process.

The educated person can produce new knowledge, products, wisdom, teamwork, understandings, or new strengths and capabilities. The educated person is better able to learn and adapt, and help others learn and adapt. The educated person has developed his or her intellectual capital—having created intellectual property and capable of producing more. The educated are more response-able, more intelligent and therefore more capable of solving problems and fashioning products. The educated understands at a higher level; most importantly, they understand that they don't fully understand the interactive whole of an endeavor, that there is always more work to be done through the application of imagination, interest, dedication, and initiative.

However, our schooling fixates on transmitting correct-answers and assessing easily-measured knowledge bits. It ignores intellectual development, for intellect is comprised of understandings, which are difficult to either transmit or measure. The result is students who understand less and less—for the present definition of learning has led them to the false conclusion that simplistic knowing is sufficient proof of capability. The process itself constantly rolls the boulder back down to the bottom of the mountain, leaving teachers and students frustrated and confused, and our potential waiting and, for the time being, wasting.

> We have schools because we hope that some day when children have left schools that they will still be able to use what it is that they've learned. And there is now a massive amount of evidence from all realms of science that unless individuals take a very active role in what it is that they're studying, unless they learn to ask questions, to do things hands on, to essentially re-create things in their own mind and transform them as is needed, the ideas just disappear. The student may have a good grade on the exam, we may think that he or she is learning, but a year or two later there's nothing left.
>
> Howard Gardner

A Cautionary Image

—Think Systemically—

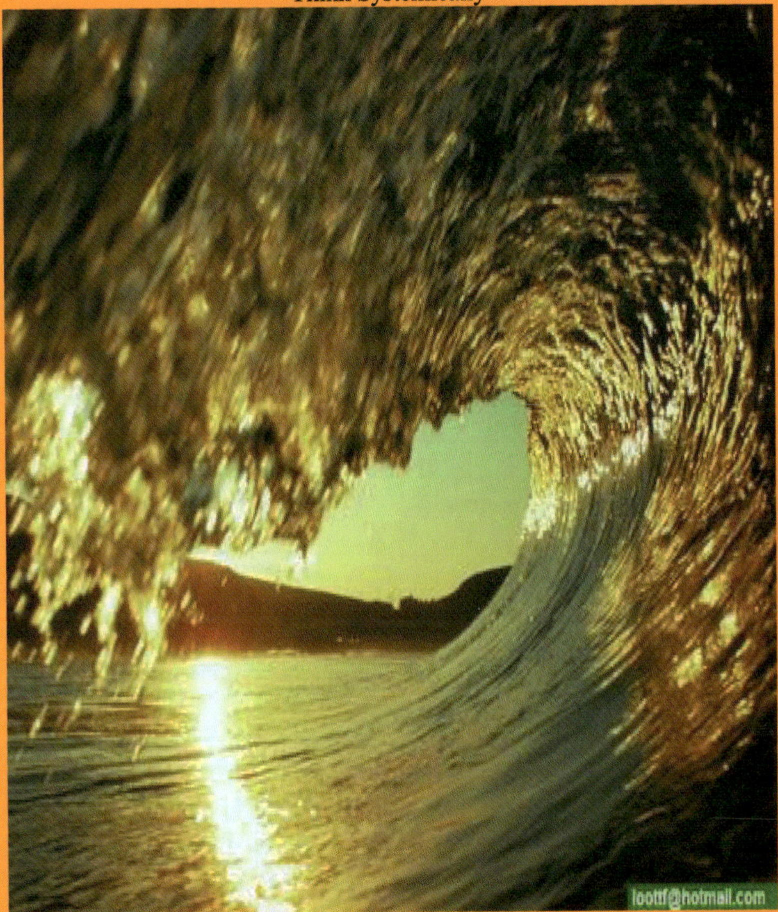

"The Moment of Drowning" by loottf

A person walking alongside a river sees someone drowning. The person jumps in, pulls the victim out, and begins artificial respiration. While this is going on, another person calls for help: the rescuer jumps into the water again and pulls the new victim out. This process repeats itself several times until the rescuer gets up and walks away from the scene. A bystander approaches and asks in surprise "where are you going?" to which the rescuer replies "I'm going upstream to find out who's pushing all these people in and see if I can stop it."

Gerard Egan and Michael A. Cowan

—11—

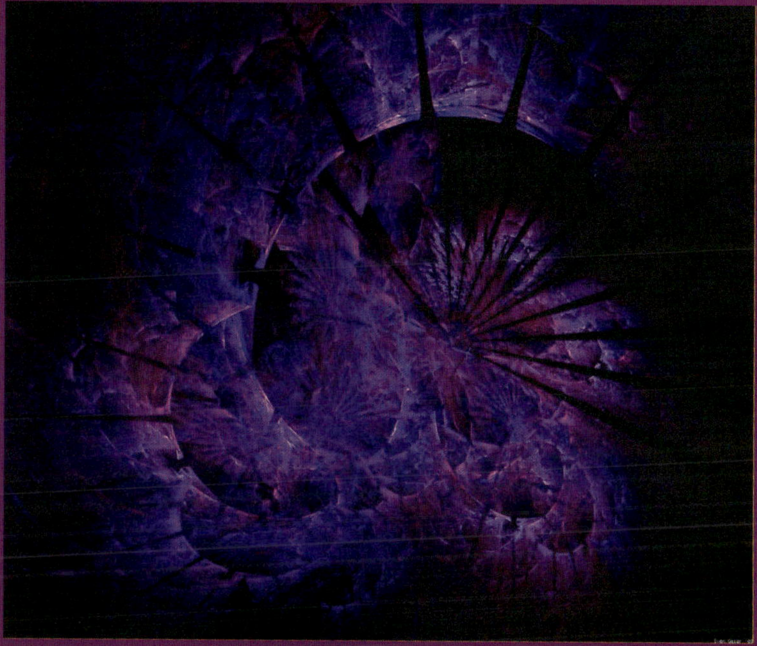

"Refocus" by Sven Geier

If a picture is worth a thousand words, a metaphor is worth a thousand pictures. We've moved from an economy built on people's *backs* to an economy built on people's ***left brains*** to what is emerging today: an economy and society built more and more on people's ***right brains***.

Daniel Pink

Perhaps one of the reasons that our schools are failing is a subconscious realization that the educational process is out of synch with the times. Perhaps people can sometimes sense relevance or the lack of it when they can't quite realize or articulate it. They don't know why something is irrelevant; they just know that it is. We can bring back an old sixties term here: Zeitgeist, the spirit of the times. Our schooling is simply not in tune with the times. Sometimes, perhaps, there is wisdom in resistance that goes beyond logic or understanding. We just somehow "know" that something is not quite right.

This is all too intuitive, perhaps, too right-brain, without the support of logic or evidence. But is it logical to teach with socialistic metaphors, methods, and materials in a democracy? Is it logical to teach in the same old ways in these dramatically changed times? How much more evidence is needed beyond the explosion of special education in public schools and remedial education in universities? Have some real conversations with students about their school lives. No more evidence will be necessary.

I sense more than resentment and resistance in many of my students to the educational process, I sense disdain. They feel like the schooling foisted upon them is like a huge day in and day out joke that they have to undergo because they lack the power to prevent it. I urge empathy here. When I attended public school over forty years ago, it too harbored the injection operating metaphor. But that metaphor was less irrelevant then than it is now. In the intervening decades left-brain learning has become less and less important to either society or the economy. But the schools have increasingly dug in their heels against that change, because assessment drives instruction, and what is increasingly assessed is the temporary ingestion of easily-measured knowledge bits. The intensity of gavaging has dramatically increased in the intervening decades, absurdly, in a negative correlation with the changing needs of the times.

Our educational system is, students can argue, simply self-serving; it only cares about itself, not them. Otherwise, why is the system so dedicated to the CYA directive, regardless of their needs? Students encounter a pervasive culture of bureaucracy, concerned only with taking care of its needs. But, even if the system did care, it is not aligned with the Zeitgeist. It is way behind the times. It is irrelevant, a feeling every teacher hates to hear. But are we not still educating for the Industrial Age? Do we not school as if the future depended upon left-brain thinking? In an absurd irony, education, the business of growth and change, is very slow on its feet. It lacks either imagination or flexibility. We keep striving to get better at educating for the left brain, preparing our students to become the managers of factories and professions that thrived a century ago. Soon, those factories and professions may no longer even exist. We are hard at work preparing people for the first part of the twentieth century.

Perhaps our students sense that truth, ahead of their teachers, and light-years ahead of the educationists and politicians in control of schooling. Students sense that the educational process, as it is now defined, is increasingly irrelevant to their future success and capability. The Zeitgeist is calling for differing capabilities than the ones demanded by the present definition of learning. Daniel Pink writes:

> When economies and societies depended on factories and mass production, R-Directed Thinking was mostly irrelevant. Then as we moved to knowledge work, R-Directed Thinking came to be recognized as legitimate, though still secondary, to the preferred mode of L-Directed Thinking. Now, as North America, Western Europe, Australia, and Japan evolve once again, R-Directed Thinking is beginning to achieve social and economic parity—and, in many cases, primacy. In the twenty-first century, it has become the first among equals, the key to professional achievement and personal satisfaction.

> But let me be clear: the future is not some Manichean world in which individuals are either left-brained and extinct or right-brained and ecstatic—a land in which millionaire potters drive BMWs and computer programmers scrub counters at Chick-fil-A. L-Directed Thinking remains indispensable. It's just no longer sufficient. In the Conceptual Age, what we need instead is a *whole* new mind.

The right brain is ignored by the present definition of learning. It must be ignored, for to recognize its importance is to pull the rug out from under the current assessment strategies and instructional directives. We need more time for instruction, the schools say, by which they mean more time to gavage, and so they push art and music out of the curriculum. (Too much hard-to-measure stuff going on in those endeavors, anyway.) And while we're at it, let's cut out recesses and physical activities. Hell, why don't we do away with playgrounds altogether whenever possible? The schools need more gavagable moments and fewer periods of time when stuff is happening that cannot be registered on the left-brain fixated assessment strategies.

Failure to redefine learning to where it incorporates metaphors, methods, and materials geared to instruction for the right brain will deserve the resentment, resistance, and even disdain of our students. When leaders or teachers generate the emergence of too much resentment and resistance, they will be removed from their positions—if not in fact, at least in influence. Disdain is an even deeper expression of disregard. We can only teach or lead those who (temporarily and provisionally) choose to give us credibility and allegiance.

Educators must understand the needs of their students in order to excite and inform their potentials. Our job, after all, is to help make possible futures more real for students. Not the futures of yesteryear—but those of tomorrow. As Aristotle stated, "Teaching is the highest form of understanding." And understanding is impossible without the proper metaphor, for it generates the constellation of pictures necessary for us to see, grasp, and comprehend such a complicated endeavor. Do we understand our students, their needs and fears, in this changing world?

Do our students sense that the system is not part of the solution—that it, in many ways, only exacerbates the problem? Dare we consider that their resentment and resistance is justified? We have a system that produces increasing numbers of dropouts and the curriculum damaged, but, so far, that only makes the system press harder in the same old ways that have previously failed. Why do we disregard facts regarding the systemic failure of our efforts provided by respected researchers such as Howard Gardner?

When the facts change, I change my mind. What do you do, sir?
John Maynard Keynes

Caution!!!

—Watch Your Metaphors—

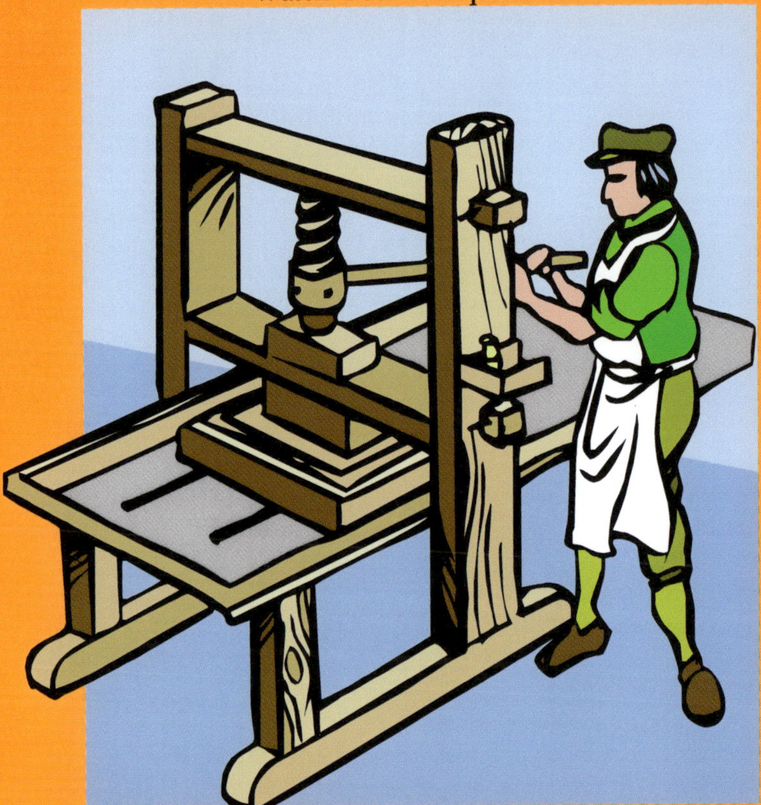

The assumption is that change comes from outside, something external has to <u>cause</u> it. Newton's first law of motion—that objects stay in their state until imposed on from the outside—reigns paradigmatic. Self-organization, a key element in complexity theory, is not considered. The curriculum counterpart of this stasis model is the student as passive receiver, moving only as moved, learning only as taught. Learning is tied directly to teaching. That we learn only that which is taught is, Dewey (1938) says, "perhaps the greatest of all pedagogical fallacies." In this stasis model, change is not only external but also causally direct. That is, there is presumed to be a one-to-one, direct relationship between the causative agent and the effected result. A typewriter or printing press, both symbols of modernist technology, are good metaphors here—the harder one presses, the greater the imprint.

William E. Doll, Jr.

—12—

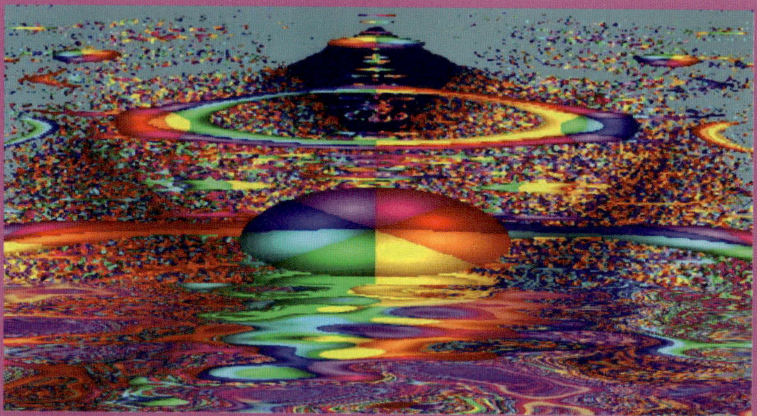

"Rainbow Way" by Judy Hart

IRIS was the goddess of the rainbow who carried messages to humans from the gods on Mount Olympus. Her name contains a double meaning, being connected both with *iris*, "the rainbow," and *eiris*, "messenger." The iris of the eye returns us to the need to revision, to see with "fresh eyes," for vision ripples through everything. Iris reminds us that image determines what we do—and that we cannot change what we do until we change what we see.

Hard to quantify qualities such as imagination, interest, initiative, and social dexterity are ignored by our schooling. Our better teachers strive to include such qualities whenever possible, to keep them alive and growing—though such teachers will not be perceived by the system as "effective," since the current operating metaphor is blind to their achievements. The present definition of effectiveness, in either teaching or learning, is locked onto the easily measured, and that blindness will continue until we achieve a revision of how and what we assess. Assessment should drive instruction, but not a simplistic assessment of a dynamically complex endeavor.

For example: an important characteristic of a successful leader is a sense of humor. Research has shown that the most effective leaders have their followers laughing three times as often as those in similar positions who were considered mere managers. But comedic ability, the capacity to suddenly leap out of a rut and spark a new perspective, is derived from the right brain. In left-brain schooling, humor is usually perceived as disruptive. And, of course, it is often employed by students toward that end. Nonetheless, humor is an important human capability that should not be ignored by our schooling. Some psychologists and educators, however, are beginning to explore assessment of right-brain qualities such as humor, imagination, initiative, and social dexterity:

> **A Hopeful Sign**—Tufts University professor Robert Sternberg heads a research team called the Rainbow Project. Designed as a supplement, if not an alternative, to the SAT, the test of right-brain capabilities has been twice as successful as the SAT in predicting student success in college. Test takers are given a series of blank New Yorker cartoons, and challenged to create humorous captions for them. They are also given titles, such as "The Octopus's Sneakers," and challenged to write or narrate a story in response. They are also given real world scenarios, such as dealing with a jerk of a co-worker, and must come up with an emotionally intelligent way of dealing with the situation.

Students who do well on the tests of their right-brain capabilities also predictably do well in college. The tests are harder to assess than multiple choice or essay, but include human capabilities presently ignored in our schooling. Some universities, tired of how ineffective the SAT is at predicting student success, and increasingly aware of its limitations regarding the capabilities of the right brain, are interested in innovative approaches such as The Rainbow Project. Scott Jaschik writes, in the magazine *Inside Higher Education*:

> This year [2006], applicants to Tufts University will also have the option of answering very different kinds of questions. They might be asked to write a short story to fit the title "Confessions of a Middle School Bully" or "The End of MTV." They might be asked to write an essay imagining what the world would have been like had Rosa Parks given up her seat on the bus or had John Paul I lived longer than a month as pope. Or they could create an advertisement or ad campaign for a product that doesn't exist. Other exercises might be timed and prompted by videos. They could watch a film about a situation they might face in college — such as going to a professor to ask for a recommendation only to realize that the professor doesn't know you — and write a short piece about what they would do.

Jaschik quotes Lee Coffin, dean of undergraduate admissions at Tufts:

> Competitive colleges have long paid lip service, of course, to the non-academic side of applicants. This is what we've always called "personal qualities." But this part of the process is doomed to be of little importance when it is so "soft" in that it hasn't been based on more than what you list on your activities. Does being student body president really mean something or was it just a popularity contest? In contrast, the "Rainbow Project" approach provides ways in theory to see how students respond to situations and how creative they can be in situations that they haven't been rehearsing at SAT camp for the last

> five summers. With a scientific basis to evaluating creativity and leadership, admissions officers are likely to put more weight on such qualities.

Also, while the SAT is not particularly effective at predicting college success for students from higher social-economic status, it is even less effective at predicting success for those from different economic and racial backgrounds. The Rainbow Project is more inclusive in its predictive abilities, uncovering capabilities that are not only more right-brain but less exclusive racially and economically. The evidence is accumulating that such right-brain focused tests are more effective than correct-answer tests at predicting success at being college students.

The name of The Rainbow Project is particularly appropriate, for it represents the widening of our eyes to become more aware. It strives to measure the hard-to-measure—ignored by our schooling because of its interactive messiness. After all, Iris is etymologically connected with eirô, "I join," whence eirênê; so that Iris, the goddess of the rainbow, would be the joiner or conciliator, or the messenger of heaven who restores peace in nature. (We can call her the Goddess of the Corpus Callosum). Also, unlike Hermes, who only did the bidding of the gods, Iris often carried messages of her own volition—advising and assisting humans of her own accord. (We can also call her the Goddess of Initiative.)

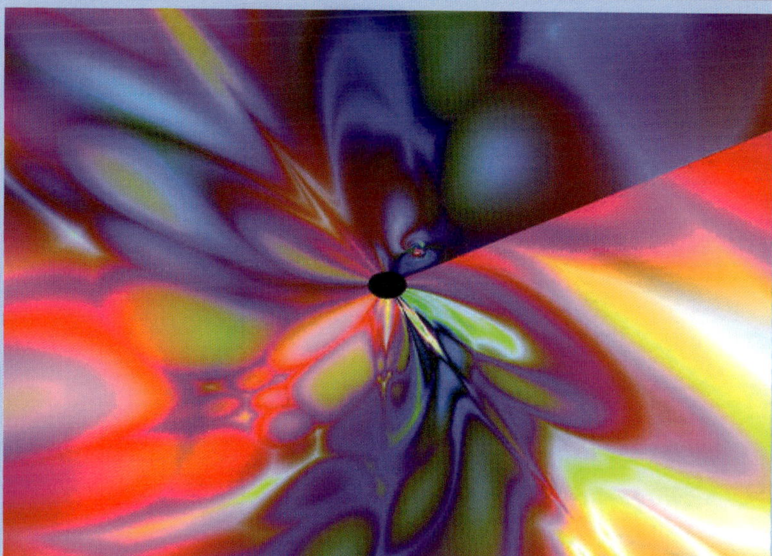

"Butterfly Song" from realeoni's photostream

Just as the rainbow displays the full color spectrum, we may be preparing to investigate and educate the full spectrum of our intelligence and capability.

Consider—the Uses of a Brick

It all has to do with the flow of those "little gray cells" made famous by Agatha Christie's Hercule Poirot. The left brain influences (affects the flow) movement toward the production of convergence (confluence into a single stream). The right brain prefers divergence (separation into different pathways). Neither type of flow of those little gray cells is either good or bad—except in relation to the demands of the situation. Convergent thinking is important to focus (or specialization). Divergent thinking is important to the exploration of alternative possibilities (new avenues of focus). Our schooling, however, is fixated on convergent thinking, the production and measurement of correct answers. It pushes convergence, regardless of the situation, regardless of the student, regardless of variation in capability or potential. It not only ignores but actively suppresses divergent thinking because it disrupts its addiction to the easily transmitted and measured. The problem is that we need divergent thinking, for two reasons: 1. the new world is calling for more right brain capabilities. 2. a culture of divergent thinking is essential to the spirit of democracy.

In his book, *Outliers: the Story of Success*, Malcolm Gladwell investigates why genius (as proven by convergence tests) isn't a good indicator of future achievements. He writes:

"...Suppose that instead of measuring your IQ, I gave you a totally different kind of test. Write down as many different uses that you can think of for the following object: **a brick.** This is an example of what's called a 'divergence test' (as opposed to a test which asks you to sort through a list of possibilities and *converge* on the right answer). It requires you to use your imagination and take your mind in as many different directions as possible. With a divergence test, obviously there isn't a single right answer. What the test giver is looking for are the number and uniqueness of your responses. And what the test is measuring isn't analytical intelligence but something profoundly different—something much closer to creativity."

Gladwell points out that Nobel Prize winning work requires both brilliance and imagination. A certain threshold of intelligence is a prerequisite, but right brain, divergent thinking, is also necessary. He compares the results of the brick test between two students: both have high IQ's but one does poorly on the test for divergent thinking. He then asks an important question: "Now which of these two students do you think is better suited to do the kind of brilliant, imaginative work that wins Nobel Prizes?"

But how do you measure divergent thinking? And how do you transmit the capability? Project-based learning, conversation, reflection, and the arts come to mind. But those approaches are anathema to a top-down, centralized-control, socialistic mindset. Still, we need to know more than one way, or even a few ways, of using a brick.

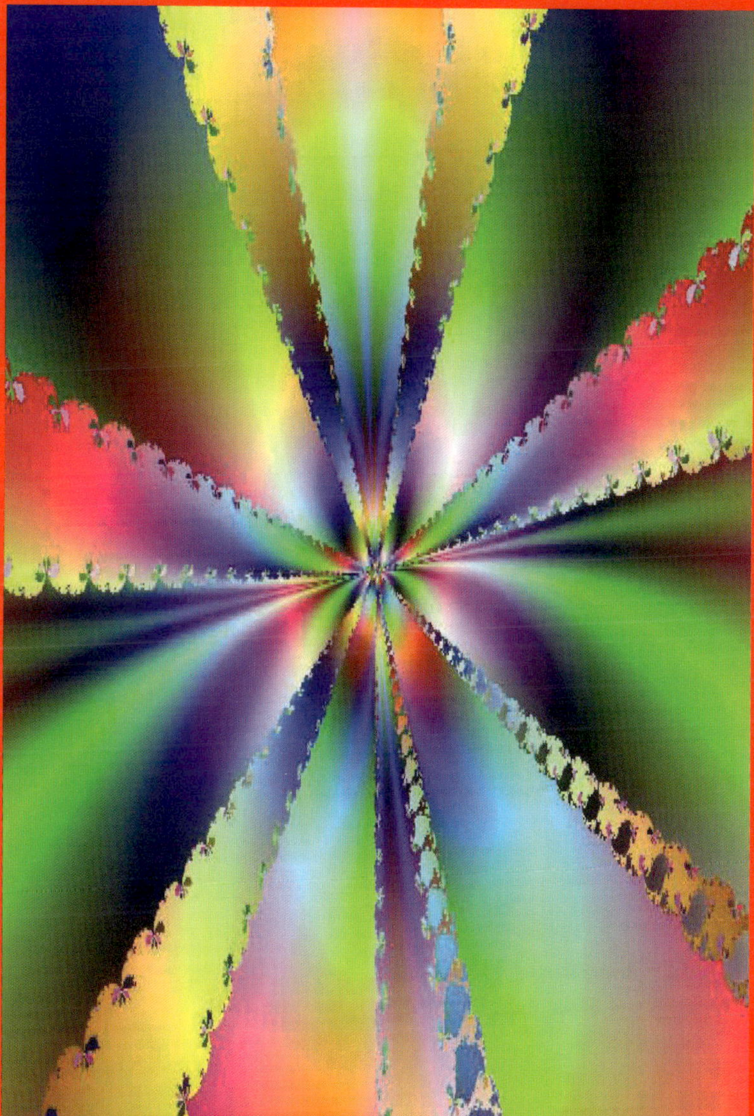

"Rainbow Ribbons—Scalloped" from Fractals by Beth

It's not that the analytical skills measured by the SAT aren't important. But they aren't enough. We have to stop putting so much emphasis on only a sliver of the abilities that kids can bring to college.

Robert Sternberg

—13—

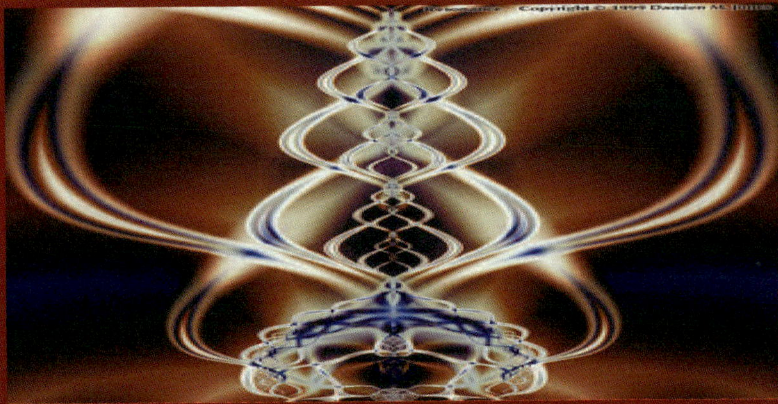

"Resonance" by Damien M. Jones

The good-to-great companies paid scant attention to managing change, motivating people, or creating alignment. Under the right conditions, the problems of commitment, alignment, motivation, and [dealing with] change largely melt away.

Jim Collins

As we better understand the nature of learning, we will forget about all this instructional methodology stuff and instead focus on developing learning environments. We will develop an ecology of education, where we better understand the conditions within the classroom that determine what grows—or doesn't grow—there. What we can and should do is design classroom conditions conducive to the emergence of imaginative and responsible learning, where intellects are developed. Present methods are formulaic at best and manipulative at worst. It's the conditions—not the machinations—that determine the presence and character of learning environments. Conditions determine whether classrooms are defined by boredom, chaos, compliance or cooperation, contribution, and worthwhile learning. A condition is defined as

Something that must exist before something else can occur.

People must trust others before they will loan them money without collateral. Mountain climbers must be in good physical condition before they tackle Mt. Everest. People must feel safe, or willing to pay the costs, before they will speak up. People generally love each other before they will get married. Fuel and oxygen must exist before fire is possible. The condition of credibility must exist before students will listen to teachers. The truly important developments are all conditions-based. Factors such as imagination, interest (and thus involvement), initiative, and, ultimately, integrity cannot be manipulated into existence. They must be grown through self-directed learning—and growth always depends upon conditions.

Intrinsic motivation, a powerful drive, is nonetheless fragile (but not always) in the face of suppressive conditions. The carrots and sticks of external control mechanisms are toxic to intrinsic motivation. The "scientific management" of a dynamically complex task, such as teaching and learning, results in the suppression of the very drive that best fuels worthwhile learning. Daniel H. Pink, in his book, *Drive: The Surprising Truth about What Motivates Us,* quotes the work of Edward L. Deci:

> Careful consideration of reward effects reported in 128 experiments lead to the conclusion that tangible rewards tend to have a substantially negative effect on intrinsic motivation. When institutions—families, schools, businesses, and athletic teams, for example—focus on the short-term and opt for controlling people's behavior they do considerable long term damage.
>
> [Pink then adds] Try to encourage a kid to learn math by paying her for each workbook page she completes—and she'll almost certainly become more diligent in the short term and lose interest in math in the long term. . . . This is one of the most robust findings in social science—and also one of the most ignored. . . . Perhaps we're scared to let go of Motivation 2.0, despite its obvious downsides. Perhaps we can't get our minds around the peculiar quantum mechanics of intrinsic motivation.

A former colleague frequently complained that she couldn't get her students to talk in class. I found out later, from different students at different times, that she had taught them to keep their mouths shut. If they dared to make a contribution and it be wrong (by her definition) or even incomplete, she would respond in such a derogatory way that the students were embarrassed and shamed. The conditions in her classroom guaranteed the suppression of any contribution. Another story illustrates the importance of conditions:

> Mr. Fogg loved history—of that there was no doubt. But it takes more than that to be a high school history teacher. He couldn't teach a motivated minnow to swim. He'd soon have it lost and confused, flopping around on the sandy floor of Death Valley. Mr. Fogg could never resist a tangent, and off he would go, until the class had no idea of what he was up to, where he was going, or even where he had been. Students got bored, then resistive. Previous students had found out that Mr. Fogg was lavish with threats but never delivered. That is a death sentence for a teacher, so the hyenas gathered. It was fun, and sad, to watch students goad him into a conniption fit. It was done easily and

> frequently. But one year, at least in one class, he became a teacher. It was a puzzle, because he was his same old confusing, ineffectual self. Nonetheless, nobody goaded him. His tortuous and never-ending lectures were not disrupted, which improved sleep patterns for many, but surprised and pleased him. He thought he had become a teacher. What he didn't realize was that conditions had changed in that one classroom. Two conditions in particular: Tootie Gorman and Donna Haynes. Both were attractive, high-status, and bright cheerleaders with high EQs. Both had ambitions, unusual in the school, of going on to college. They therefore wanted a real history class, so they went to the usual "goaders," the athletes, and requested that they not only behave but compel other rascals to toe the line. So Tootie and Donna, and maybe two or three others, paid attention; the athletes slept or looked at Tootie and Donna, unless it was necessary to stare threateningly at a disrupter, and the class went like clockwork. Poor Mr. Fogg probably saw that one class as evidence of his teaching ability, "If only they would listen!" He never knew the conditions that had caused the emergence of a learning community (well, sort of) that year.

Teaching is a leadership position—but poor Mr. Fogg had no leadership ability. He lacked the emotional intelligence. His inability to resist a tangent, a mind-numbing delivery, and making constant but empty threats were the dominant cultural conditions preventing him from teaching what he truly loved. Therefore, learning communities never developed in his classrooms—under his leadership.

The present definition of learning *pushes* learning with coercive and manipulative mechanisms, instead of designing conditions that *pull* learning through appeals to student interest, imagination, and initiative. It is the difference between management and leadership: managers push while leaders pull. Policies guided by the operating metaphor of management generate conditions that invite compliance at best and resentment and resistance at worst while those guided by the operating metaphor of leadership trust the power of intrinsic motivation to excite initiative in pursuit of our best selves.

Rexford G. Brown, in *Schools of Thought: How the Politics of Literacy Shape Thinking in the Classroom*, writes:

> Again and again, we saw that the difference between a school or district that offered conditions hospitable to thoughtfulness and a school or district that did not was a difference in the kind, quality, and coherence of the conversations that were taking place there. What good policy can do is stimulate, legitimate, and sustain healthy conversations and literate discourse. It can assemble people to inquire into the most fundamental matters, to argue about them and use the very skills and dispositions they want to develop in students: problem solving, reasoning, analysis, questioning, collaborating, democratic decision making, and all the rest. Bad policy either does nothing to the system, in which case its natural

> entropy grows, or it stimulates unhealthy conversations and resistance. It shuts discourse down, rather than opening it up.

Policies often mindlessly generate conditions that prevent the delivery of what we most value. Andrea Batista Schlesinger, in *The Death of Why: The Decline of Questioning and the Future of Democracy,* discusses Susan Engel's "Open Pandora's Box: Curiosity and Imagination in the classroom:"

> In a telling experiment, teachers were presented with a list of twenty-five goals for their teaching and asked to circle the top five. "Curiosity" was circled by a majority. But when teachers were asked to name the top educational goals without reference to such a list, there was almost no mention of curiosity. Engel concluded that "teachers may passively endorse curiosity, but we have evidence that they do little to actively promote it."

Teachers know that the present definition of learning does not support conditions conducive to curiosity, imagination, initiative, and inquiry, which are all inimical to coverage-fixation and test scores. They, and we, wish to design and deliver classroom conditions that excite and inform such factors, but the system dictates otherwise.

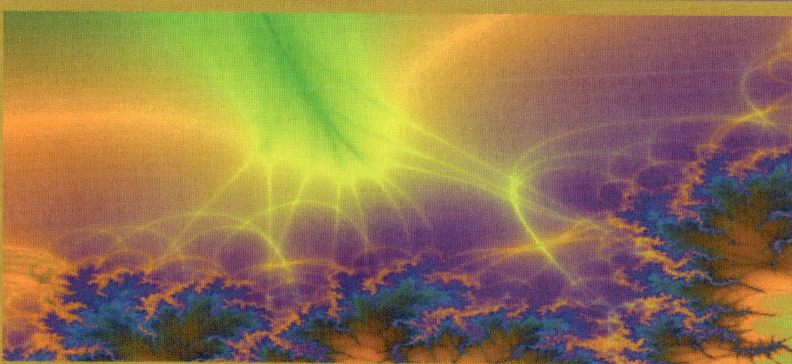

"Synapse Attack" by Noel Clark

We should ditch the word policy and replace it with **delivery plan.** The word policy does not project a clear image of its function. It also carries the onerous connotation of unthinking adherence to procedures-in-place regardless of their impact on effectiveness. Whenever policy impedes delivery, the plan needs to be changed. The word itself impedes its function by establishing conditions that suppress individual judgment and personal initiative and, therefore, response-ability as well as responsibility. Instead of asking, "What's the policy?" we should ask, "What's the delivery plan?" There is a world of difference in the mindsets behind those two questions. For one thing, delivery plan is more mindful of conditions.

Policy is the wrong word for the job.

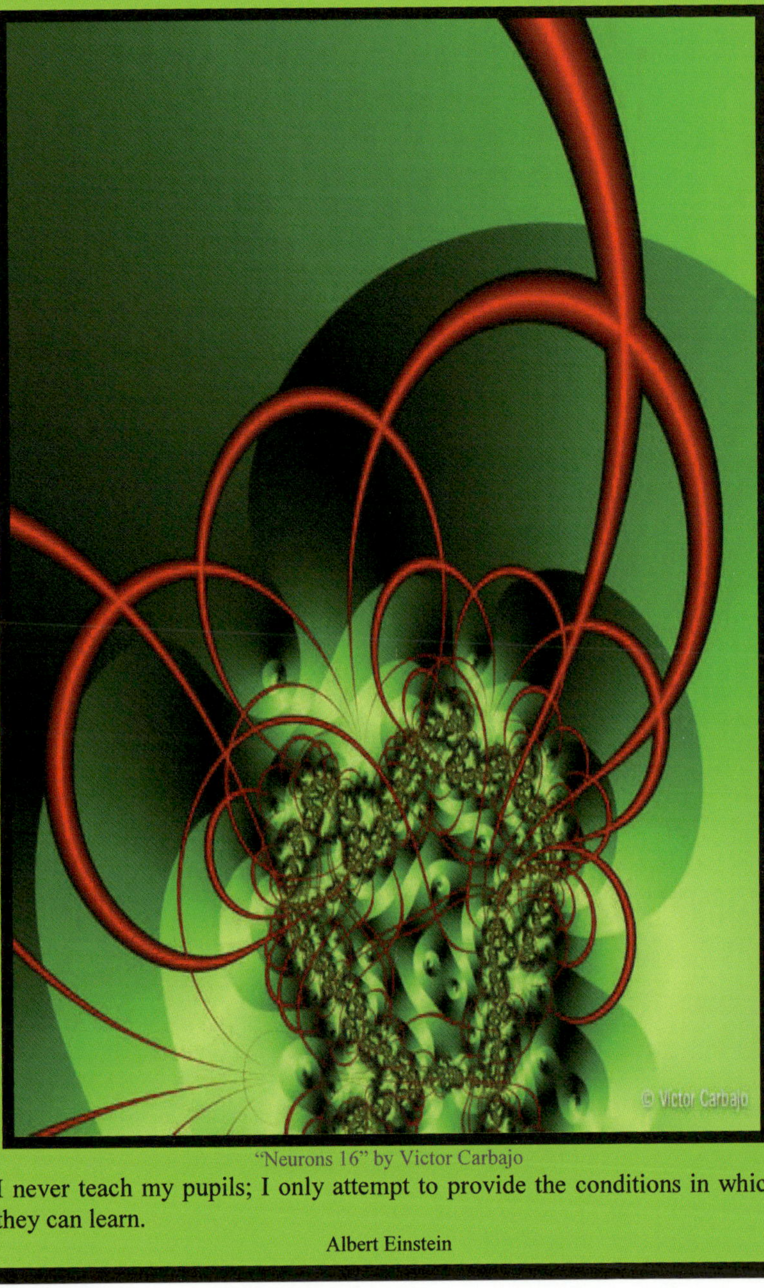

"Neurons 16" by Victor Carbajo

I never teach my pupils; I only attempt to provide the conditions in which they can learn.

Albert Einstein

—14—

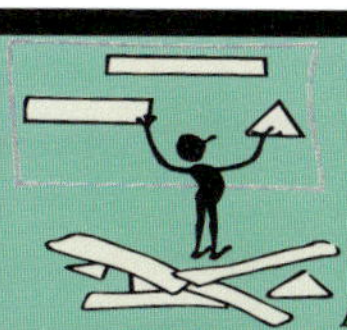

All thought is a feat of association: having what's in front of you bring up something in your mind that you almost didn't know you knew. Putting this and that together. That click.

Robert Frost

In order to construct an association, a learner must have the energy of initiative. Thinking is a personal act, one that develops from the desires for understanding, ownership, and self-expression. Thinking is always an adjustment to the situation, in the perspective, in the approach, in the understanding. It is the click that changes the picture. Training can and should inform the act of thinking but, in our imbalanced schooling, training discourages thinking by persistently implying it is unnecessary. Schooling becomes a process where students are not challenged to construct associations. They are instead fed a steady stream of disconnected knowledge bits. As initiative is crowded out of the educational process, so is thinking.

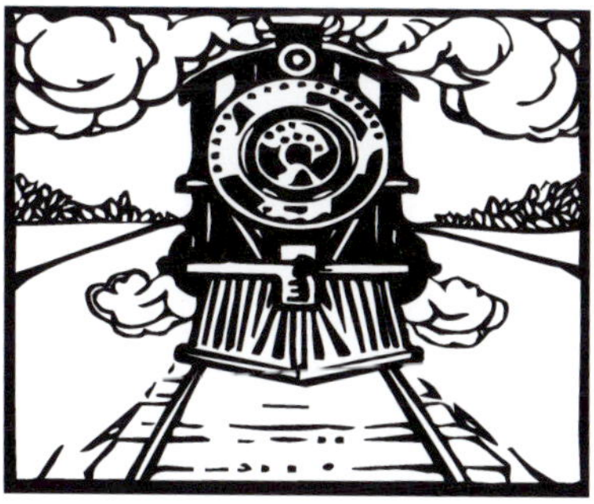

Training, as *The Oxford Universal Dictionary* informs us, is etymologically related to the locomotive device that drags things down a laid-out track: from the Latin *trahere*, to draw, drag. To draw or pull along after one; to drag, haul, trail.

The locus of control in training is the curriculum (a sputum-sounding disease-looking word related to the circular track around which Roman chariots raced). The curriculum (or track) is pulled by assessment strategies, or locomotive (locus of motives?). Some years ago I attended a workshop on "calibrated curriculum." The premise was that a truly well-constructed curriculum would guarantee specific (and I mean specific) learning outcomes. We spent a weekend calibrating curriculum, laying out the track so well that no student's learning could deviate from the design or be derailed by even their own hesitations or resistance. They would be "gavaged" whether they liked it or not.

However, the locus of control—of whether learning occurs and how it develops—resides in the learner. Initiative is integral to the constructive nature of the educational process. It comes from antithetical origins:

Initiative—from the Latin *instiare*, to begin, commence, enter upon, introduce, set going, originate—the function, power, or faculty of beginning or originating something.

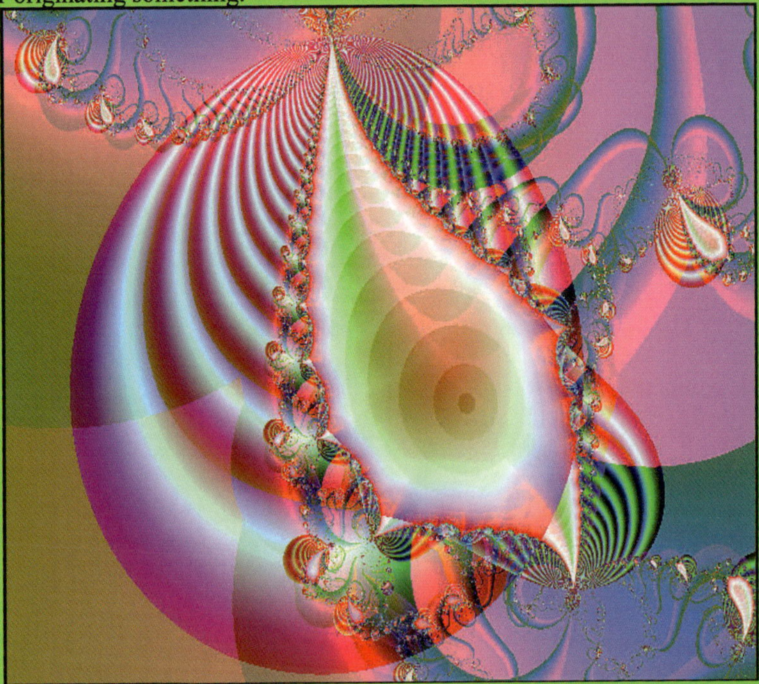

"Opening Seeds" by Ken Keller

The energy of initiative is at the core of all effective teaching and worthwhile learning. It is a cardinal strength. Without its confident and vigorous presence, the development of other strengths, such as thinking, is not possible. It is the energy behind the construction of associations indicated by Robert Frost. Initiative cannot be dragged forth by training. It must emerge of its own volition. We can establish conditions that encourage that emergence, but we cannot make it happen. When we intentionally ignore that bothersome truth, we neglect the heart of education.

The worst systemic effect of training crowding initiative out of schooling is the loss of the arts in the curriculum. The arts encourage and inform initiative, but they are harder to measure and supervise than the transmission of facts. The arts have been treated as the bathwater, when they are essential to imagination, interest, intelligence, intellect, and integrity—when they are the baby. Without the arts, students are more often disinterested and disengaged; they lack initiative and therefore responsibility. Every culture realizes the fundamental importance of art to our humanness and potential—except that of our schools.

Knowledge not allowed to be turned into a gift by the unwrapping done by initiative becomes a curse. Knowledge not given life by initiative becomes nothing more than a collection of "inert ideas." Knowledge is a gift, but only if it is unwrapped by thinking, application, and utilization. Learning redefined will bring the arts back into our schooling by understanding its integral role in holistic (left and right brain) worthwhile learning.

Here is a secret suppressed in a culture of prediction and control, real learning is dependent upon the **freedom** of individual teachers—and students—to engage their initiative. As Donald W. Oliver and Kathleen Waldron Gershman write, in their book, *Education, Modernity, and Fractured Meaning: Toward a Process Theory of Teaching and Learning*:

> We would suggest that the secret of learning also lies in its freedom. Learning that stops in the memorization stage does little to deserve the name. What activity there is usually compelled by the teacher [in the name of the system], and yet we know that true creativity is self-compelled.
>
> . . . Knowledge, treasured as the gift of education, is really only useful as a catalyst for the active use of the student's creativity. Not used for this purpose, knowledge simply amounts to inert ideas, Alfred North Whitehead's definition of the most useless thing in education. "What is wanted is activity in the presence of knowledge, novel viewpoints, knowledge applied to experience."

Correct-answer schooling crowds out initiative through training, as well as interest through coverage, imagination through, again, coverage, and intellect, through testing for temporarily memorized knowledge bits. Correct-answer schooling fears the messiness of freedom even though freedom is necessary for intellectual development, for how can the intellect grow without interest, initiative, and imagination? Without freedom, ideas, no matter how important or even inherently interesting, are inert.

The education world constantly trots out rhetoric calling for self-directed learners while it pushes correct-answer schooling and suppresses the arts. Real learning, and, ultimately, real teaching cannot be forced. Freedom to self-direct and self-engage individual initiative is essential. Creativity can only be produced by the interactive dance within the individual or social corpus callosum; our fixation on the left brain diminishes both innovation and ownership.

> If we value independence, if we are disturbed by the growing conformity of knowledge, of values, of attitudes, which our present system induces, then we may wish to set up conditions of learning which make for uniqueness, for self-direction, and for self-initiated learning.
>
> Carl Rogers

–15–

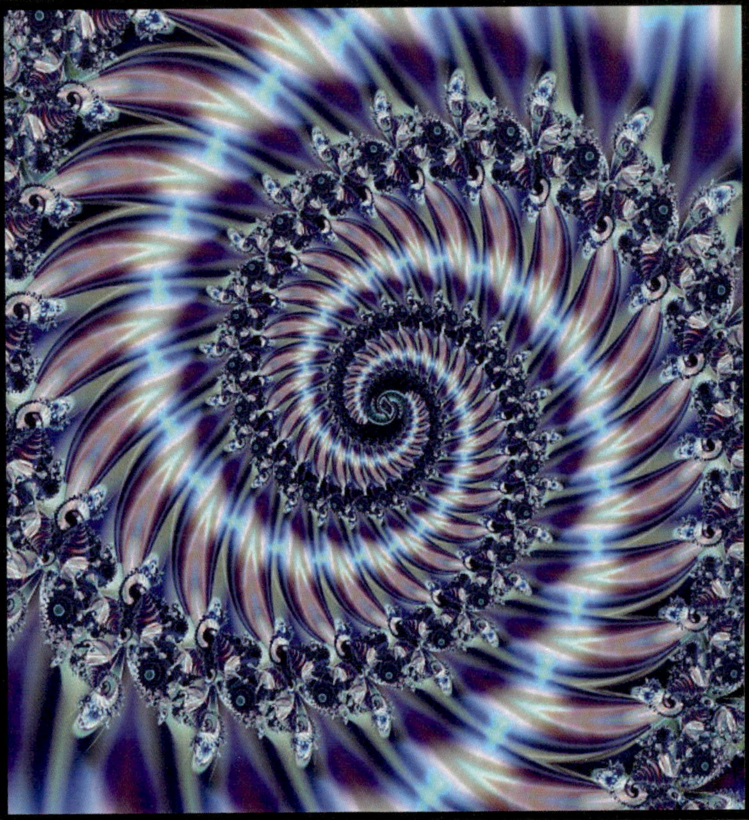

"Hypnotic Blues" by Donna Casey

Those who seek to label a swirl in the river are condemned to be identified with it and to be imprisoned by their attachment to it—a frozen moment in the dance with reality.

Anthony Judge

Learning as it is presently defined is fixated on **Congelated Knowing**:

> Congeal means to convert from a fluid to a solid state (*Oxford English Dictionary*). The congelation of knowledge occurs when it is presented with its shape and substance "frozen" in meaning and separated (or curdled) into compartmentalized lumps.

Congelated knowing forgets about the river. It focuses on the easily measured swirls, the parts frozen from the messy, complicated dynamics of the whole. It ignores the fluid nature of reality—and learning. That is why it systemically pushes "inert ideas"—which accounts for the "inert atmospheres" of most classrooms. It suppresses opportunities for imagination, interest, and initiative, though they bring life and flow to the learning, because they cause messiness in transmission and assessment. Learning redefined will be more focused on **Narrative Knowing**:

> Understanding, the product of narrative knowing, is produced by awareness of the story in both its process and its completeness. The best questions are: What is the story? How does this fact or factor fit in with the story? How does this new knowledge or reality affect the story? What do we want to happen next in developing our understanding of the subject under study? Narrative knowing indicates the presence of personally constructed thought about ecological relationships. Narrative learning perceives the interconnected fluidity of situations—its flow.
>
> Narrative Knowing addresses flow realities while Congelated Knowing strives to disconnect variables from their ecological situatedness. This makes them easier to measure at the same time it makes them less meaningful, for meaning resides in the evolving context of story. Dynamic complexity is beyond the capacity of congelated knowing to either envision or measure. Therefore, both its reality and importance are denied. Because of this systemic approach to learning, we gather knowledge at the same time we lose understanding. It is possible, after all, to know everything and understand nothing. It is not just the dots, it's also their connecting; no matter how much we measure otherwise.

Narrative knowing—and developed intellects—will be a key aspect of Learning Redefined. The increasingly dynamic complexity of our challenges and opportunities demands that we increase our capacity for perceiving and dealing with ecological realities. A fixation on freezing, labeling, and testing the swirls in the river will not help us understand the river. It is increasingly necessary for us to encourage, inform, and assess the capabilities of the right brain—since it takes imagination, interest, and initiative to construct the comprehensions, the pictures that provide the story. An educational system fixated on "correct-answer schooling," as Gardner warned us, cannot support the "risks for understanding" necessary for dealing with a dynamically complex world. Congelated knowledge-bits not woven into the flowing fabric of a narrative bed contribute nothing to the development of intellect—and are thus meaningless noise and distracting static.

> It is a well-known scandal that our whole educational system is geared more to categorizing and analyzing patches of knowledge than to threading them together.
>
> Harlan Cleveland

—16—

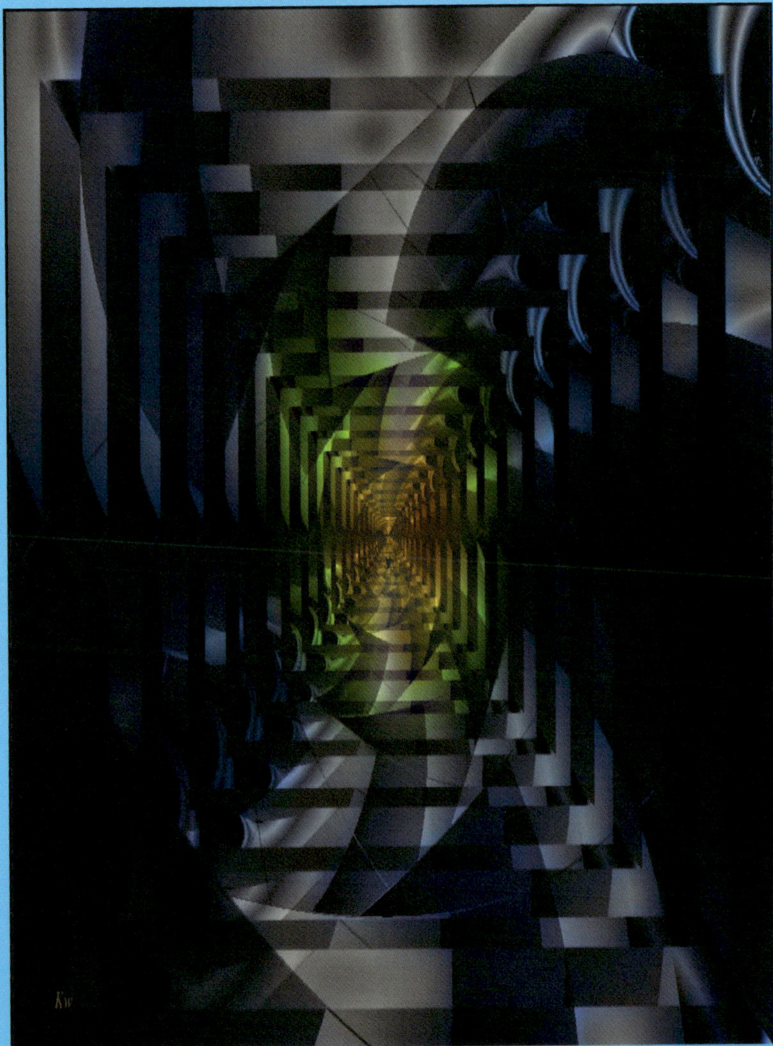

"Hall of Mirrors" by Ken Worden

The philosophy of the schoolroom in one generation will be the philosophy of government in the next.

Abraham Lincoln

> The ideal of democracy is continuously taught in American schools. But it is taught through lecture, workbooks, homework, and the occasional (usually canned) discussion. It is not modeled. The habits of democratic thinking are suppressed by the designs of our schooling. The conditions underlying the way we school our children are antithetical to the emergence of democratic habits and responsibilities. Philosophy begets methods and materials, and, as Lincoln pointed out, future conditions.

There is little about the structure of our schools that promotes and extends the democratic way of life. As we have discussed, present schooling is philosophically based on the work of Frederick Taylor, an American economist much beloved by Lenin, who incorporated his views into the Soviet economic and educational systems. Regrettably, our educational system also bought the Tayloristic operating metaphor. Our schooling is not aligned with our democratic values. It is, however, aligned with the socialistic metaphors of the educational bureaucrats, who, through on-the-same-page training and centralized assessment impose socialistic methods and materials.

James A. Beane and Michael W. Apple write, in their book, *Democratic Schools*:

> If people are to secure and maintain a democratic way of life, they must have opportunities to learn what that way of life means and how it might be led (Dewey 1916). Although common sense alone tells us this is a true statement, there is perhaps no more problematic concept in education than that of democratic schools, a concept that some consider almost an oxymoron. How can this be so? Simply put, many people believe that democracy is nothing more than a form of federal government and thus does not apply to schools and other social institutions. Many also believe that democracy is a right of adults, not of young people. And some believe that democracy simply cannot work in schools.

As John Dewcy said, "Democracy has to be born anew in each generation, and education is its midwife." The times call for the strengths of a democratic citizenry, who have the individual initiative, desire for personal ownership and dedication, and the contributing individuality coupled with collaborative synergy to meet the challenges of tomorrow. It would be a deep irony if our educational practices failed to accomplish that, despite the advantages of our history and our ideals.

Apple and Beane are concerned that America is suffering from a lack of what Dewey and other thinkers have referred to as "democratic faith." We have somehow allowed the spirit of democracy to be suppressed within the development of ourselves.

They write:

Democratic faith is the fundamental belief that democracy has a powerful meaning, that it can work, and that it is necessary if we are to maintain freedom and human dignity in our social affairs.

It is hard to find evidence of democratic faith in the metaphors and methods of most of our educational organizations. Socialistic faith is more common, more often at the core of the procedures and policies that govern schooling in this, in essence, democratic nation. The conditions of American schooling are more conducive to developing the kind of passive and compliant citizens desired by non-democratic countries.

Two Cautionary Tales

A lady asked Benjamin Franklin after the convention, "Well, Dr. Franklin, what have we got, a republic or a monarchy [or a dictatorship]?" "A republic," replied one of our wisest founding fathers, "if you can keep it."

We have reason to fear!

Alfie Kohn writes: "Some years ago, a group of teachers from Florida traveled to what was then the USSR to exchange information and ideas with their Russian-speaking counterparts. What the Soviet teachers most wanted from their guests was guidance on setting up and running democratic schools. Their questions were based on the assumption that a country like the United States, so committed to the idea of democracy, surely must involve children in decision-making processes from the earliest years. The irony is enough to make us wince."

The systemic ramifications of the present educational process could be severe. If Lincoln is correct and the philosophy of the schoolroom in one generation is the philosophy of government in the next, then we have good reason to fear for the future of our democracy.

As James Madison, father of the Constitution and fourth president, warned us,

> **A well-instructed people alone can be permanently a free people.**

The problem lies within the definition of "well-instructed," for it has come to indicate the successfully gavaged and tested. The current mandarins of the educational process are addicted to the easily measured, claiming it to be proof of instruction, when the hidden curriculum is passive learning. The systemic result of education that trains learners into being passive recipients of transmitted data is ignored—to our peril.

Have we lost our democratic faith?

Yong Zhao, now at Michigan State University, grew up in China, and experienced its educational process both as a student and teacher. He set out to write about education in China but changed his focus to the puzzle of why American education seems to be losing its faith in itself. *In Catching Up or Leading the Way,* he writes: ". . . the U.S. has been trying hard to implement what China has been trying to get rid of. An increasing number of states and the federal government have begun to dictate what students should learn, when they should learn it, and how their learning is measured through state-mandated curriculum standards, high school exit exams, and NCLB. There are calls for even more centralization and standardization through national standards and national testing, as well as through rewarding or measuring schools and teachers based on test scores.

"I find this trend in American education perplexing. If China, a developing country aspiring to move into an innovative society, has been working to emulate U.S. education, why does America want to abandon it? Furthermore, why does America want to adopt practices that China and many other countries have been so eager to give up? But most vexing is why Americans, who hold individual rights and liberty in the highest regard, would allow the government to dictate what their children should learn, when they should learn it, and how they are evaluated?"

What <u>are</u> we doing?

A Cautionary Thought

Thomas Jefferson observed that America, alone of all the nations, has its coherence centered upon its ideas. Other countries have ethnicity to cohere their identities, to bond their citizenry, but ours is a hodgepodge of nationalities held together by principles. This wonderful uniqueness, however, makes our nation inherently fragile. Ours is a patchwork heritage held together by ideals. If we fail to educate our citizens to the worthiness of our ideals, we will perish. The future of our integrity depends upon the strength of our principles to weave us together—a future current schooling ignores and even degrades.

Ideals appeal to and depend upon the strength of the right brain. The left brain likes the easily tangible connections of ethnicity, sectarianism, or party loyalty. The right brain more often resonates with principles. The left-brain simply doesn't get them—for they are holistic and spiritual rather than tribal or legalistic. We cannot ignore the right brain in our schooling—and expect to remain a democracy.

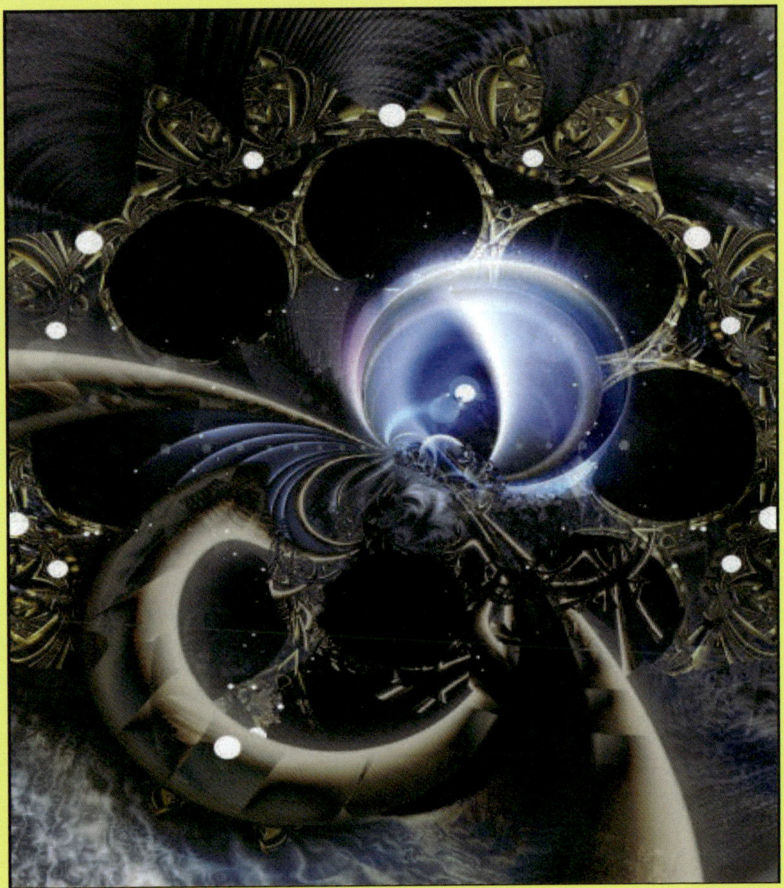

"Circle of Trust" by Cynthia Pedrosa

Becoming American is less a function of birth or blood and more a function of embracing a set of ideas. It is only for this reason that terms like "un-American" and "anti-American" make sense. You could not accuse someone of being "un-German" or "un-Pakistani." They would not know what you were talking about.

Dinesh D'Souza, *What's So Great about America*

In *The American Democrat*, published in 1838, James Fenimore Cooper argued that the word "American" was synonymous with the habit of telling the truth.

Lewis H. Lapham

The democratic process demands a true and vital conversation, where every stakeholder feels free to "turn" the flow of attention and endeavor into a different consideration or effort. When individual uniqueness and ownership are respected, disorder logically ensues. However, the strength, flexibility, and creativity of democracy—coupled with the power of personal ownership and responsibility—are considered worth the messiness by those with democratic faith. Our system has fixated on educating the left brain because it has an affinity for convergent thinking. Democratic education, on the other hand, is sympathetic to divergent thinking. Socialism likes to train its teachers and students to adhere to centralized definitions of productivity; democracy likes to encourage the emergence and development of initiative within its teachers and students.

It takes a mature community, one with the integrity of shared principles and tolerant if not affectionate connections to live the democratic process. It takes a mature teacher, confident with his or her ability to deal with tangents, messiness, and sometimes damnable truths to allow democratic conversation in the classroom. But the healthy educational process, as Whitehead understood, requires both order (training) and disorder (initiative). Training strives to prevent messiness within the educational process while initiative invites it.

But here is the rub: reality is messy, especially in dynamically complex times. This is why we need more right brain thinking, i.e. such factors as imagination, interest, and initiative. The left brain is uncomfortable with messiness and will try to avoid it, even to the point of intentional ignorance. The right brain is more accepting of disorder, and is continually following its curiosity in search of dangers and opportunities.

American democracy took root within the context of the frontier, unknown territory with unknown (for the most part) dangers and unknown opportunities. It took the imagination, interest, and initiative of individual community members to deal with the dangers and seize the opportunities. Geographical frontiers are now pretty much gone—but cultural, technological, and economic frontiers are constantly emerging. The world is getting messier—whether we like it or not. American education is therefore on the horns of a dilemma. If it continues with its current fixation on educating the left brain, it will fail to provide citizens with the necessary capabilities to deal with an increasingly messy world. If it strives to educate the right brain, the resulting unleashing of imagination, interest, and initiative in both teachers and students will destroy the present paradigm governing its day-to-day practice.

Faith in democracy invites disorder in the belief that initiative is essential to both creativity and ownership. It believes in the power of conversation, that individuals have the freedom, and the responsibility, to turn the flow of attention and endeavor when, in their judgment, it is necessary. Democracy depends upon right-brain factors such as the imagination, interest, and initiative of its citizens. That faith is well-founded, especially in messy times.

Convergent thinking calls for everyone to get on the same page. Divergent thinking also calls for everyone to get on the same page—the Democratic Page—which recognizes the interactive power and potential and beauty of individual ownership and responsibility.

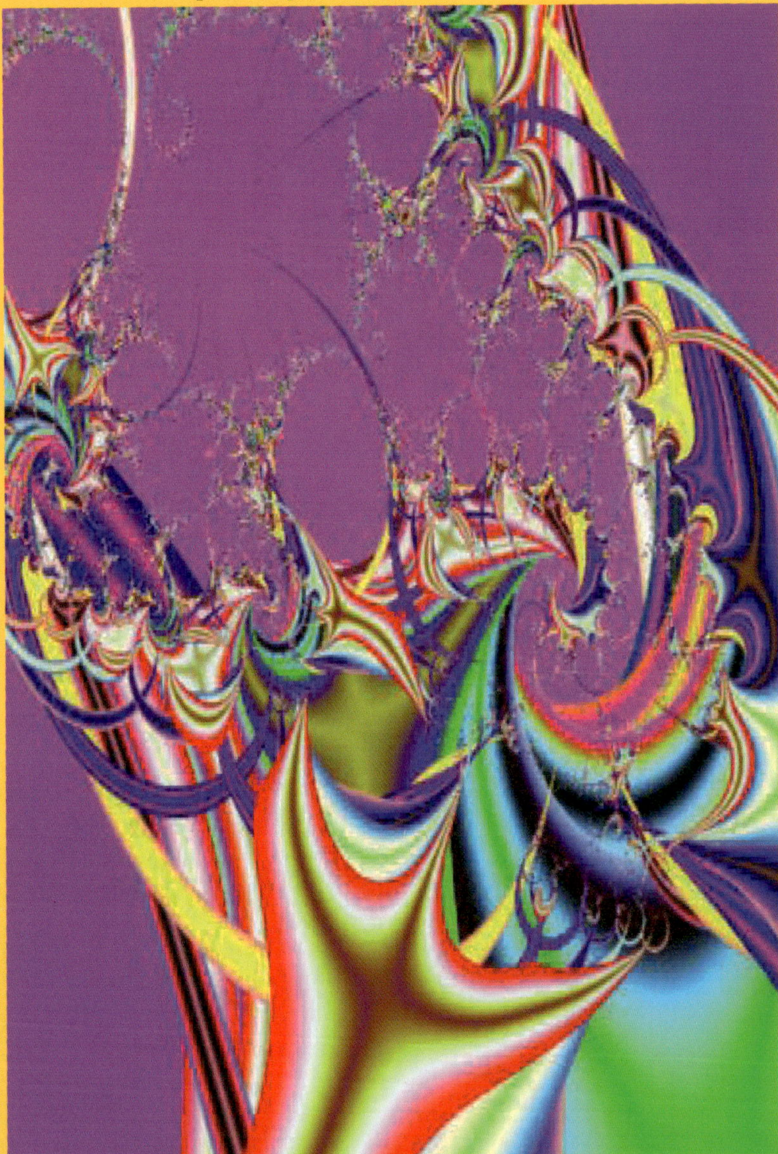

"Dancers" by Judy Hart

The Best Way to the Moon

Years before the moon landing, Abraham Maslow was at a dinner where the discussion revolved around who would get to the moon first. "Don't worry," Maslow said. "The Russians will not get there for twenty years." With the triumph of *Sputnik* so recent, everyone wondered how he could count the Russians out with such certainty. With prodding, he went on. Maslow described a countdown he had witnessed at Cape Canaveral. Twenty-four hours before the scheduled launch he listened to the countdown.

"General Electric!"
"All systems go!"
"Rockwell!"
"All systems go!"

And so it went until one of the many vendors had a glitch.

"Consolidated Hydraulics!"
"We have a problem."

Then the countdown paused while the people involved, and anyone else who could help, worked out the bugs.

Maslow explained that though the Soviets could succeed with a brute task like building rockets with the huge throw weight and orbital velocity to launch a *Sputnik,* the task of landing on the moon and returning safely was too complex for their bureaucratic systems. In the Soviet system, Maslow suggested, the person buried in some functional hierarchy who suspected a glitch would be likely to cover it up rather than disgrace his boss and destroy his career. Maybe he could fix the problem in time, or maybe the blame would fall elsewhere if the fault caused a major problem. In the Soviet Union it was more dangerous to tell the truth.

Our early space program was full of feisty iconoclasts of a type unlikely to rise in a mature bureaucracy. The program depended on the goodwill and competence of a myriad of companies, large and small, working together creatively and in extraordinary coordination. As Maslow predicted, no system created by a hierarchy of bureaucrats has yet succeeded in landing on the moon. It was accomplished by dedicated people working in networks of trusted collaborators, all doing what they did best. The collaborations crossed boundaries of business and government, and linked groups of subcontractors from organizations that might also have directly competing products. Since then, more time and a larger budget have allowed bureaucracy to creep into NASA, resulting in less for more—for example, the disastrous suppression of concerns about the *Challenger's* seals.

Gifford and Elizabeth Pinchot
The End of Bureaucracy and The Rise of the Intelligent Organization

–17–

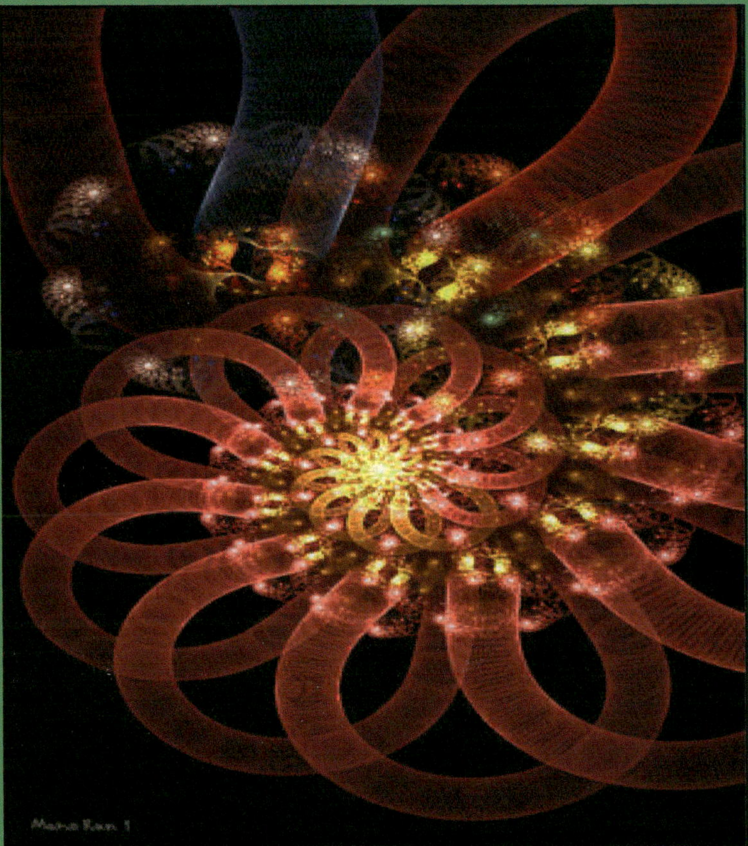

"Hermes Orbit" by Mano Geranis

I think I grok that my people—Martians—are man. Not shape. Shape is not man. Man is grokking. I speak rightly?

Robert A. Heinlein

The present definition of learning is anti-hermeneutic; it prevents the spiraling circle of interpretations that lead us toward deeper, more comprehensive understandings. The term of hermeneutics is derived from Hermes, the messenger god who not only brought us messages from the gods but helped us understand them. The mathematician and chaos theorist Ralph Abraham suggests that we replace the awkward term of hermeneutics with the writer Robert Heinlein's "grok." As he says, "We grok something (an archaeological find, artifact, art work, text, poem, letter, natural process, and so on) by a cycle of observing, thinking, poking, and once again observing."

The big questions, the really worthwhile questions, are always open to interpretation. The world is neither simple nor black and white. When we stop trying to understand and instead trap ourselves in simplistic knowing, we lose something essential. The hermeneutic—or grokking—process is integral to the definition of ourselves. This was understood by the Martian speaking in Heinlein's *Stranger in a Strange Land*: "Shape is not man. Man is grokking." The present definition of learning implies that there is no need to grok; an interpretation of the knowledge will be provided—if one is needed. The personal effort of observing, thinking, and poking is unnecessary. The danger in this perspective is deep and pernicious, for it degrades the essence of ourselves.

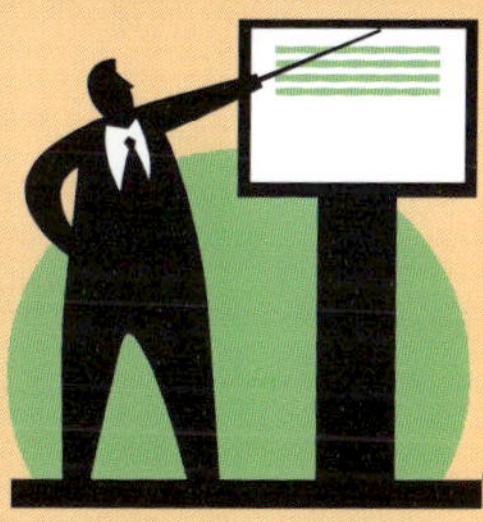

The man stood in front of the class. "Now learn this," he said, writing an equation on the board. We wrote it in our books. Three months later we wrote it out again in an examination paper. If the second writing was the same as the first, we had learnt it. I exaggerate, but only a little. That was my early concept of learning. Later on, I came to realize that I had learned nothing at school which I remember except this—that all problems had already been solved, by someone, and that the answer was around, in the back of the book or the teacher's head. Learning seemed to be transferring answers from them to me.

Charles Handy

Charles Handy is a British business consultant, and the author of *The Age of Unreason*. The quote perfectly illustrates the old definition of learning. He had learned that the answers already existed somewhere, either in the back of the book or in the teacher's head. Thinking was not necessary; just gather the knowing together and keep track of it. This truth is succinctly illustrated in Helen Boyden's (a teacher at Deerfield Academy) admonishment to one of her students:

> Victor, when will you stop trying to remember and start trying to think?

Poor Victor could have justifiably complained that he was curriculum damaged, a victim of our school system. What right did Boyden have to come in at this late date and demand that he think when all that had been developed by his schooling was his memory? A passive attitude and good memory are the desired attributes, with an occasional need for research skills. We have systemically transmitted that message to millions of students for over a century. Is it any wonder that Victor believes thinking unnecessary?

When we neglect the fluid and contextual capabilities of intellect and understanding in fixation on "skills training" and "knowledge acquisition," we diminish our capacity to perceive and respond to the conditions underlying our predicaments. We believe a good curriculum is a hard one, full of stuff to memorize and be tested. We forget or disbelieve Dewey's insight that the value of schooling "resides in its connection with a stimulation of greater thoughtfulness—not in the greater strain it imposes."

We have chosen the strain, even if it's at the cost of thought. In a curious irony, we call for a hard curriculum, when thinking is much harder on the student, as well as the teacher, who must keep growing in order to provide the conditions in the classroom that encourage thinking. However, though thinking is harder, it is more rewarding, for it engages the power of intrinsic motivation. It is also more effective in the long run, for thinking produces both innovation and engagement.

The times are changing. We are beginning to remember that the life of the mind, and therefore the life in the classroom, consists of students striving, through their thinking, to develop their webs of understanding—their groks. There is, after all, despite the present definition of learning, a lot to think about.

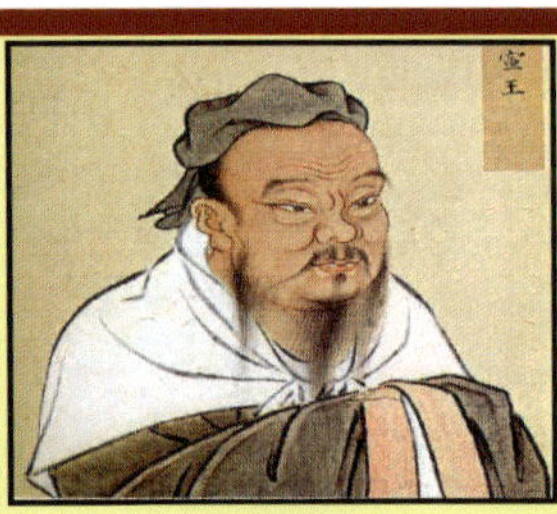

Confucius

Learning without thought is labor lost.

Capability comes not from memorization and tests, but from the accomplishment of significant tasks. The word "significant" is important: students who are not engaged with their learning will perhaps comply with the demands of schooling but they will not commit their interest and initiative—their ownership. They will not think about what they are learning; it will therefore not become part of their developing intellect.

Learning must have true significance to learners in some emotionally important way if they are to learn effectively. Unless the learning process engages the thinking of learners, the labor is lost. Or worse, the students learn that learning is the passive reception of transmitted knowledge—that need not be thought about. We continually neglect the essential connection between learning and thinking:

> Thinking is how individuals establish ownership of their learning—and themselves. If students do not think about their learning, its potential to give meaning, to nourish, is lost. Learning not owned by thinking does not permeate the self and intellect of the learner. It does not become a substantiating part of the person. That is why learning without thought is labor lost—and democratic potential is squandered.

Learning that is not an active expression of self is a passive negation of self, a surrendering of identity to manipulative external forces. It is possible to learn at the cost of both education and maturation. Learning without thought is more than labor lost. It is irresponsible, both to self and to a democratic community. Learning that is not a pathway of personal initiative, but merely another example of passivity, diminishes individual and, eventually, social integrity. It constricts both capability and potential.

The problem with external motivation is that, as a process, it works to a degree that allows a shallow feeling of effectiveness. The effectiveness is short-sighted, however, for it systemically addicts people to external rewards, thus making them subject to whoever has control of the compensations they have been programmed to desire. It conditions students to accept their learning without thought. Instruction addicted to external motivation also sets up a general climate of manipulation. It pushes teachers and administrators to depend on manipulative techniques, which systematically removes them from genuine interaction with students. Conversations between teachers and students are rare because the schooling environment harbors conditions antithetical to them.

Also, such an external motivation process, when successful, tends to addict people to external rewards—which suppresses not only intrinsic motivation but the development of such conditions as trust, credibility, and personal integrity. Worse, it diminishes the soul, for the life and health of the soul depends upon intrinsic motivation. Thus it not only suppresses the effectiveness of innovativeness and engagement that are best borne intrinsically, it also degrades our spiritual health.

> Socrates and the men of the Renaissance did so much because the rewards were intrinsic, i.e., the enlargement of the soul.
>
> Brenda Ueland

The cultural habit of external motivation sets up a "field" where such attributes as caring, contribution, generosity, and self-directed learning are squelched. It also discourages personal initiative and responsibility. We are presently (as we do periodically) increasing our concern for such strengths as character and creativity, but we do not understand how the philosophy behind our instructional practices sets up conditions which discourage their emergence. Such strengths cannot be manipulated, or trained, into existence; initiative is essential to their emergence.

Learning without thought is not only labor lost, but potential squandered. The result is a possibly fatal (in a democracy) systemic cost because **learning with thought** is essential to the development of such factors as initiative, capability, and integrity. Programmed instruction ignores the ingredient of thinking within the learning process because of its unpredictability and immeasurability. This is short-sighted and stupid behavior. There is a lot we need to grok.

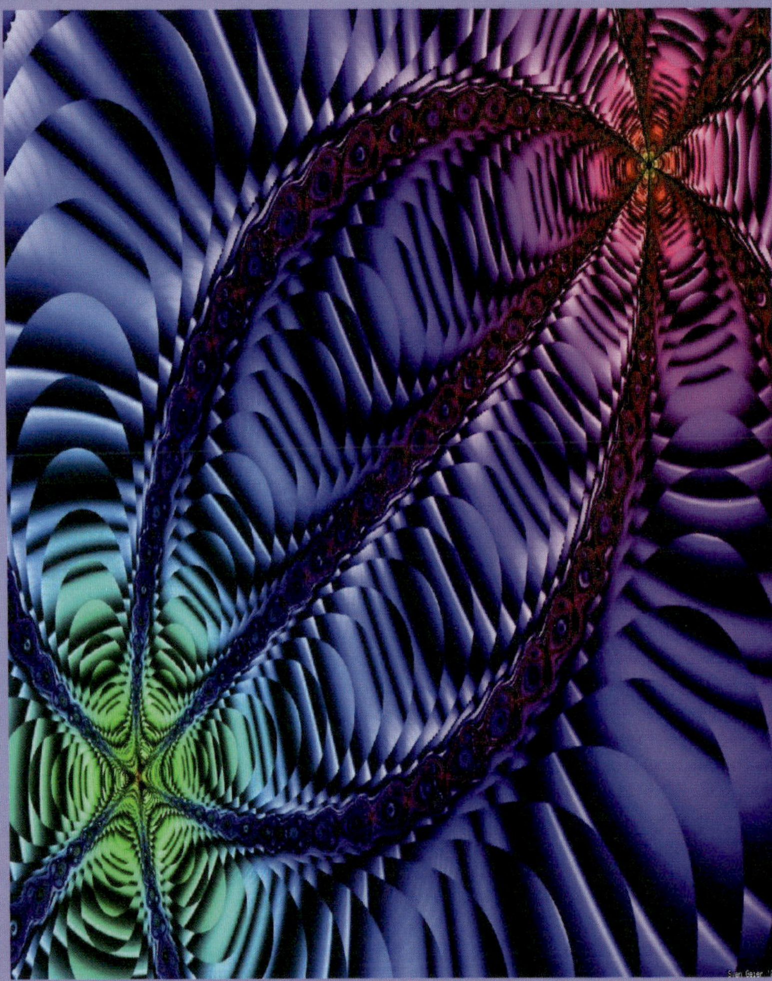

"Transmission" be Sven Geier

The mind is like the stomach. It is not how much you put into it that counts, but how much it digests.

Alfred J. Nock

—18—

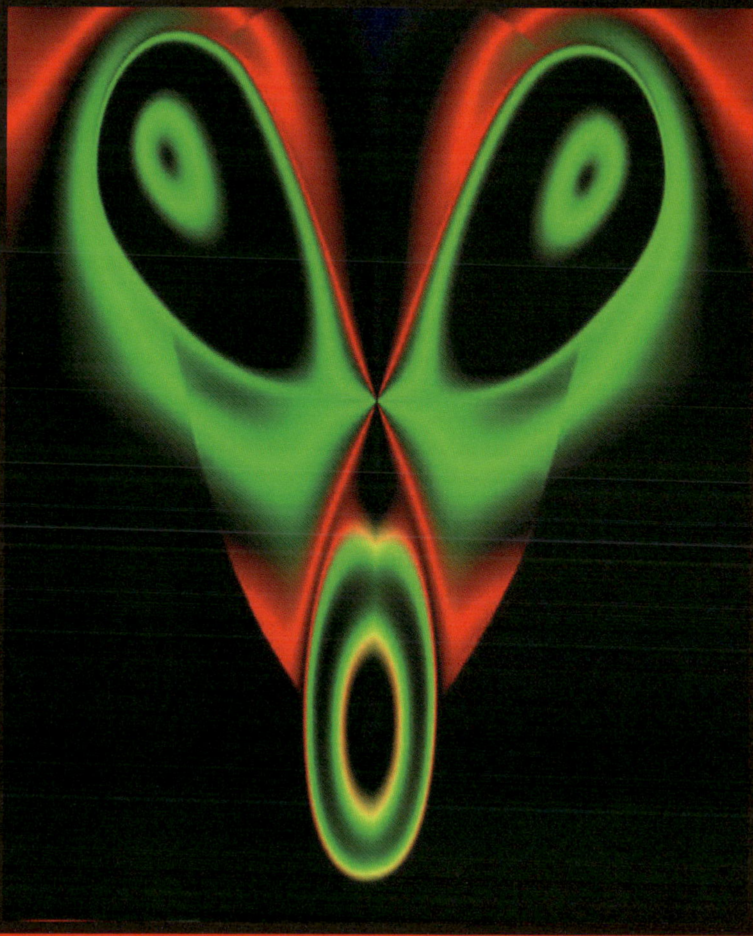

"Oh No!" by Marie Luise Schmidt

Librarian:	*Ava, you seem far away. Is anything wrong?*
Ava:	*Why do we have to spend so much time talking about this?*
Librarian:	*We're talking about it so that you'll understand it better. I want you to learn about it.*
Ava:	*We don't have time to learn it. We have to get the assignment done. Mr. Smith is going to collect it.*

Jacqueline Grennon Brooks and Martin G. Brooks

As far as Ava was concerned, the librarian was wasting her time. There was no need to either talk or think about the assignment. The task was just to get it done; learning about it was not part of the equation. However, learning is, at its best, messy, because it invites in such unpredictable factors as conversation, thinking, reflection, and imagination. Brooks and Brooks, in their book, *The Case for Constructivist Classrooms: In Search of Understanding,* write:

> Schools throughout America are filled with students like Ava, students who have been acculturated to devalue thinking, to feel uneasy about in-depth analysis, and to view anything other than rapid coverage of the curriculum as wasting time. These students are frequently successful in school. They study, complete their assignments, pass their tests, and receive good grades. Yet, these are not meaningful victories. They are victories of form over substance, of superficiality over engagement, of coverage over depth.*

Students like Ava are damaged by schooling driven by the present definition of learning. She has been systematically taught not to think about her assignments. There is no time for substantial investigation, one that engages her imagination, interest, and initiative. The task is to complete the assignment, period.

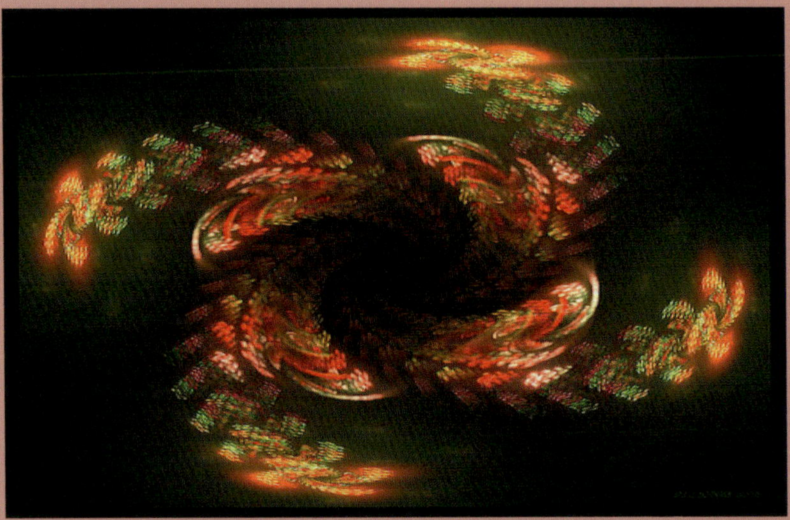

"Snake Oil" by Sue Jones, found at sue tortoise's photostream

*A useful word in the struggle to redefine learning is sciolism, defined by the O.E.D. as a noun meaning superficial knowledge. The adjective form is sciolistic. We need antidotes, or better yet, vaccinations against the spread of sciolism. Without either reflection or conversation, all learning is sciolistic to the learner—and therefore worthless.

A Cautionary Tale

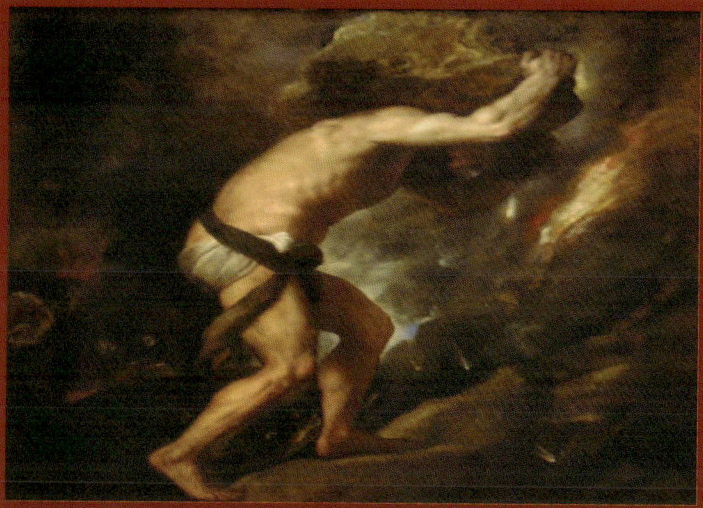

"What are you doing in my class?" I asked a student who was reading out of a book instead of attending to the conversation.

"Don't worry. I am a multi-tasker. I can do two things at once."

"Really, so what were we talking about?"

She gave an accurate and succinct rendition of the conversation to that point. I complimented her or her ability to multitask but still wanted to know what she was reading. She answered that it was a short story that she was going to have a quiz on in the next class. I pointed out that she should have read it the night before.

I can't do that," she answered.

"Why not?"

"Because I forget everything I read the night before. I always have to read something just before the test. Otherwise, it's all gone."

"And how long does it last after the test?"

"Pssst," she said, or something akin to that, with a quick wave of her hand to help communicate that it would be flicked out of her memory (and intellect) almost immediately.

Sisyphus Trudges On.

—19—

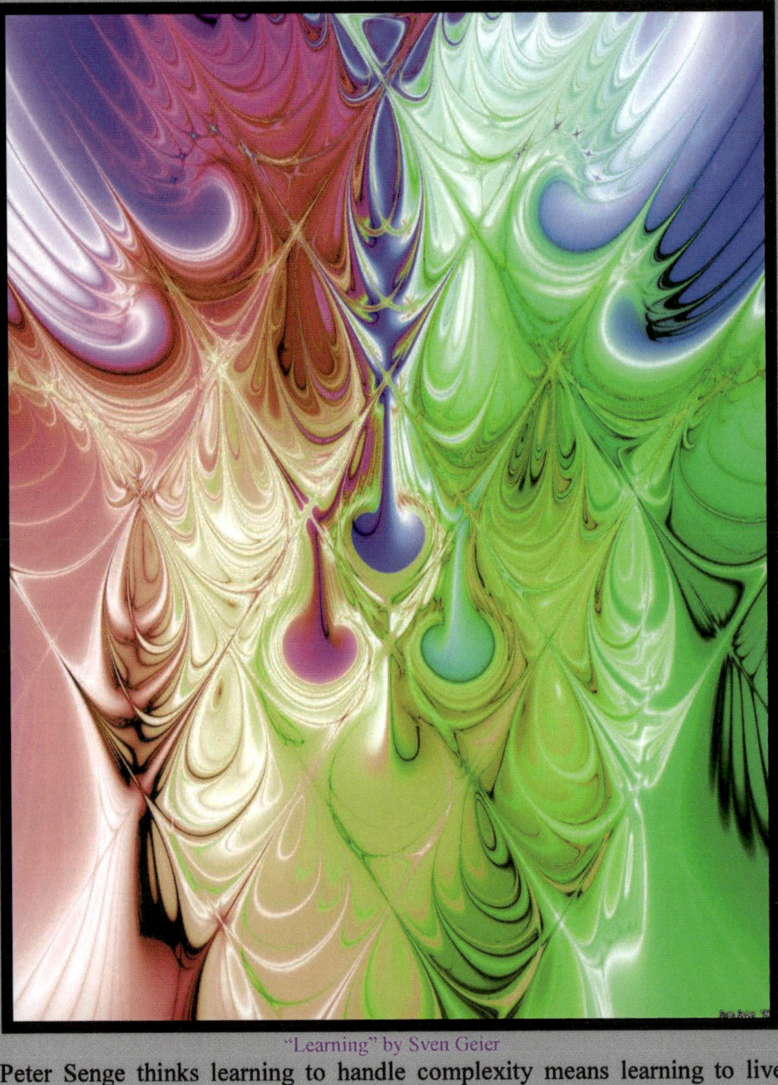

"Learning" by Sven Geier

Peter Senge thinks learning to handle complexity means learning to live more intuitively, because intuition is the key to making significant changes in complex systems, helping them evolve, and evolving with them.

John Briggs and F. David Peat

Intuition, the often puzzling ability to not only see but understand what is seen while others do not, is a non-linear, right brain capability. It may seem to come from nowhere but it doesn't; it comes from past attention and constructed understanding resulting in wisdom about dynamically interactive relationships. The "eyes in the back of the head of the experienced teacher," for example, are not gifts from some god, but grown by the courage and concern and creativity of a persistent, professional practitioner. Intuition is constructed by interest, imagination, and, most importantly, initiative; all right brain capabilities. Intuition is a special kind of intellect, an understanding about dynamically complex endeavors.

The transmission of knowledge-bits is only a small part of intellectual development; without the synergy of imagination, interest, and initiative, intellect does not and cannot grow. The absence of intellect in our students is alarming. And lack of intellect translates into lack of curiosity and engagement. Why be curious and engage your efforts if you don't have a scaffold of understanding with which to make meaning of the new learning?

Peter Senge adds the following perspective on learning:

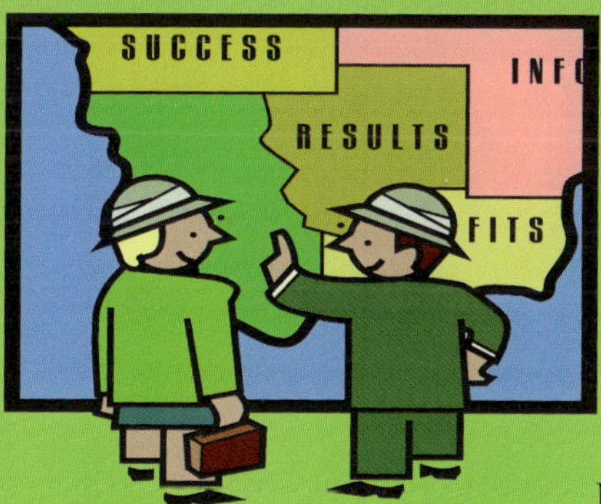

Learning does not mean acquiring more information but expanding the ability to produce the results we truly want in life.

Senge's definition of learning helps us recognize and reorganize our values. What are the results we truly want in life? The simple accruing of knowledge bits is not learning, unless you wish to be a professional Jeopardy contestant. Learning is increasing our capability to be effective at what we believe to be worthwhile accomplishments.

> Shouldn't "educated" mean, "able to make more sense of self, of others, of the world, of experience, of life?"
>
> Marion Brady

–20–

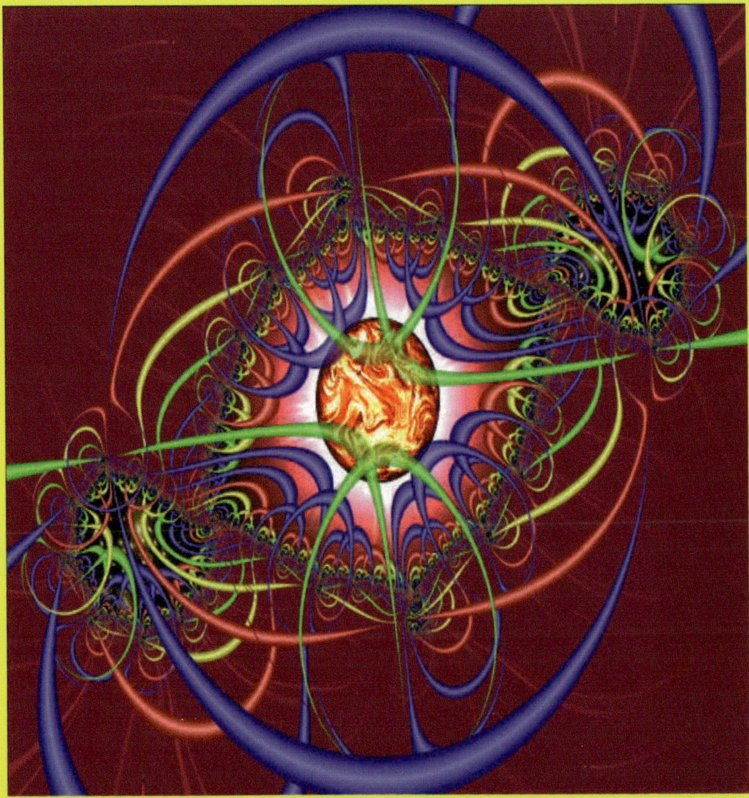

"A Stitch in Time and Space" by Dale Adcock

I teach history to smart students at a good college, who, it is often said, know less when they graduate from secondary school than their counterparts of years past. In fact, I think they have more knowledge. But they can do less.

Carol Gluck

A systemic cause of students who know more but can do less is our addiction to standardized tests. Students, after all, who do well on standardized tests, have learned. Have they not? The current definition of learning thinks so. Otherwise, why would we spend so much time in teaching to the tests and money in their administering? Standardized tests, however, are focused on what students don't know, not on what they can do. Peter Sachs, author of *Standardized Minds: The*

High Price of America's Testing Culture and What We Can do to Change it, quotes Bob Zenhausern, professor of psychology at St. John's University:

> Get rid of standardized tests, period. What you put in its place is an evaluation that makes sense. . . . These standardized tests evaluate what somebody can't do [well on the "objective" tests]. That's because it's easier to find out what somebody doesn't know. They give you a bunch of questions and count how many mistakes you make. We need instead to measure what somebody can do.

We need students who can do more—not just know more. Our current fixation on standardized tests serves educators desperate to prove they are accomplishing something in our schooling. They do not serve our learners. Nor do they serve our future as a society comprised of citizens who can do more. The capacity to do is pleasurable. We want to feel effective, capable, and productive. But the capability must be real, not a sham. Accomplishment, confidence, and potential are intimately intertwined, a truth frequently ignored by fads such as the self-esteem movement. True capability provides poise, the sense of sitting deep in the water, and openness to future challenges.

Eric Jensen, author of *Teaching with the Brain in Mind,* writes:

> When students feel more capable of solving a problem, their thoughts change their body's chemistry. Stanford University's Albert Bandura found that when the feelings of competence increased, the subjects in the test released fewer catacholomines, the body's natural response to stress.

Stress can be defined as the fear people feel that they may not be capable of dealing with whatever is happening to them. The feeling of stress is tightly bound with the feeling of capability. We should ask: what is the relationship between the prevalence of stress and the educational process? We should also ask: what kind of capability does our schooling produce in order to alleviate the stress? Many of my fellow professors often ask the following questions:

> What is happening to intrinsic motivation? Where are the students who not only want to learn, but take ownership of their learning? Where are the self-directed learners, who are energized by personal interest and curiosity, who take responsibility for their own learning?

The answers to our questions reside in the educational process, one that systemically insists on extrinsic motivation. In her book, *The Death of Why: The Decline of Questioning and the Future of Democracy*, Andrea Batista Schlesinger discusses how the educational system degrades intrinsic motivation by focusing on the "smartness" of students instead of effort. She discusses the work of Stanford psychology professor Dr. Carol Dweck:

> For the next round of the exam, the children were given a choice: either stay at the same level of difficulty or increase it. Group A, praised for its intelligence, opted for the same level of difficulty. Group B, praised for

its effort, opted for a harder exam. The children who were praised for being smart did not want to take a risk that they would fail. When faced with a challenge, they were more interested about losing their standing as "smart" than interested in what they could learn from the exercise to make them even smarter. The children, however, looked forward to the challenge. In their view, the process of learning was what counted, and the challenge of learning brought them reward.

Dweck believes that there are two mind-sets when it comes to intelligence. Those with a fixed mind-set (an outgrowth of the messages children are sent about their value) "shun effort in the belief that having to work hard means they are dumb." Those with a growth mind-set, on the other hand, believe that one can work hard and get smarter. They enjoy challenges. According to Dweck's studies, students with a growth mind-set are those most likely to succeed.

Simply by signaling what we think is most important, therefore, we can change a person's motivation. Our children can be *intrinsically* motivated to take action that is rewarding in itself—such as thinking critically about a new and harder task. But our answer-obsessed society is organized to cultivate *extrinsic* motivation—rewards, such as the praise earned from getting the right answer, even on a simpler question.

Intrinsically motivated students enjoy the learning process. They are therefore more resilient learners, more likely to be life-long, and more likely to achieve. They may know less, as far as the standardized tests indicate, since their relative lack of extrinsic motivation will interfere with test preparation and memorization, but they will be able to do more. This is because intrinsic motivation generates a more unique individuality that is more capable of unique contribution, which is at the core of today's necessary skills. C. Lemke, E. Coughlin, V. Thadani, and C. Martin list those skills in *enGauge 21st century skills: Literacy in the Digital Ages*:

•**Digital Age Literacy** (basic scientific, economic, and technological literacies; visual and information literacies; multicultural literacy and global awareness.

•**Inventive Thinking** (adaptability, managing complexity; self-direction, curiosity, creativity, and risk taking; higher order thinking and sound reasoning)

•**Effective Communication** (teaming, collaboration, and interpersonal skills; personal, social, and civic responsibility; interactive communication)

•**Higher Productivity & Quality, State-of-the-Art Results** (ability to prioritize, plan, and manage for results; effective use of real-world tools; the ability to create relevant, high–quality products)

A cardinal component of the capacity to do something is self-reliance—the strength to go beyond the given (pre-directed and pre-masticated) to self-direction (self-guided attention and interpretation). We are, of course, talking about imagination, interest, and initiative.

A recent movement in the education world is "Cash for Classes," where students are paid to attend classes, where they are paid to learn. God help us! What if this notion really takes hold and dominates our schooling? Competence begets competence, but what about the issue of intrinsically-based doing as opposed to extrinsically-based doing? Doesn't a democratic community depend upon those who do for intrinsic reasons?

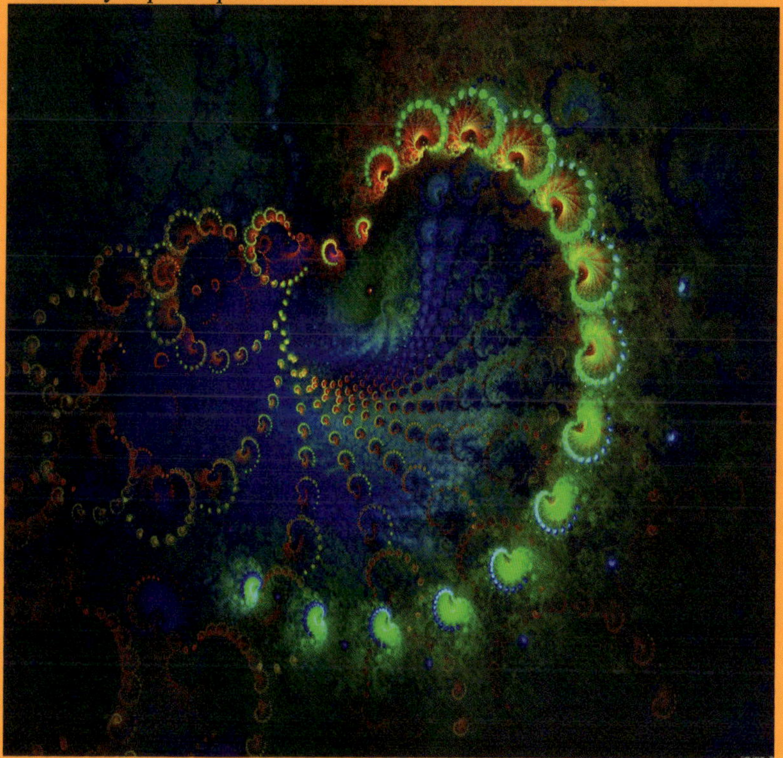

"Deeper Dive" by Sven Geier

Students rarely bring themselves as individuals—and can we not assume a positive correlation between individuality and intrinsic motivation?—to the learning table; they arrive as "products of schooling" prepared for further instruction. Too often, students have the attitude of "Tell us what you want us to know," instead of "This is what I am interested in and puzzled about." Schooling is perceived by them as the attachment of additional knowledge parts. They have been sold into the factory metaphor, where they are merely "products" of a process (The curriculum demands that we attach the prescribed parts, though we sometimes wonder about the wisdom of attaching windshield wipers to products lacking windshields.)

Initiative, the energy that gives us ownership and traction, is a characteristic of intrinsic motivation, so it is suppressed by a prediction and control image that places its focus on extrinsic motivation, which prefers training. Intrinsic motivation is too idiosyncratic, too messy, and too divergent.

The present definition of learning therefore prefers extrinsic motivation. Intrinsic motivation, because it generates inquiry and initiative and imagination, disrupts curriculum coverage and the almighty tests. That is why the current process systemically crowds out conditions for intrinsically-guided learning, even if it decreases individuality and capacity for achievement, for doing. However, as Pink pointed out, we increasingly need the capabilities of the right brain: which means factors such as imagination, interest, and initiative. Holistic capabilities rarely emerge and flourish in conditions of extrinsic motivation. Intrinsically-based doing is the kind of competence called for by these challenging times—and by the spirit of democracy.

The human brain, by the way, prefers learning within a healthy educational process over the supposed products of the easily measured. Jensen writes:

> Surprisingly, it doesn't matter to the brain whether it ever comes up with an answer. The neural growth happens because of the process, not the solution. A student could go to school for 12 years, rarely get right answers, and still have a well-developed brain. Some learners simply choose harder and harder problems to solve. That may stimulate the release of noradrenaline and also create dendritic growth.*

The intrinsically motivated learners described by Jensen have a rough time in our schools. The present operating metaphors controlling the schooling process push learning as stuff to memorize and regurgitate, not as harder and harder problems to solve. Their fellow students, who acquiesce to the image of correct-answer schooling, will have their brains undeveloped by the process responsible for it, making them incapable of constructing useful understandings of what they supposedly know. On the other hand, they will more likely be able to do well in whatever way they are instructed by a perceived authority. (Something to consider is that a high GPA is not necessarily an indicator of a good learner.)

*I love studying. The harder I study, the more confused I get. The more confused I get, the deeper I want to dig. The deeper I dig … the better questions I ask. I've been doing my "thing"—worrying in one way or another about business and management—for 35 years. Fact is, I'm more confused now than I was when I began. And yet I hope, and believe, that I'm asking better questions now than when I started out. Maybe somebody will put that on my tombstone, come to think of it:

Thomas J. Peters (1942-????)
He Kept Asking Better and More Annoying Questions

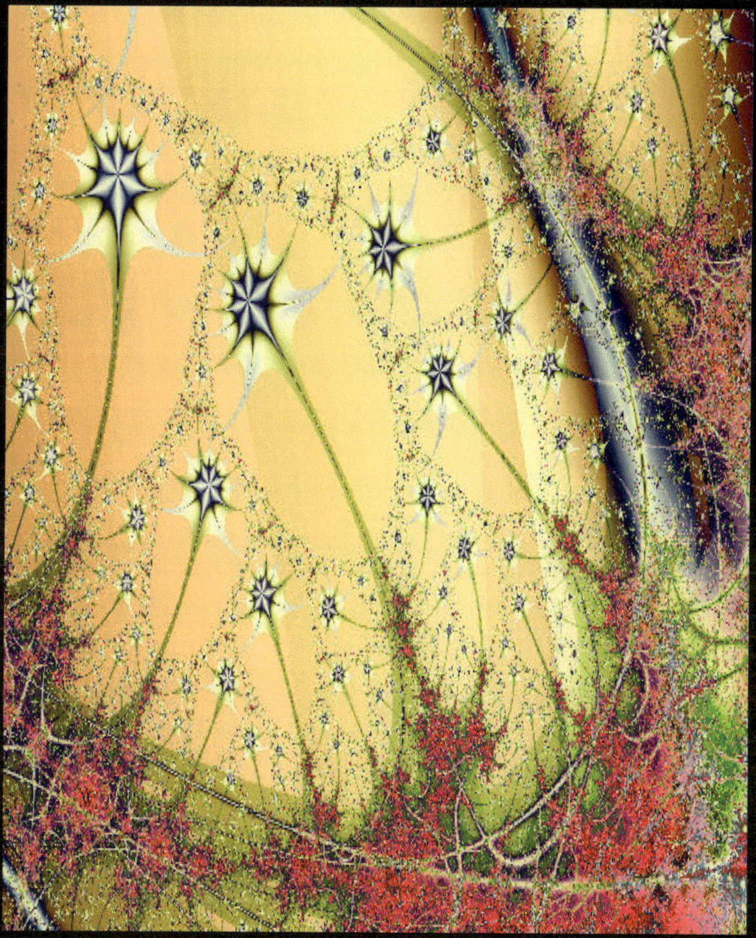

"Release the Spores" by Ken Keller

A fundamental reason our students can do less is that they don't understand the need to mull and muck—or even that it's necessary to give life to their learning. In a culture of correct-answer schooling, our students have learned that, if they don't know, what's the use? And, if they do know, what's the need? Conjecture, consideration, and conversation are not required—but the life of the mind consists of mulling and mucking.

The competence of the extrinsically motivated is not what a democracy needs. Our democratic future depends upon the competence of the intrinsically motivated.

—21—

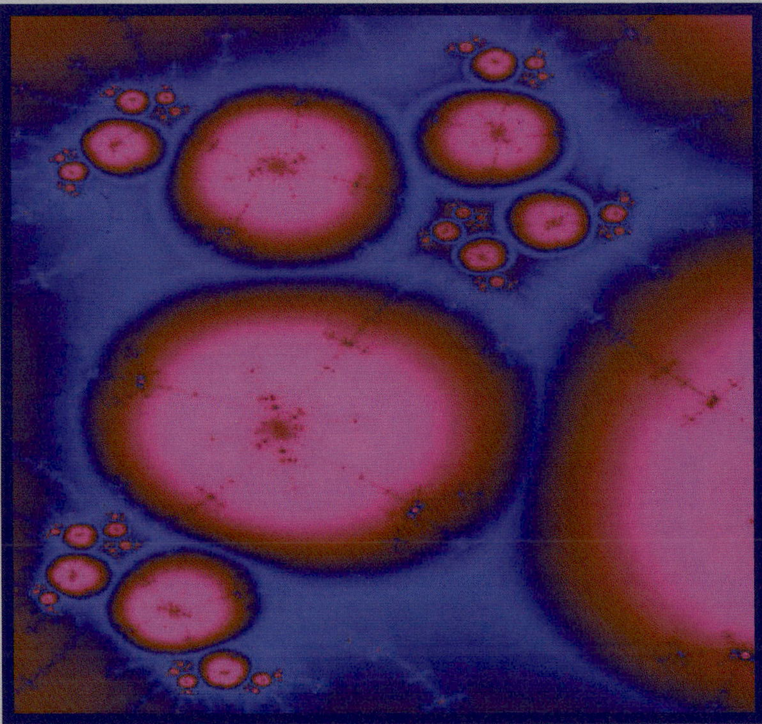

"Boils" by Ken Keller

Students, however, are not only asked to learn useless information, they are pressured to learn it through the threat of punishment and are severely punished with low or failing grades if they refuse to make the effort to memorize what to them is useless. This is a high price to pay for retaining the destructive tradition that for centuries has made memorizing an important component of education. It may have been important before Gutenberg, but not since then.*

William Glasser, M.D.

In Glasser's work on developing quality schools, he advocates that teachers concentrate on teaching useful skills. He defines information as what you know; skills are what you use, or what you can do. There are five basic skills: speaking, reading, writing, calculating, and problem solving. Information should be taught, according to Glasser, only if it falls into at least one of the following four categories:

1. **Information directly related to a life-skill.** Grammar is essential to reading and writing. The times table is important to math problems. Such information need not be memorized; incorporating it into the development of skills will embed them.
2. **Information that students express a desire to learn.**
3. **Information that the teacher believes is especially useful.** Even if the teacher believes that memorizing Shakespeare is essential, then that information should be taught. [This relates to teacher initiative, ownership, and responsibility.]
4. **Information required for college.** It is okay to teach for the tests, as long as that is made clear to the students. The students and teacher together determine how much information (even if useless) to learn in order to punch the college ticket.

Respect for both learners and teachers are reflected in Glasser's priorities. He is less concerned with the system of schooling taking care of itself, which is the current value-in-place. Learning should increase intelligence, the capability to solve real problems and fashion useful products. It should also reflect the interest and judgment of learners and teachers. Glasser's operating metaphor, as reflected in his categories, dramatically changes the methods employed and materials used. He envisions the task of learning constructively. It is action on the part of learners and teachers, not the passive reception and forced ingestion of predigested information.

Glasser has been hard at work redefining learning for a long time. Skills acquisition, however, is not as easily measured as information acquisition. Skill development also demands learning environments that encourage and inform initiative. That runs counter to the culture of training that needs prediction and control. In his Quality Schools, the initiative, as well as the responsibility, of both teachers and students are encouraged and reinforced. The result is ownership and commitment.

Glasser understands that if we let go of control, we gain the power of engaged and committed learners.

*According to Glasser, we haven't needed all this focus on memorization since the life of Gutenberg, and he died in 1468.

—22—

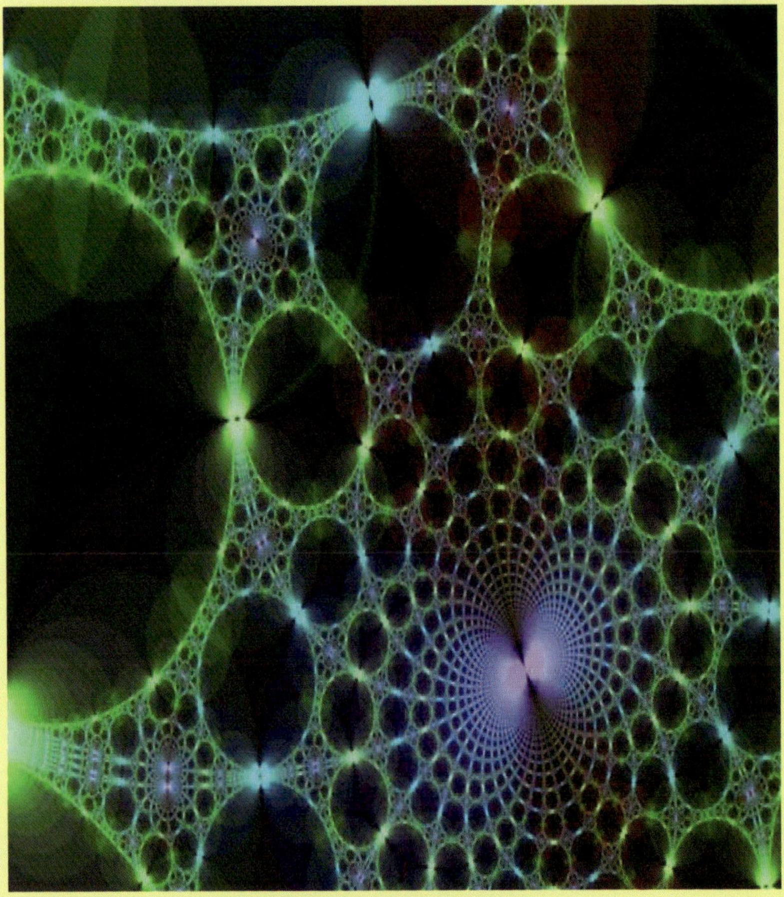

"Spider Web" by Dave Massey

God sends threads to webs begun.

A wise old teacher

The image of threads moving toward evolving webs illustrates intellectual development. The job of a teacher is to help students design and construct their webs of understanding, their intellects. The necessary threads will then, with the help of student interest and initiative, accumulate to elaborate and nourish the evolving intellects. Learning as it is now defined and practiced in our schooling rarely nourishes intellectual development.

Learning redefined will move toward a more constructionist perspective. The job of a teacher is to establish the conditions conducive to the emergence of student-constructed learning (as opposed to manipulatively transmitted and passively received or actively resisted) in classrooms. Teachers should develop the interactive conditions in the student/teacher relationship conducive to the development of initiative, since it is essential for the construction of learning.

Note

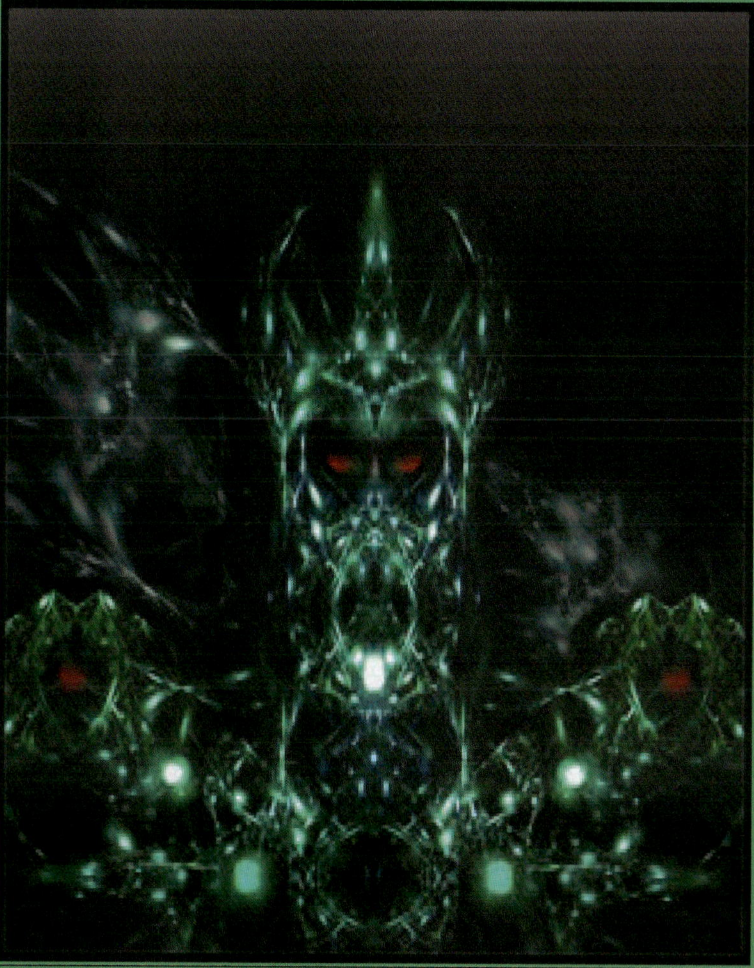

Art by Jacob Laren

If God sends threads to webs begun, then it must be the devil that sends threads to webs not begun.

–23–

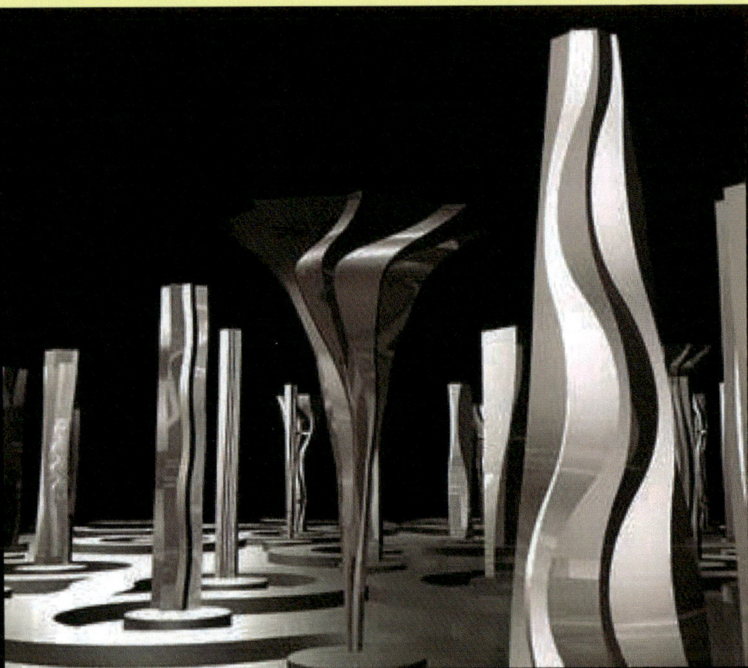

"Column Museum" by Haresh Lalvani*

Learning is a genuine **making**, an act of gathering and forming, by persistence and struggle. Each act of learning reorganizes reality, each is an act of creation.

Louise Cowan

What does learning do, anyway? This is an important question to ask. It is, as Cowan indicates, the making of something, but the making of what? The quick answer is that learning makes awareness and interpretation, which is the meaning constructed to explain a new awareness. There is a dialectic between awareness and interpretation. (Picture Gregory Bateson's analogy defining dialectic: the river forms the banks while the banks guide the river.) Awareness demands interpretation which then expands awareness. Ultimately, we can only see what we can understand—though we must understand that understanding is itself a construction that can be shoddy or built on swamp land.

Awareness and interpretation comprise intelligence, the capacity, as Howard Gardner tells us, to solve problems and fashion products. Bear in mind that wisdom, the product of awareness and intelligence, is informed and expanded by learning. What else does learning do—other than improve awareness and interpretation and therefore intelligence—and thus expand wisdom?

Learning can merely entertain and, sometimes, simply feed our delusions. We can also learn ourselves into traps and dead ends. Learning can develop us—or diminish us. Like evolution, it is not always positive, though the overall direction, we can optimistically assume, is an upward spiral of attention and capability. Humans are specialists in learning for a reason, because it usually, and on occasion, exponentially, expands our intelligence. We become more response-able.

Learning can be envisioned as the cobbling together of insights in the process of developing understanding, an image of the endeavor. The cobblestones of insights then form pathways to interpretation and utilization and, eventually, to experience and wisdom. Conversation (and reflection) is how we "cobble" those pathways into existence. Without it, learning does not contribute to either personal or social understanding of the subject.

This thought is key: Learning is constructed by learners—not transferred by teachers or curriculum. As Donald Block says:

Learning is not a spectator sport.

Teachers are the leaders of the mind's activities in their classrooms. The working relationships they forge—or fail to forge—determine the presence and vitality of learning environments. The importance of teaching to our awareness and intelligence as individuals, as a culture, is rarely considered. If it were, we would channel our resources to the education and support of our teachers. However, our teachers are compelled to transmit correct-answers, not help students construct understanding, even though, as Gardner realizes, understanding, not the acquisition of correct answers, develops intelligence. It also expands awareness, for the more we understand, the more we realize that we don't know, and that makes us both curious and determined to find out more.

> Any kind of significant learning is a kind of discovering: a "seeing" of how things fit together, of what meaning they have, a "seeing" which for the student involves something new, unforeseen, even unexpected. Either that, or we have mere rote learning: memorization followed by the writing out of what is remembered.
>
> Pete A. Y. Gunter

*The Column Museum is a virtual environment of all possible architectural columns of the past, present, and future. Haresh Lalvani, is a self-described "architect morphologist" at Pratt Institute.

—24—

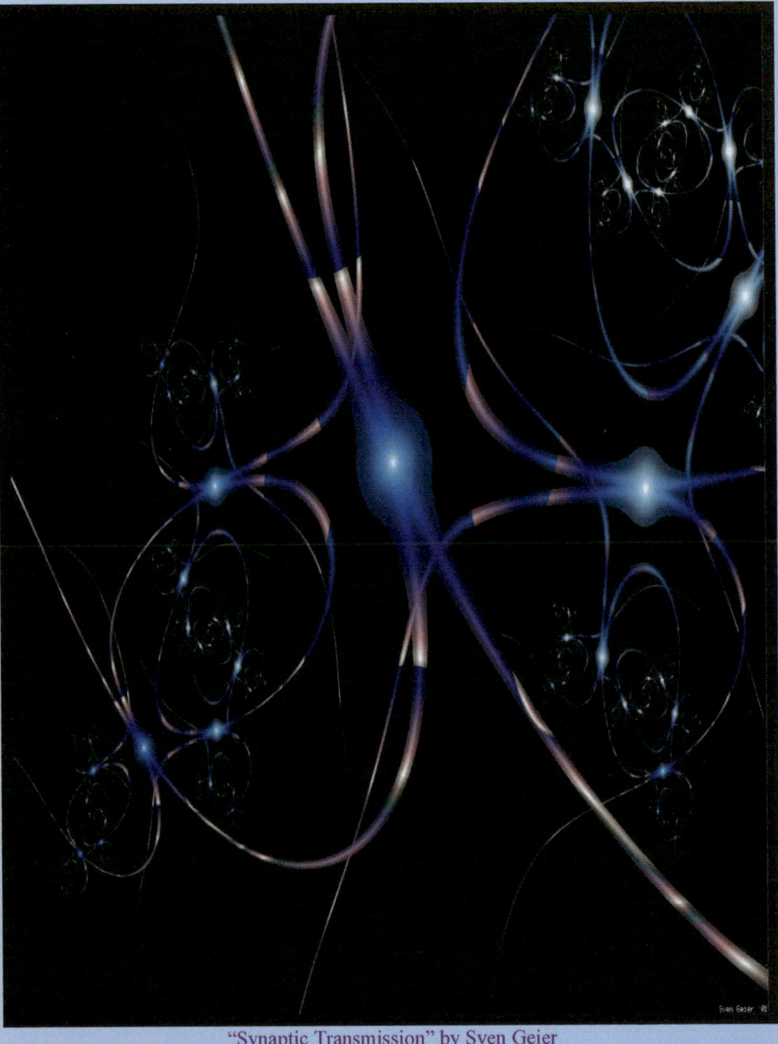

"Synaptic Transmission" by Sven Geier

Among the features of brain-based learning are active uncertainty or the tolerance for ambiguity; problem solving; questioning; and patterning by drawing relationships through the use of metaphor, similes, and demonstrations.

Renate and Geoffrey Caine

The brain prefers projects over lectures. It resents and resists prediction and control machinations, finding them boring, insulting, and meaningless. It prefers real problems and authentic projects. The brain wants to engage, exercise, and inform its initiative. The healthy brain is always looking for problems and puzzles to solve. Ambiguity and uncertainty, though anathema to our socialistic schooling metaphor, excite the healthy brain.

Thinking, the way we make adjustments to our knowing, is essential to worthwhile learning, but it is disruptive to the current definition of schooling, and it is damned hard to measure. The root of thinking is individual choice, and that plays havoc with curriculum.

Paul Kussrow writes, in his article, "Brain-Based Leadership:"

> For over thirty years authors such as Mager and McCann (1963) have reported that when learners are afforded some control over the process and content of the learning experience that their motivation significantly goes up. When the learner sees ways to move toward their own personal and professional agenda they are more willing to work toward the leader's goals. Learners with a strong locus of control are more open to feedback and are looking for clues to improve their performance (Clark, 1986).

Thinking and knowing are an interdependent dynamic. The health of either is dependent upon the growth of the other. Without co-evolutionary development of thinking and knowing, the necessary balance between tension and resolution—the rhythm between confusion (the new, disorder) and comprehension (the old, order)—is disrupted. This is what Whitehead understood when he warned us not to let training crowd out initiative.

It can also be argued that the thinking individual is essential for democracy, As Paulo Friere said, in *Learning to Question: A Pedagogy of Liberation:*

> Any educational practice based on standardization, on routine in which everything is predetermined, is bureaucratizing and thus anti-democratic.

Correct-answer schooling is also stultifying. It is thinking that breathes life into knowing while the gaining of knowledge keeps thinking from stewing within itself. Acquired knowledge provides thought with new foundations from which to expand. But it is thinking that gives learning its aliveness with the energy of initiative. Thinking constructs new understandings from the acquisition of new knowledge, for, as knowledge is born it must be fused into the developing intellect; otherwise, the brain discards it. Kussrow writes:

> It would behoove the leader (classroom, building, district, corporation) to allow humans great flexibility to affirm, bond, connect, and relate to

others around their topic, vision, or goal(s). Supportive relationships and group interaction build a sense of belonging, cohesiveness, and community that increases learning (Cohen, 1984). Increased communication, networking, and bonding through social/emotional interactive opportunities create new patterns of thought and neuronal connections. Just as the brain doesn't like isolated bits of information, or someone else's logic pattern, it prefers to create its own relationships (patterns) and make sense out of its surroundings.

Regardless of systemic pressures to teach to the tests of the easily measurable, teachers who really want to teach must engage their students in projects, either in the form of conversations or real life problems and constructions. This of course goes against the grain of the present operating metaphor. If teachers really want to teach, however, they must escape the compulsion to constantly lecture. Transmitting easily measured but congelated knowledge bits—which are just as easily regurgitated from the minds of students—with no chance of sticking to the frames of their intellects, is not teaching.

Brain-based education calls for increased recognition of the central role teachers play in establishing learning environments. Teachers with their initiative suppressed, their judgment disrespected, and their experience disregarded will not be able to convey the model of capable and responsible individuality so essential to a democracy.

Teachers can take heart from the explosion of practitioners in the field of neuroscience—and those scientists increasingly provide the evidence necessary to eradicate the absurdities borne, ironically, of our scientism. Science, real science, is increasingly on the side of real teaching. As the neuroscience revolution takes hold, lecturing and correct-answer schooling will eventually give way. Teachers will then be expected to develop their intellects as teachers; their judgment will become increasingly respected; classrooms will become smaller as the science proves it necessary; and new assessments of teacher effectiveness will be created. The central role of teachers in the learning process will be supported by neuroscience. Correct-answer schooling will not hold up to neuroscientific scrutiny; education for understanding will therefore become the focus and value. And the development of understanding depends upon the imagination, initiative, and capability of individual teachers.

To many, the term "brain-based learning" sounds redundant. Isn't all learning and teaching brain-based? Advocates of brain-based teaching insist that there is a difference between "brain-compatible" education, and "brain-antagonistic" teaching practices and methods which can actually prevent learning.

Lisa Chipongian

—25—

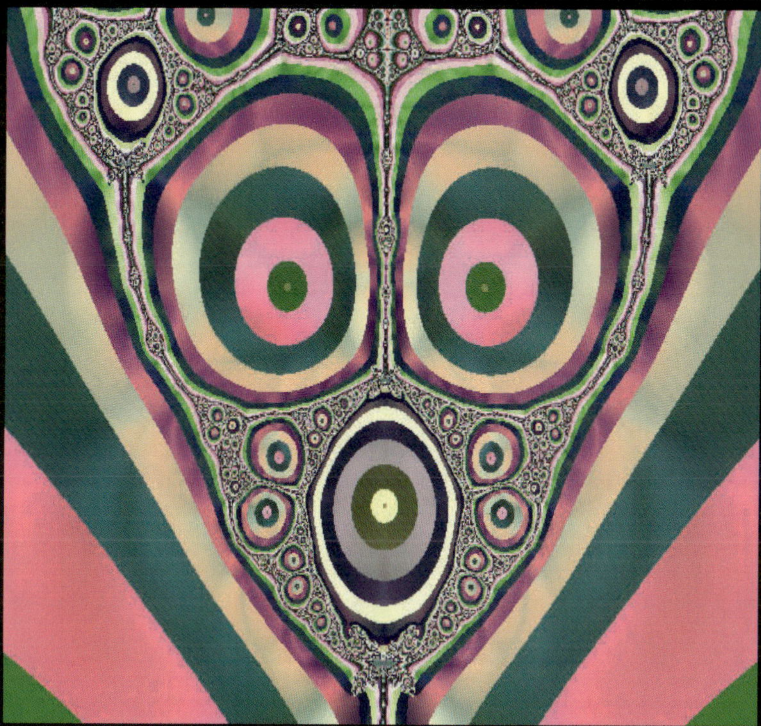

"What?!" By Ken Keller

Only the curious will learn and only the resolute overcome the obstacles to learning. The quest quotient has always excited me more than the intelligence quotient.

Eugene S. Wilson

We call for life-long learners and critical thinkers. But our educational system is one crammed with answers, not opportunities for questions. We present learning as the ability to provide answers, when real learning is closer to improving our capacity for asking questions. The learned person, to a redefined definition of learning, is not someone filled to the gunwales with data, but someone with a high and growing higher quest quotient. The word "quest," after all, has always had the connotation of a sacred search.

Do we want life-long learners—or life-long knowers?

Life-long learning presupposes the habit of and capability for critical thinking. But how can you develop critical thinking within an environment that suppresses questions? Not just questions about what will be on the test, but real questions, ones that search for the significant, the meaningful, the insightful, the ones that increase understanding. In her book, *Teaching Critical Thinking*, bell hooks writes:

> The heartbeat of critical thinking is the longing to know—to understand how life works. Children are organically predisposed to be critical thinkers. Across the boundaries of race, class, gender, and circumstance, children come into the world of wonder and language consumed with a desire for knowledge. Sometimes they are so eager for knowledge they become relentless interrogators—demanding to know the who, what, when, where, and why of life. Searching for answers, they learn almost instinctively how to think.
>
> Sadly, children's passion for thinking often ends when they encounter a world that seeks to educate them for conformity and obedience only. Most children are taught early on that thinking is dangerous. Sadly, these children stop enjoying the process of thinking and start fearing the thinking mind. Whether in homes with parents who teach via a model of discipline and punish that it is better to choose obedience over self-awareness and self-determination, or in schools where independent thinking is not acceptable behavior, most children in our nation learn to suppress the memory of thinking as a passionate, pleasurable activity.
>
> By the time most students enter college classrooms, they have come to dread thinking. Those students who do not dread thinking often come to classes assuming that thinking will not be necessary, that all they will need to do is consume information and regurgitate it at the appropriate moments. . . .

Bell discusses the work of Richard Paul and Linda Elder, who, in their book *The Miniature Guide to Critical Thinking: Concepts and Tools,* elaborate that critical thinking is self-directed, self-disciplined, self-monitored, and self-corrective. Underpinning those self-authoring constructions is the habit of and capacity for quality questioning—which presupposes a primarily intrinsic rather than extrinsic motivation. The necessary initiative, after all, is intrinsically generated. The extrinsically motivated are not very interested in critical thinking. They look for training. For them, the self-constructed stuff is unnecessary bother and even a danger—and the present definition of learning agrees with them. Bell calls for genuine learning communities in our schooling: "The most exciting aspect of critical thinking in the classroom is that it calls for initiative from everyone, actively inviting all students to think passionately and to share ideas in a passionate, open manner." Such a community finds significance and builds understanding. However, the necessary initiative plays havoc with standardized curriculum and assessments. Here is the paradox:

While quality questions are the best way to expand knowledge, especially the kind we call understanding, they disrupt the transmission of easily assessed knowledge-bits—even if worthless from a critical thinking perspective. So we school and test for them, uncritically.

As the image of conversation replaces that of presentation, the capacity for questioning will become increasingly recognized as essential. Questions, after all, further the "quest." They excite and express thinking rather than follow the habit of knowing into simplistic answers. Real questions exercise the right side of the brain; they strive for perspective, comprehension, and understanding; ultimately, they also encourage connection and responsibility.

The capacity to question is increasingly recognized in the business world as essential to the best kind of leadership. Jim Collins, in *Good to Great: Why Some Companies Make the Leap ... and Others Don't,* writes:

> Leaders in each of the good-to-great transitions operated with a somewhat Socratic style. Furthermore, they used questions for one and only one reason: to gain understanding. They didn't use questions as a form of manipulation ("Don't you agree with me on that? …") or as a way to blame or put down others ("Why did you mess this up? …"). When we asked the executives about their management team meetings during the transition era, they said that they spent much of the time "just trying to understand."…Leading from good to great does not mean coming up with the answers and then motivating everyone to follow your messianic vision. It means having the humility to grasp the fact that you do not yet understand enough to have the answers and then to ask the questions that will lead to the best possible insights.

Questioning not only feeds the right brain, it fits in with the business world's changing understanding of leadership. Questions, however, derail the curriculum for they interfere with knowledge installation. They disrupt the "proper" business of schooling, the transmission of knowledge-bits. Such derailments can only have negative impacts upon traditional assessment strategies. After all, the results of investigating such questions will not be on the tests.

The educator S. Snyder writes:

> The title of this essay is "How to Ask a Smart Question" and I have tried to lay out some general guidelines and pitfalls to avoid when you pose questions to gain a greater understanding. I wish I could tell you that asking such questions comes easily; it doesn't. Rather, it's an intellectual habit or a disciplined way of thinking that you can only learn by doing. After all, an expert can give you pointers on shooting a free throw or hitting a golf ball, but you only get good at it with practice.

> I also wish I could promise you ample opportunity to learn this skill in life, but it is one of the great ironies of the modern world that we spend a lot of time thinking about Powerpoint presentations, web search engines, electronic databases and no end of splashy technological gimcrack, yet spend almost no time thinking about the nature and structure of questions. I am not sure why this is, but I suspect it may have something to do with the way good questions unsettle the certainty of what we think we know.
>
> I also wonder to what degree society really wants people to ask a lot of questions. Let's face it: questions are dangerous to those who think they have the answer. And when the powerless begin to put questions to the powerful, look out. World's may change, empires may topple. And maybe, friends, this is why many colleges and universities are more likely to offer you free laptops than lessons in how to use the single most powerful learning tool that humanity has ever devised: a smart question.

In today's schooling, so fixated on the Test it ignores the Quest Quotient, where are the opportunities to learn the habits and skills of questioning? Do we really want people to ask serious questions? If not, we have a problem because the world insists on making its demands—and what of our democratic faith?

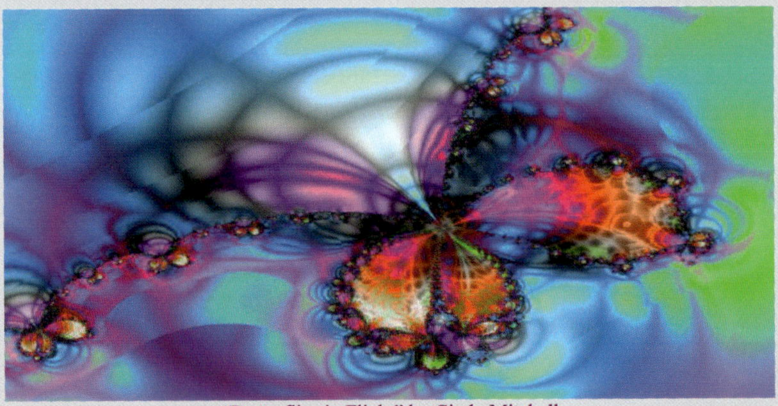

"Butterflies in Flight" by Cindy Mitchell

John Naisbitt, in his book, *Mindset!,* comments that sequence is the enemy of making connections: "Sequence originates from the Latin *sequo,* meaning 'to follow,' . . . But to explore, we have to make connections between things that seemingly don't fit, are not obviously related, and sometimes seem to contradict common sense or formulas." Naisbitt then asks: **"Who has ever solved a picture puzzle by first putting the pieces in a straight line?"**

Did you ask a good question today?

—A Mother's Wisdom—

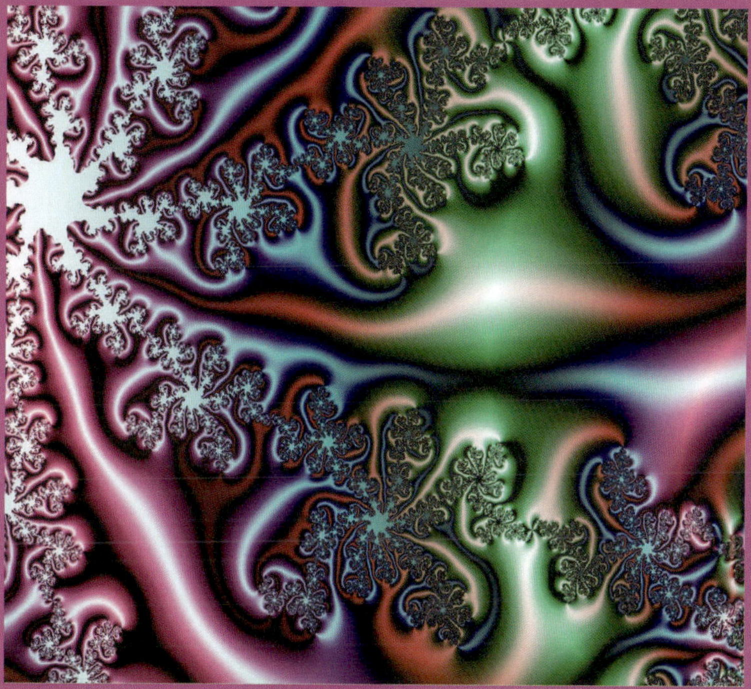

"Deceptively Simple" by Sven Geier

Isidor I. Rabi, the Nobel laureate in physics, was once asked, "Why did you become a scientist, rather than a doctor or lawyer or businessman, like the other immigrant kids in your neighborhood?" His answer has served as an inspiration for me as an educator, as a credo for my son during his schooling and should be framed on the walls of all the pedagogues, power brokers and politicians who purport to run our society. The question was posed to Dr. Rabi by his friend and mine, Arthur Sackler, himself a multitalented genius, who, sadly, also passed away recently. Dr. Rabi's answer, as reported by Dr. Sackler, was profound: "My mother made me a scientist without ever intending it. Every other Jewish mother in Brooklyn would ask her child after school: 'So? Did you learn anything today?' But not my mother. She always asked me a different question. 'Izzy,' she would say, 'did you ask a good question today?' That difference—asking good questions—made me become a scientist!"

Donald Sheff

The Death of Why

A bright young man recently contested my classroom leadership:

> "Is this going to be on the test?"
>
> I replied, "No, it's not."
>
> To which he responded: "Then why are you wasting our time with it then?"

His disrespect aside, he had an argument. After all, the information and conversation were not going to be useful to him, given his definition of learning. In his eyes, I was failing to do my job, which was to gavage him; therefore he couldn't do his job, which was to regurgitate the correct answers on the test. Real questions are rare these days. Teachers get plenty of "hoop questions," such as that young man's, those required to get through—or avoid—the hoops, but where is the habit of mind that inquires, that strives to understand? That habit of mind has found the schooling environment antithetical to its health and vitality, so it has withered and, in many cases, died, at least in relation to formal education.

Andrea Batista Schlesinger, in her book, *The Death of Why: The Decline of Questioning and the Future of Democracy,* writes:

"Inquiry is more than an act; it is a value deeply embedded in our notions of democracy. Democracy—which I use to mean not only our representational form of government but also a system that values equality, justice, and the idea that each member of the group has something worthy to offer the whole—requires citizens who pay attention, who synthesize and analyze, who evaluate the information they have uncovered, and who are discerning about its source. Democracy needs citizens who can inquire. When I look at contemporary culture, however, I see an obsession with answers, not questions. I see an environment that prizes projections of certainty over the wisdom gained from questioning, and questioning again. I see us asking our media, our politicians, our self-help gurus for the answer, any answer, to help us understand the world around us.

"Our schools send the message to children that the answer is all that counts. We test students to death, conveying the idea that correctly filling in the bubbles is the same as learning. Our classrooms become dedicated to the cause of test preparation, as science and its guiding philosophy—that we must discover, ask questions, accumulate evidence, make determinations—become optional.

"It is in our schools that the lack of questioning should trigger the greatest alarms about the future of our democracy."

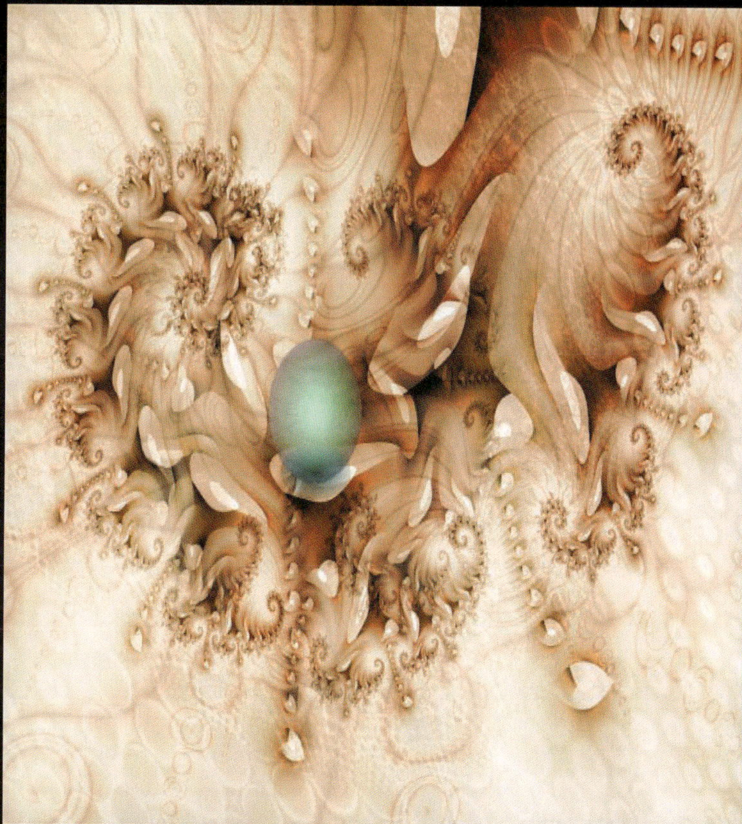

"A Wary Curiosity" by Helen Grainge

The great pleasure of ignorance is the pleasure of asking questions. The man who has lost this pleasure or who has exchanged it for the pleasure of dogma, which is the pleasure of answering, is already beginning to stiffen.

Robert Lynd

In our schooling, knowledge doesn't have dynamic complexity or interactive context. Knowledge is presented as clear, unmuddied, and static, not subject to change or interactive influences. And that static, mess-free knowledge will be on the test. Students who do well under this guiding image of learning take pleasure in the clarity and sureness of their answers. Students who ask questions, however, frequently get into trouble. If they question the curriculum as given, they will certainly get into trouble. Teachers who question will also get into trouble. Thus teachers model an absence of initiative, as well as a lack of personal responsibility.

> By engaging students only in a quest for the correct answer rather than for the interesting question, we condemn them to live inside other men's discoveries.
>
> Priscilla Vail

The systemic suppression of student and teacher initiative by programmed instruction is articulated in the movie *Dead Poets Society*. The "learning as passive reception of pre-packaged material" mindset of Mr. Nolan, the headmaster of Welton Academy, is clear when he reprimands Mr. Keating for unorthodox teaching methods:

"What was going on in the courtyard the other day?"

"Courtyard?"

"Boys marching, clapping in unison."

"Oh that, that was an exercise to prove a point—the dangers of conformity."

"But John, the curriculum is set, it's proven, it works. If you question it, what's to prevent them from doing the same?"

"I always thought the idea of education was to learn to think for yourself."

"At these boys' age, not on your life."

The boys were of high school age. When were they supposed to learn to think for themselves, to develop the habit of initiative? With the kind of perspective illustrated by the headmaster, not uncommon in educational experts and administrators, is it any wonder that student initiative is suppressed? Mr. Nolan wanted to install training while Mr. Keating wanted to inspire initiative. Here lies the crux of the debate:

Which do we value most—training or initiative?

Both are valuable, but only in tandem. A balanced rhythm is necessary between the two energies. Our addiction to prediction and control machinations causes an excessive focus on training and the easily measured. However, that compels us to exclude the energy of initiative from the practice of our teachers and the schooling of our students. As a result, our students question less, about themselves, about what they are learning, about life.

A tension exists between trainers and teachers. Trainers want everyone to be "on the same page," to be, in essence, clapping in unison. They want their students to have the answers. Teachers, on the other hand, want their students to be capable of "marching to a different drummer." They want their students to have the perspective and the strength to be capable of either choosing to commit to the agreed upon rhythm or finding their own way through situations. They want their students to be able to question, habitually and effectively.

There are no whole truths: all truths are half-truths. It is trying to treat them as whole truths that plays the devil.

Alfred North Whitehead

A Cautionary Thought

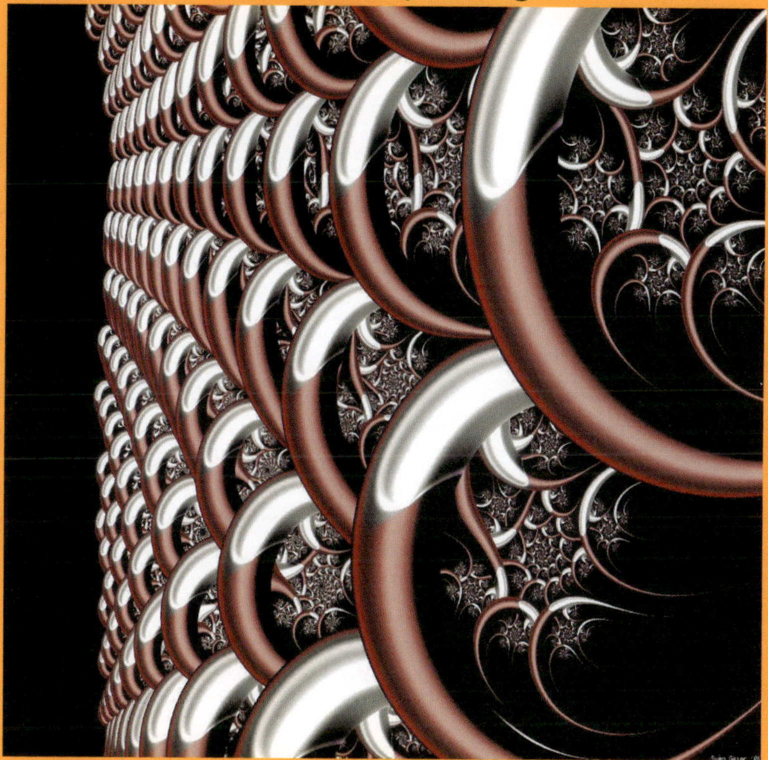

"Chainlink" by Sven Geier

As we shove both teacher and student initiative out of the curriculum, we crowd in the pleasure of answering. Trainers (not teachers—as redefined) provide a steady diet of answers and students dutifully accept them. We systematically portray learning as the successful ingestion of answers, which students can then proudly display during class "discussions" and regurgitate at testing time. Students are led, by the systemic effects of the learning environment, away from the joy, and power, of asking questions. Are we predisposing our students to closed-mindedness, to the predilection for grabbing and adhering to dogmas?

Are we working hard to forge the conditions for fundamentalism?

—26—

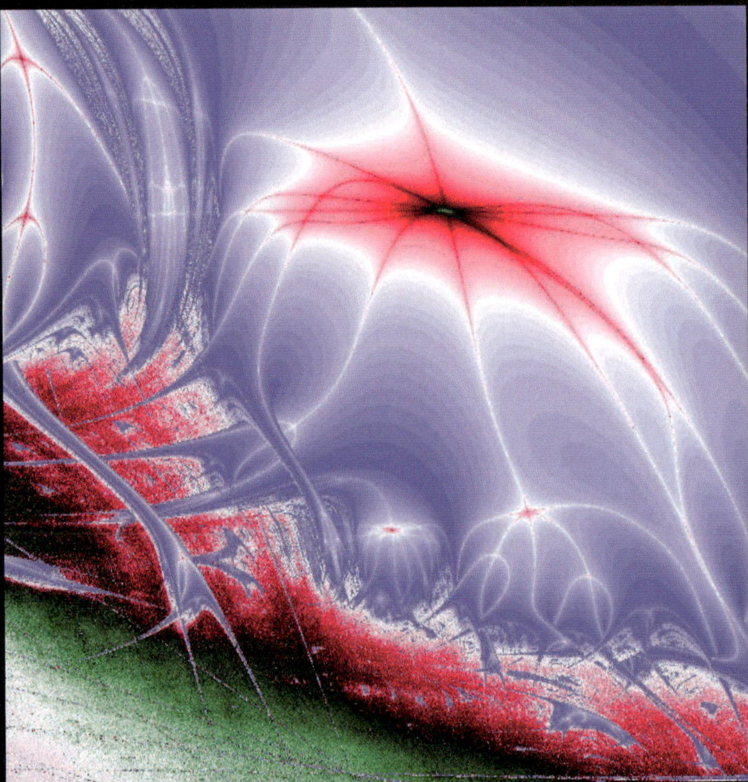

"Probing the Bottom" by Ken Keller

One of the reasons I haven't chosen to present one idea at a time has something to do with my sense that maybe learning—real learning—is not clean and simple, that it does involve messing around with a couple of ideas at once, that it does mean bouncing one concept off of another in an attempt to look at both their relationships and their individuality.

Susanne M. Wilson

Curiosity is characterized by messiness. Albert Einstein's desk, by all personal accounts and photographic evidence, was one of stupendous, serendipitous disarray. The following photograph of his messy desk was taken on the last day of Einstein's life, when the energy of his curiosity, imagination, and life was at low ebb—we can only imagine the mess at the height of his productivity:

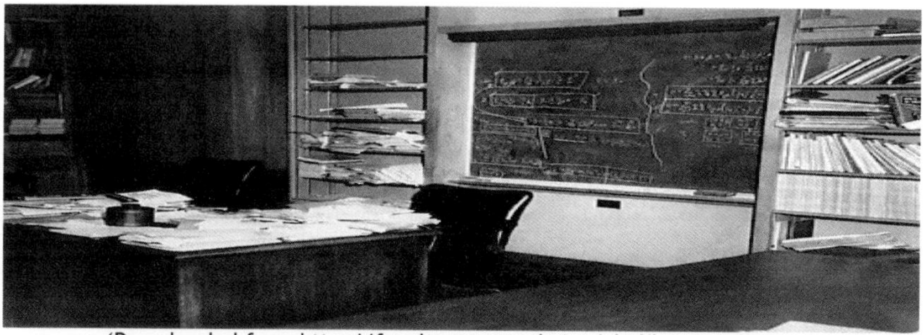

(Downloaded from http://faculty.rmwc.edu/tmichalik/einstein.htm).

Good conversations are often messy: "Oh, we talked about everything under the sun." Creativity, almost by definition, involves messing around with several ideas at once. Mulling and mucking are essential to worthwhile learning. Learning redefined would incorporate the benefits of messiness to the process. Initiative messes with curriculum. It messes with the prediction and control machinations of educationists. It messes with coverage. So many students have heard: "We don't have time to talk about that now, Johnny. We have to get back to the lesson." Johnny's concern and curiosity are shoved aside, and then we wonder why he becomes disengaged.

Training crowds out initiative by treating it as messiness. Curricular presentations should not be interrupted by conversations. The lecture must go on. The material must be covered—because the tests will be administered. Interaction, however, is at the heart of the educational process, and any interaction, by definition, will contain messiness because no two people are always on the same page. No two people—if they are individuals—can ever really be on the same page. If we are going to increase the Quest Quotient of our students, then we must allow more conversations, real conversations, to develop in our learning environments. Then we will have the educational process called for by the postmodern world.

At a performance of a jazz pianist in Louisville last year, a member of the audience gave an impassioned approval of the artistry and creativity of the performer's rendition of "Imagine" by John Lennon:

"He's messing with it! Messing with it!"

The appreciative listener was saying that the artist was putting his creativity and capability into the curriculum, into the established composition. He was making it his own. He was fusing his own engagement into the creation of John Lennon. Jazz both adds and reminds; it adds to the old melodies and rhythms. That is the essence of Jazz, the bringing of unique, idiosyncratic creative aliveness into a prior composition. Every performance is a renewal of the life force.

Curiously, or perhaps, tellingly, a concurrent travesty, along with the left-brain driven fixation on easily tested transmission of knowledge bits in the present definition of learning, developed in the music world; it lost its appreciation for messiness. Improvisation used to be the hallmark of a professional musician. It was the inferior musician who was micro-managed by the composition, who did not mess with the program as given.

In *A Perfect Mess: The Hidden Benefits of Disorder*, Eric Abramhamson and David H. Freedman talk about how one superstar musician [and composer] who "may be the greatest improvisationalist of all time is well known to the public for everything *except* his improvisation:"

> The irrepressible improviser was Johann Sebastian Bach. If you're wondering how Bach managed to reconcile improvisation with the highly ordered, intricate, precise domain of baroque music, consider that in the eighteenth century improvisation was regarded as an integral component of serious music. It would have been a second-rate performer indeed who thought to limit recitals to prescribed notes. The opportunity—the imperative, really—for improvisation was explicitly written into baroque compositions and in more than one way.
>
> ...Bach and his colleagues could not have predicted that by the middle of the twentieth century the improvisational elements of their compositions, and of all classical music, would have been gradually and thoroughly excised. Composers had later filled in the bass lines and cadenzas with note-for-note versions, so that today musicians play only what's on the page, and every performance is melodically identical to every other.

The left brain, in the spirit of the times, filled in the blanks. Compositions that encouraged, that even called for, improvisation, invited too much messiness. The Zeitgeist called for programmed playing, not improvising. Initiative on the part of performers was to be replaced by doing as trained. Abrahamson and Freedman add these thoughts:

> Taking it on oneself to add off-the-cuff flourishes to the music in the middle of a performance would be seen not as an exhibition of musicianship and creativity, but as a career-ending stunt that violated the music—even though to do so would be far more in keeping with the composer's intentions than the frozen-in-place versions we hear today. It has been a centuries-long organizing project that almost certainly would have appalled some of the very composers we most ardently lionize.

What if this freeze-drying of the music had not happened? What if the juice, and the messy aliveness, had been left in? What would have been the effects on our thinking, on our consciousness over the years, decades, and centuries? What were the deadening impacts of all the regimentation that took place despite the imagination and intentions of the original composers?

Our schools need to be messier, in both process and curriculum. Order is a characteristic of left-brain operation. Right-brain thinking is always jumping out of the set-in-stone boxes. Just as modern musicians are compelled to suppress their initiative in a mistaken allegiance to the old masters, our teachers are coerced into a regimen of orthodoxy. We need more improvisation across the board, in our schooling, in our thinking, in our music, in our culture.

Abrahamson and Freedman talk about the leadership and initiative of Gail Leftin, the founder and director of the Little Red Wagon school, famous for its creative students and lack of discipline problems—but also its messiness. The school has escaped the dictates of correct-answer schooling and test-fixation, prefering the organic aliveness of placing its trust in interest, imagination, and initiative. Abrahamson and Freedman write:

> The Little Red Wagon's disordered, curriculumless approach seems especially risky at a time when states have rushed into standardized testing for elementary school students, leading to more sharply defined, rigid curricula as early as kindergarten. But Leftin has tracked Little Red Wagon graduates and found they generally score well above average on standardized testing in early grade school. Still, the real advantage to the Little Red Wagon approach, she says, is the creativity, confidence, and boldness that it imparts—the school's messy approach to education instills an intellectual robustness that holds up in any classroom or testing situation. Children who are exposed to more focused curricula specifically geared toward testing, in contrast, often have difficulties with creative exercises and even with new curriculum.

If we are to develop right-brain capabilities, then we must set up conditions conducive to the emergence of the necessary mess. That way we will bring life into our schooling.

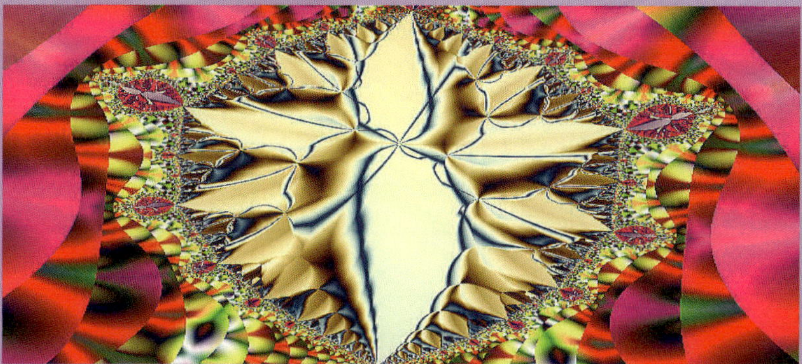

"Fractured Facets" by Ken Keller

I love playing with ideas, looking at something from as many sides as possible, lifting up an observation and shaking it to see if a revelation might fall out.

Diane Ackerman

This book messes with the image of learning. It bounces one concept off another in an attempt to arrive at some real learning about learning. Comprehension, after all, is the construction of meaning upon a previously perceived mess, an enlightening picture of the interconnected whole. We must grok our way toward that awareness and understanding. That is why the book is a mosaic—a hodgepodge of small pieces cemented (or patched) together in order to picture a larger, dynamic whole.

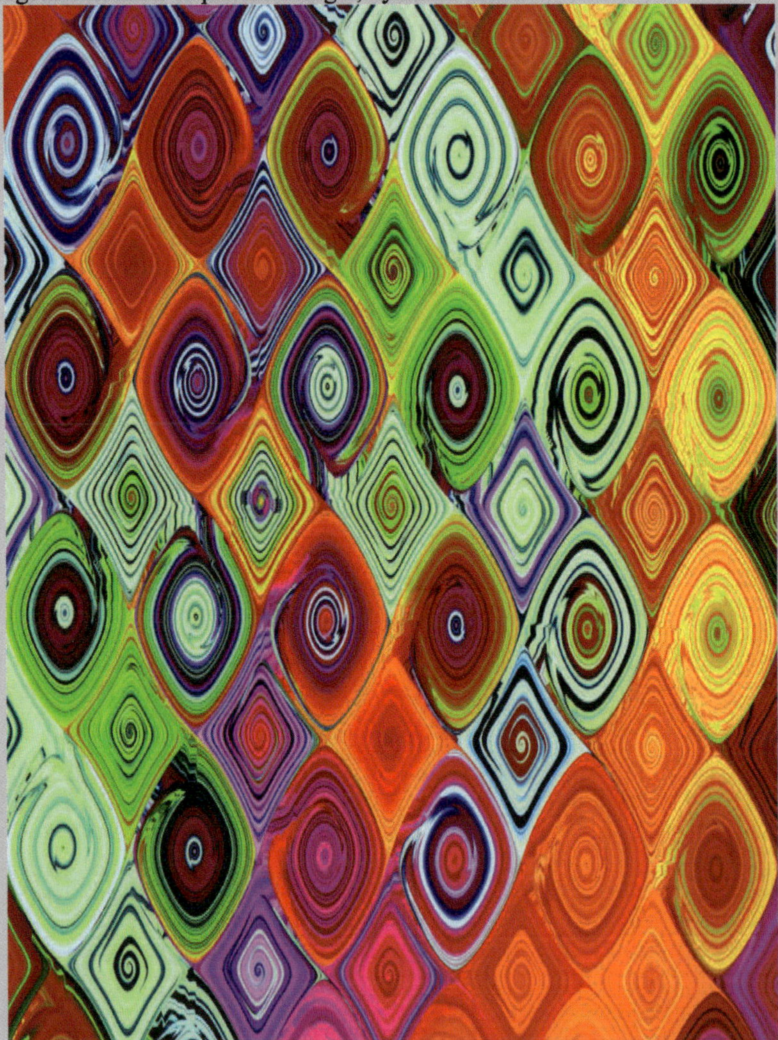

"Mosaic" by Vicky Brago-Mitchell

–27–

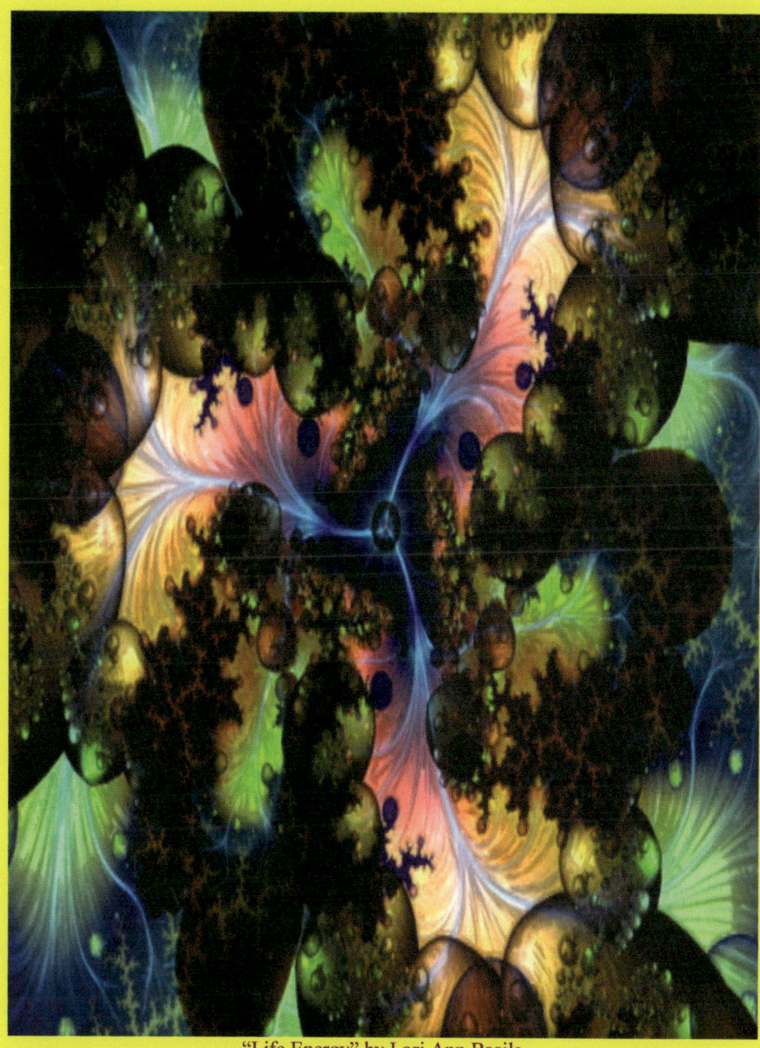

"Life Energy" by Lori Ann Basile

We need to develop new approaches to information—not management but encouragement, not control but genesis. How do we create more of this wonderful life source?

Margaret J. Wheatley

Wheatley understands that it is no linguistic accident that the word "information" is the same as the phrase "in formation" as in a marching band or flight of planes overhead. Information is the construction of meaningful patterns. A fact or an idea is not information until placed into a pattern of understanding, until it is made meaningful. Information cannot be transmitted, or managed into the mind of learners, because it is a construction that must be made by the learners. Therefore, while the transmission of data and ideas can be controlled, the construction of information cannot be controlled. Such construction can only be encouraged and environments conducive to their emergence developed. But information construction is a messy process, for it requires periods of reflection and conversation that mess with the prediction and control of curriculum.

Wheatley envisions the construction of information as a wonderful life source. She is talking about the business world and how the aliveness of an organization depends on the organization's ability to get employees to construct information, but the same challenge holds for our schools: How can we encourage and help students construct information, their own patterns of understanding? What does learning do if it does not expand awareness and construct information? Is that not the ultimate purpose of learning? Can it accomplish that goal, given its present definition, which perceives information (and even awareness) as something to manage and control?

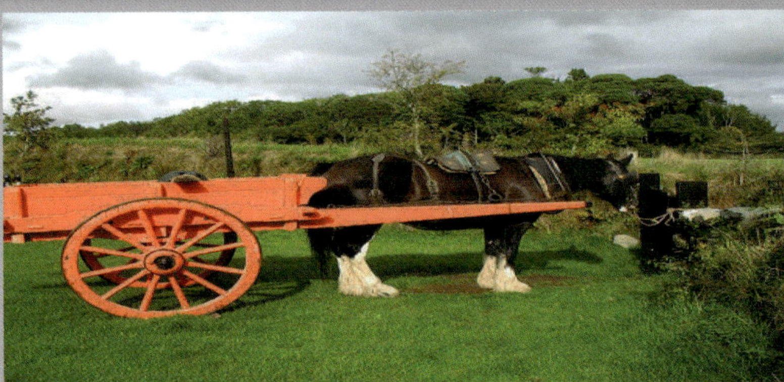

From www.flickr.com/photos/g9g/253329527/

The current definition of learning doesn't realize that simplistic transmission of knowledge bits is neither the cart nor the horse. True: learning is the horse, the motive force, but it must have a stout back (meaningfulness and engagement), good teeth (interpretation) and strong legs (interest and initiative). The cart is expanded awareness (removed ignorance) and developed intellect, (information constructed by interpretation). Transmitted knowledge bits are useful only when they fill the cart or excite the horse.

—28—

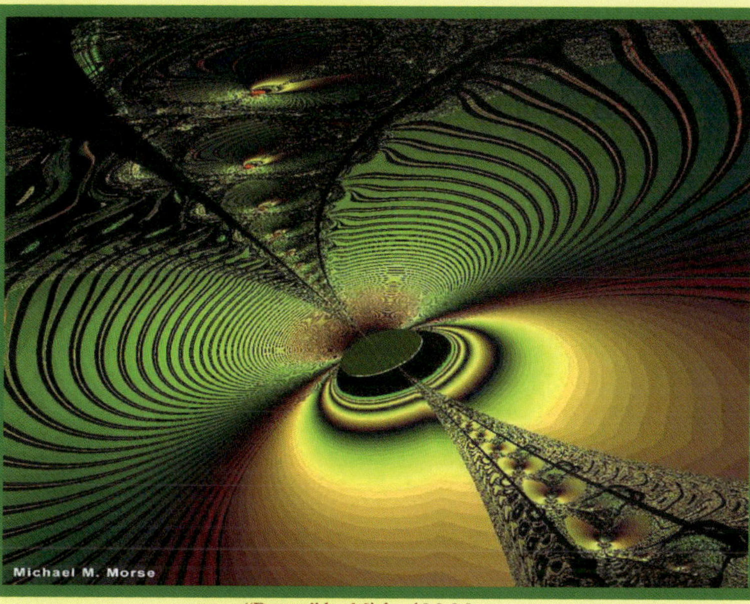

"Button" by Michael M. Morse

Learning is like Velcro. An unfiltered fact is not a complete fastener. Only one side of learning is made up of facts; the other consists of stories, i.e. ideas and images.

Richard Saul Wurman

Wurman's analogy gives us another perspective on the importance of learning's constructive nature. We need more stories and images in our schooling, especially if they are brought in by the students themselves. Facts have to be filtered through imagination, conjecture, and experience before they are worthwhile. Their meaning and utilization must be constructed. Thus interpreted, they become a complete learning. They are "buttoned" (or velcroed) into place in the mind of the learner.

Gary Marcus writes in, *Kluge: the Haphazard Construction of the Human Mind*:

> Consider our outmoded system of education, still primarily steeped in ideas from nineteenth-century pedagogy, with its outsized emphasis on memorization echoing the Industrial Revolution and Dickens' stern schoolmaster, Mr. Gradgrind: "Now, what I want is, Facts. Teach these boys and girls nothing but Facts . . . Plant nothing else, and root out everything else."

Mr. Gradgrind's perspective dominates the operating metaphor for our schooling. Training has crowded out initiative. The left-brain has starved the right-brain. The easily measured Facts rule the day, every day, and have for the past century or more. "But," as Marcus points out, "it scarcely does what education ought to do, which is to help our children learn how to fend for themselves." Marcus quotes Deanna Kuhn, author of *Education for Thinking*:

> A seventh-grader at a considerably above average school asked his (well-regarded) social studies teacher, "Why do we have to learn the names of all thirteen colonies?" The teacher's answer, delivered without hesitation, was, "Well, we're going to learn all fifty states by June, so we might as well learn the first thirteen now." Clear evidence that the memorization cart has come before the educational horse . . . The result, in the words of one researcher, is that:
>
> > Many students are unable to give evidence of more than a superficial understanding of the concepts and relationships that are fundamental to the subjects they have studied, or of an ability to apply the content knowledge they have acquired to real-world problems . . . it is possible to finish 12 or 13 years of public education in the United States without developing much competence as a thinker.
> >
> > In the information age, children have no trouble *finding* information, but they have trouble *interpreting* it.

Without the stories, ideas, and images behind the memorized facts, thinking is not done and the learning—no matter how much "knowledge" is memorized and measured—is not complete. Without initiative, interpretation is not constructed. Without the capacity for interpretation, individuals are unable to expand and control their awareness. They therefore cannot form the foundation necessary for a democracy, people who can think for themselves—who are self-reliant.

Educational psychologist David Perkins asked high school and college graduates to evaluate social and political questions, such as "Does violence on television significantly increase the likelihood of violence in real life?" or "Would restoring the military draft significantly increase America's ability to influence world events? Responses were evaluated in terms of their sophistication. How many times did people consider objections to their own arguments? How many different lines of argument did people consider? How well could people justify their main arguments? Most subjects settled for simplistic answers no matter how much the experimenters tried to push them—and the amount of education made surprisingly little difference. As Perkins put it, "Present educational practices do little to foster the development of informal reasoning skills."

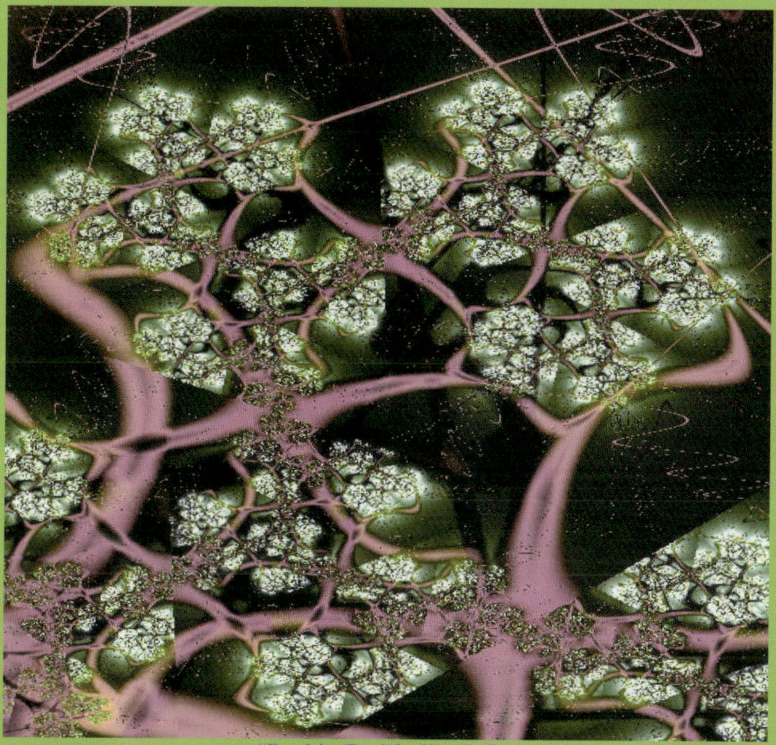

"Dendrite Tree" by Ken Keller

Kluge (klooj) is a slang term for a clumsy or inelegant solution to a problem—a cobbled-together contraption, a mess of often contradictory beliefs, thoughts, and emotions. Marcus proposes that the human mind is often more klugey than logical in its design, and thus more quirky and imperfect. Our thinking is more contextually-dependent than previously considered: "Another lab studied people as they played a trivia game. Those briefly primed by terms like *professor* or *intelligent* outperformed those prepped by less lofty expressions, such as *soccer hooligan* and *stupid*." Another study asked undergraduate students to unscramble a series of sentences. But the real experiment was their walking speed when leaving the task. Those who had unscrambled sentences with words such as retired, elderly, and Florida ambled more slowly than those who didn't. The few words intimating old age embedded in the study affected their mood and energy. Our mind is more of a haphazard hodgepodge of interacting influences than we would like to assume. Learning Redefined will take the idiosyncratic quirkiness of the human mind into consideration as it constructs learning environments—leaving more room for curious playfulness, unusual projects, and joyous discoveries.

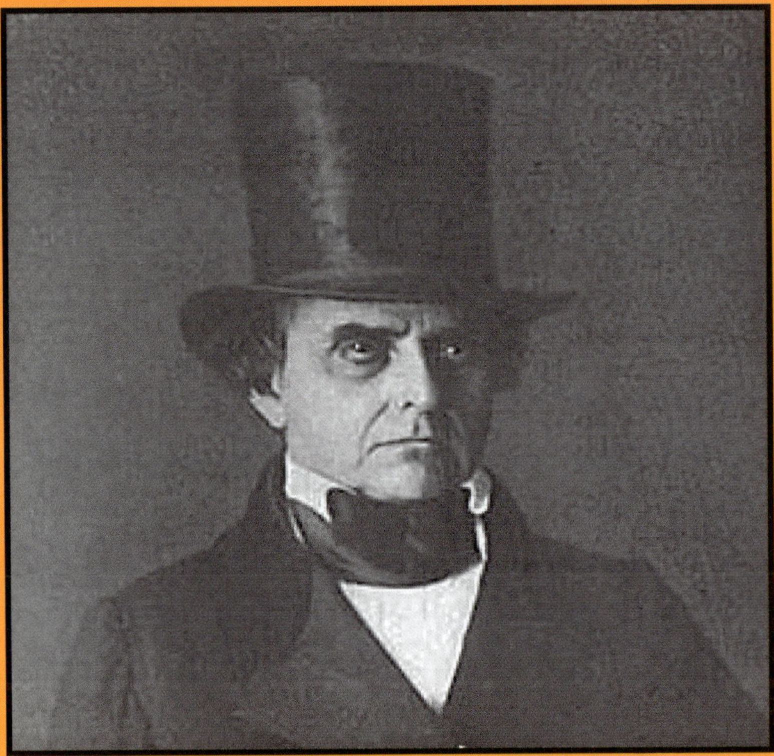

Image of Gradgrind from www.wsu.edu/~brians/gradgrind.html

MR GRADGRIND walked homeward from the school, in a state of considerable satisfaction. It was his school, and he intended it to be a model. He intended every child in it to be a model — just as the young Gradgrinds were all models. There were five young Gradgrinds, and they were models every one. They had been lectured at, from their tenderest years; coursed, like little hares. Almost as soon as they could run alone, they had been made to run to the lecture-room. The first object with which they had an association, or of which they had a remembrance, was a large black board with a dry Ogre chalking ghastly white figures on it. Not that they knew, by name or nature, anything about an Ogre. Fact forbid! I only use the word to express a monster in a lecturing castle, with Heaven knows how many heads manipulated into one, taking childhood captive, and dragging it into gloomy statistical dens by the hair.

Charles Dickens
Hard Times

—29—

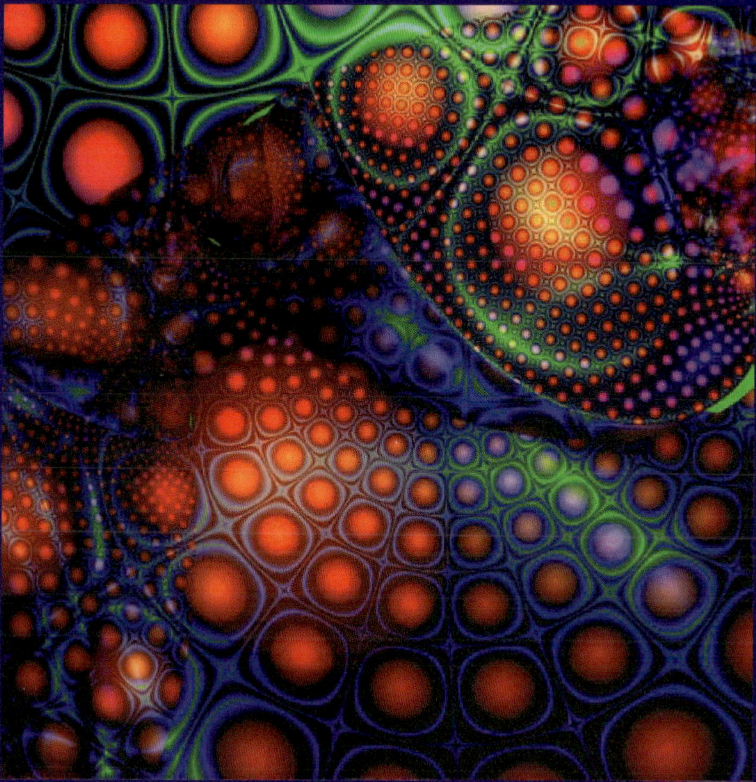

"Composition" by Titia

What we do as teachers is orchestrate the dialogue moving from one side of the room to the other . . . The teacher reads the qualitative cues of the situation as it unfolds and thinks on her feet, in many cases like a stand-up comedian. Reflection is not absent, theory is not irrelevant, even research conclusions might be considered, but they provide guidance, not direction. They are more in the background than the forefront of the action.

Eliot Eisner

The image of teaching provided by Eisner is much closer to the kind of teaching we will need for educating students capable of dealing with the dynamically complex challenges of the future. In order to encourage more of this kind of teaching, the tasks are clear:

> We must fundamentally alter the philosophical assumptions presently underlying educational practice and construct new operating metaphors that are more organic and less mechanistic. We must wean ourselves from the compulsion to instruct for the easily measurable and seemingly predictable and design learning environments that encourage the development of thinking, ownership, initiative, responsibility, and maturation.

Teaching is the constructing and melding of temporary webs of connection between developing intellects. It is not the building of permanent architectures, brick by packaged brick, until supposedly firm and stable structures are in place. Learning is too alive and dynamic to be adequately reflected by that image of teaching. Good teachers are much closer to improvisational jazz musicians than they are to brick-layers. Elliot Eisner writes, in "The Art and Craft of Teaching:"

> We need to give the piccolos a chance—indeed to encourage them to sing more confidently—but we also need to provide space for the brass. And as for the violins, they always seem to have a major part to play. How is it going? What does the melody sound like? Is the music full enough? Do we need to stretch the orchestra further? When shall we pause and recapitulate the introductory theme? The clock is reaching ten and we have not yet crescendoed? How can we bring it to a closure when we can't predict when a stunning question or an astute observation will bring forth a new melodic line and off we go again? Such are the pleasures and trials of teaching, and when it goes well, there is nothing more that we would rather do.

Only teachers who understand and appreciate this jazz-like truth of the teaching endeavor can really succeed at generating conversations and encouraging learning communities. As long as teachers buy into the assembly line metaphor, they will push their students around with mechanisms of prediction and control instead of gently pulling forth the emergence of learning and maturation. When teachers escape notions of prediction and control, they best develop their capacities to lead students toward ownership of what they know, who they are, and who they can become. The best professionals rely less on formulas learned in school and from books than on the kind of improvisational skill learned from gaining the experience of surviving the predicaments of actual practice. They constantly reflect on their professional actions, often reflecting while immersed in action. This capacity to adjust while on stage, so to speak, is what separates excellent practitioners from the ordinary. They become adept at improvising upon their formulas within the turmoil of the endeavor.

Donald A. Schon, in *The Reflective Practitioner: How Professionals Think in Action,* elaborates:

> When good jazz musicians improvise together, they also manifest a "feel for" their material and make on-the-spot adjustments to the sounds they hear. Listening to one another and to themselves, they feel where the music is going and adjust their playing accordingly. They can do this,

> first of all, because their collective effort at musical invention makes use of a schema—a metric, melodic, and harmonic schema familiar to all the participants—which gives a predictable order to the piece. In addition, each of the musicians has at the ready a repertoire of musical figures which he can deliver at appropriate moments. Improvisation consists in varying, combining, and recombining a set of figures within the schema which bounds and gives coherence to the performance. As the musicians feel the direction of the music developing out of their interwoven contributions, they make new sense of it and adjust their performance to the new sense they have made. They are reflecting-in-action on the music they are collectively making and on their individual contributions to it, thinking about what they are doing and, in the process, evolving their way of doing it.

Elliot W. Eisner, in *The Educational Imagination: On the Design and Evaluation of School Programs,* talks about how teaching is an art:

> 1. It is an art in that teaching can be performed with such skill and grace that, for the student as well as the teacher, the experience can be justifiably characterized as aesthetic.
>
> 2. Teaching is an art in that teachers, like painters, composers, actresses, and dancers, make judgments based largely on qualities that unfold during the course of action.
>
> 3. Teaching is an art in that the teacher's activity is not dominated by prescriptions or routines but is influenced by qualities and contingencies that are unpredicted.
>
> 4. Teaching is an art in that the ends it achieves are often created in process. . . . teaching is a form of human action in which many of the ends achieved are emergent—that is to say, found in the course of interaction with students rather than preconceived and efficiently attained.

Margaret J. Wheatley, in *Leadership and the New Science: Learning about Organization from an Orderly Universe,* comments:

> Those who have used music metaphors in describing leadership, particularly jazz metaphors, are on a quantum track. Improvisation is the saving skill. As leaders, we play a crucial role in selecting the melody, setting the tempo, establishing the key, and inviting the players. But that is all we can do. The music comes from something we cannot direct, from a unified whole created among the players—a relational holism that transcends separateness. In the end, when it works, we sit back, amazed and grateful.

Barzun and Eisner (and others) have been trying to tell us for years that teaching is more of an improvisational art than a "scientifically rational" endeavor. We will achieve restructuring (in the purest sense of the word) when we stop seeing the endeavor from a static, linear assembly-line perspective and understand the ebb and flow of symphogenetic education. The best, most alive, learning process is always symphogenetic (interactive, improvisational, and emergent).

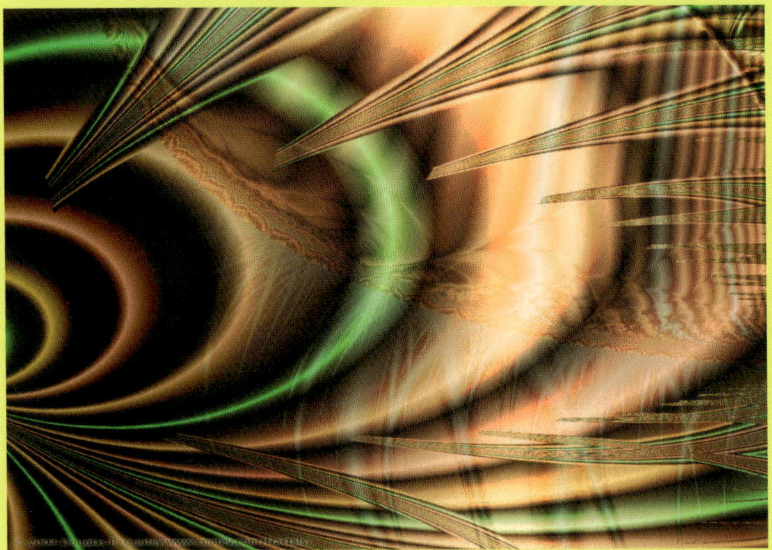

"Orbital Convergence" by Douglas Cootey

Symphogenesis (from sympho; to fuse together, and genesis; to be born) is related to the concept of symphony. The Oxford English Dictionary defines the symphogenetic process as "the union of previously separate elements." The image of symphogenesis needs to replace the banking metaphor in order to redefine learning. Symphogenesis is creativity in action, where divergent (right brain) and convergent (left brain) thinking weave and dance. It illustrates a neurogenic process.

Symphogenesis depends upon the confidence necessary for inclusiveness. It encourages rather than suppresses imagination, interest, and initiative, or counter-examples and disagreements. The symphogenetic teacher is confident of his or her capability to forge music from any messiness that may emerge from the unpredictable contributions. They know they can improvise; they can forge new patterns of meaning from the initiative of the learners; they are jazz teachers.

Symphogenesis is a messy, idiosyncratic, emergent, constructive, juicy, and exhilarating process. It carries the life of the mind toward intellectual, emotional, and spiritual growth. It is in every worthwhile conversation, every nourishing reflection. It is what gives every relationship innovativeness, vitality, character, momentum, vividness, interestingness, flow, and resiliency. It is the confluence of synergizing relationships, the connecting between the developing new and the existing whole capable of expanding itself and its capabilities. It is at the core of all worthwhile learning.

Symphogenesis indicates a process that can be summed up in the phrase,

As they are born—they are fused together.

The absence of symphogenesis is characterized by weakness, brittleness, resentment, resistance, boringness, and "death in life." The relationship without symphogenesis is doomed to emptiness, stagnation, loss of potential, and "making do" until the opportunities are lost. The term symphogenetic education recognizes the messy, improvisational nature of real learning. The process of teaching and learning is not simply one of assembling skills or data. It is more like a jazz ensemble, where elements merge idiosyncratically and unpredictably and are then fused into a new emergence into the evolving harmony of the whole.

Perhaps the most important operating metaphor we need to change in order to redefine learning is the one that guides teacher education. The present system, through education professors, professional development consultants, and school administrators, communicates that teachers are "curriculum implementation specialists." Harboring such a guiding metaphor, practitioners will never develop the necessary leadership ability to practice symphogenetic teaching. Teachers must recognize that they are artists—not curriculum implementation specialists, but artists dedicated to helping others learn and develop. Teachers who identify themselves as curriculum implementation specialists can easily be replaced by computers—and should be.

Symphogenetic education succinctly illustrates the interactive, interweaving relationship between knowing and thinking. It is also a helpful metaphor for imaging the maturational process. Symphogenesis images the developmental process of how both learning and maturation unfold—sometimes in fits and starts—but always by melding the new into the old.

Learning changes—sometimes transformationally—old understandings. As we redefine learning, we will increasingly image it as a symphogenetic process. This will inspire and inform the initiative of both teachers and students. The best learning and teaching are symphogenetic. A good conversation is symphogenetic. Good thinking is symphogenetic. Creativity is symphogenetic. Life itself is symphogenetic. We need more of it in our classrooms and schools.

Both Schon and Eisner understand the symphogenetic process—that learning relationships are always growing and changing in context. This is especially true—or should be—during the heat and juice of classroom life. The essential difference between managers and leaders is the type of metaphors that determine and guide their methods. Management assumes the effectiveness (and desirability) of prediction and control sets. Leadership understands the realities of emergence and interaction. Therefore, leaders (especially those informed by symphogenetic images), utilize methods that are less manipulative—that are more closely aligned with recognizing and encouraging the expression of mutually desirable potentials.

Symphogenesis occurs and grows when we have the strength and vitality of love—for learning, for students, for relating—to transform ourselves beyond the will to control to the will to connect.

The Improvising Brain

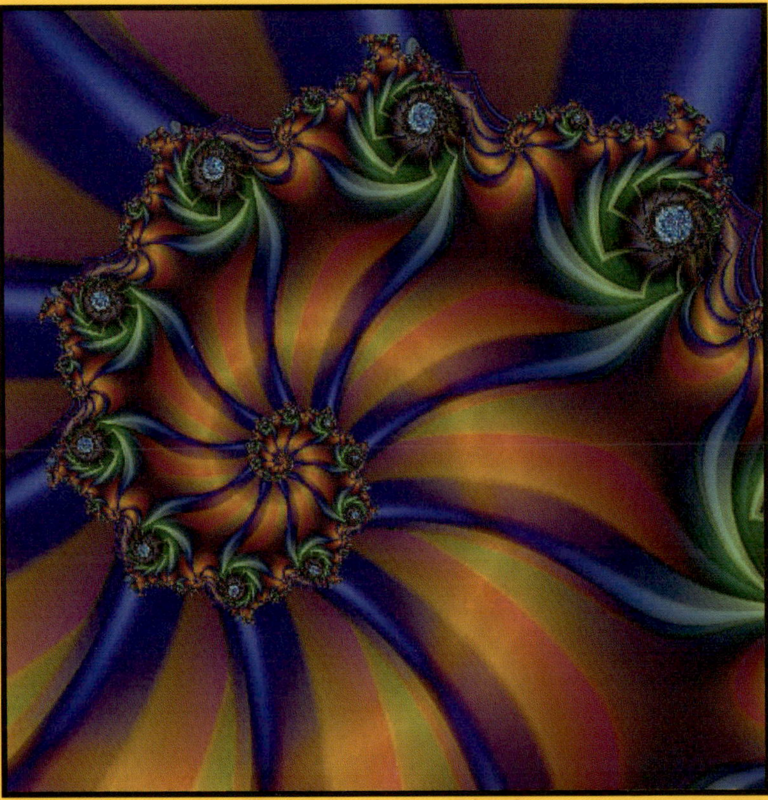

"Smooth Jazz" by Dawn Edwards

The brain also operates symphogenetically. Diane Ackerman, in *An Alchemy of Mind*, writes: "When shocked, refreshed, or just learning something, neurons grow more dendritic branches, increasing their reach and influence even more. It's as if a neuron sends scouts to many outposts to gather news. The scouts gossip among themselves, too. Based on their reports, a neuron passes messages to other neurons, using its axon, a fine branching limb anywhere from a few millimeters to a meter long. As the axon's tip grows, it senses its environment, getting cues on which direction to turn. Somehow all that nosing around, connecting, and networking orients personality, chisels character."

–30–

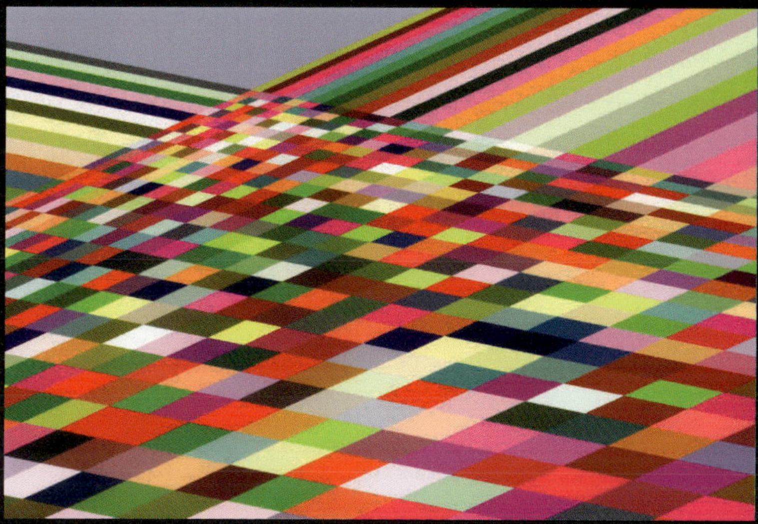

"Weave 12" by Ken Keller

Symphony is the ability to put together the pieces. It is the capacity to synthesize rather than analyze; to see relationships between seemingly unrelated fields; to detect broad patterns rather than to deliver specific answers; and to invent something new by combining elements nobody else thought to pair.

Daniel H. Pink

Present schooling essentially gavages. Rarely does the creative spirit of symphogenesis develop, for it must emerge despite the conditions of coverage-fixation and assessment by the easily measured. Symphony depends upon initiative in both teachers and students. While training can inform it cannot compel symphony—and distilled to a toxic dose will suppress it. The educational profession must reach a new realization:

> **No amount of gavaging will prepare us for the future that is unfolding. A symphogenetic educational process is required.**

So what is the future going to look like? That is, as always, hard to say. But we can safely assume that more and more left-brain functions will be taken over by computers. Correct answers are easily accessible now. Understanding, however, the capacity to interpret knowledge and construct a new interpretation, is increasingly necessary. Daniel H. Pink, in his book, *A Whole New Mind: Why Right-Brainers will Rule the Future,* argues that we are moving from the left-brain, data-driven, number-crunching, sequential world that has dominated the economy for the past several hundred years to a new economy, the Conceptual Age. This different kind of future will call for different kinds of capabilities if people are to survive and flourish. Pink calls these capabilities senses:

1. **Not just function but also DESIGN.** It's no longer sufficient to create a product, a service, an experience, or a lifestyle that's merely functional. Today it's economically crucial and personally rewarding to create something that is also beautiful, whimsical, or emotionally engaging.
2. **Not just argument but also STORY.** When our lives are brimming with information and data, it's not enough to marshal an effective argument. Someone somewhere will inevitably track down a counterpoint to rebut your point. The essence of persuasion, communication, and self-understanding has become the ability also to fashion a compelling narrative.
3. **Not just focus but also SYMPHONY.** Much of the Industrial and Information Ages required focus and specialization. But as white-collar work gets routed to Asia and reduced to software, there's a new premium on the opposite aptitude: putting the pieces together, or what I call Symphony. What's in greatest demand today isn't analysis but synthesis—seeing the big picture, crossing boundaries, and being able to combine disparate pieces into an arresting new whole.
4. **Not just logic but also EMPATHY.** The capacity for logical thought is one of the things that make us human. But in a world of ubiquitous information and advanced analytic tools, logic alone won't do. What will distinguish those who thrive will be their ability to understand what makes their fellow woman or man tick, to forge relationships, and to care for others.
5. **Not just seriousness but also PLAY.** Ample evidence points to the enormous health and professional benefits of laughter, lighthearted-ness, games, and humor. There is a time to be serious, of course. But too much sobriety can be bad for your career and worse for your general well-being. In the Conceptual Age, in work and in life, we all need to play.
6. **Not just accumulation but also MEANING.** We live in a world of breathtaking material plenty. That has freed hundreds of millions of people from day-to-day struggles and liberated us to pursue more significant desires: purpose, transcendence, and spiritual fulfillment

Symphony is a cardinal capability; without it, nothing else follows. All the other capabilities called for by the Conceptual Age hinge upon the health and vitality of its existence. Symphony can be thought of as the ability to create a new, or more comprehensive, picture. It is the constructive energy that makes new connections. It is creative power. The poet Edna St. Vincent Millay warned us about this need for context and symphony in order to avoid contextual blindness and metaphorical incompetence:

> **Upon this gifted age, in its dark hour,**
> **Rains from the sky a meteoric shower**
> **Of facts . . . they lie unquestioned, uncombined.**
> **Wisdom enough to leach us of our ill**
> **Is daily spun, but there exists no loom**
> **To weave it into fabric.**

Symphony underlies empathy, meaning, design, and story, and fuels curiosity, creativity, and imagination. Symphony supports the work of play—which provides the relaxation necessary for seeing new connections. The sense of symphony is also essential for thinking. As Robert Frost informed us previously: "All thought is a feat of association. . . . Putting this and that together. That click." Symphony also guides and informs initiative in an interactive dialectic; they co-evolve each other. Symphony is particularly important in a world where butterflies are increasingly busy flapping their little wings.

The sense of symphony is the creative power that carries systems thinking, the search for seeing things whole. "It is all about relationships—even at the subatomic level," physicists now tell us, enlightened by Quantum Physics. Previous schooling has focused on developing habits of mind that separated realities from their contextual beds. We now need more systems thinking, in order to find the new contextual realities. Pink talks about the work of Daniel Goleman, who studied executives at fifteen large companies:

> "Just one cognitive ability distinguished star performers from average: pattern recognition, the 'big picture' thinking that allows leaders to pick out the meaningful trends from a welter of information around them and to think strategically far into the future." These star performers, he found [again quoting Goleman], "relied less on deductive, if-then reasoning" and more on the intuitive, contextual reasoning characteristic of Symphony.

Symphony is not only essential for creativity but integral to leadership. The time of matrix-driven micro-managers is past. The kind of leaders we now need will have the capabilities outlined by Pink. Symphony will be especially important. The question is: can we change the operating metaphors guiding education to those conducive to the emergence and development of the necessary capabilities? Solving the problems and fashioning the products of the future calls for a dramatic redefinition of learning as well as teaching. Is that task beyond our intelligence? Pink is hopeful:

> Design. Story. Symphony. Empathy. Play. Meaning. These six senses will increasingly guide our lives and shape our world. Many of you no doubt welcome such a change. But to some of you, the vision might seem dreadful—a hostile takeover of normal life by a band of poseurs

> in black unitards who will leave behind the insufficiently arty and emotive. Fear not. The high-concept, high-touch abilities that now matter most are fundamentally human attributes. After all, back on the savannah, our cave-person ancestors weren't taking SATs or plugging numbers into spreadsheets. But they were telling stories, demonstrating empathy, and designing innovations. These abilities have always comprised part of what it means to be human. But after a few generations in the Information Age, these muscles have atrophied. The challenge is to work them back into shape.

We need to exercise those atrophied muscles—not perpetuate and exacerbate the atrophy, as we do now. Can we make the necessary adjustments? Do we have the symphony within us to construct the new connections? Can we strengthen our corpus callosum, metaphorically—maybe even literally?

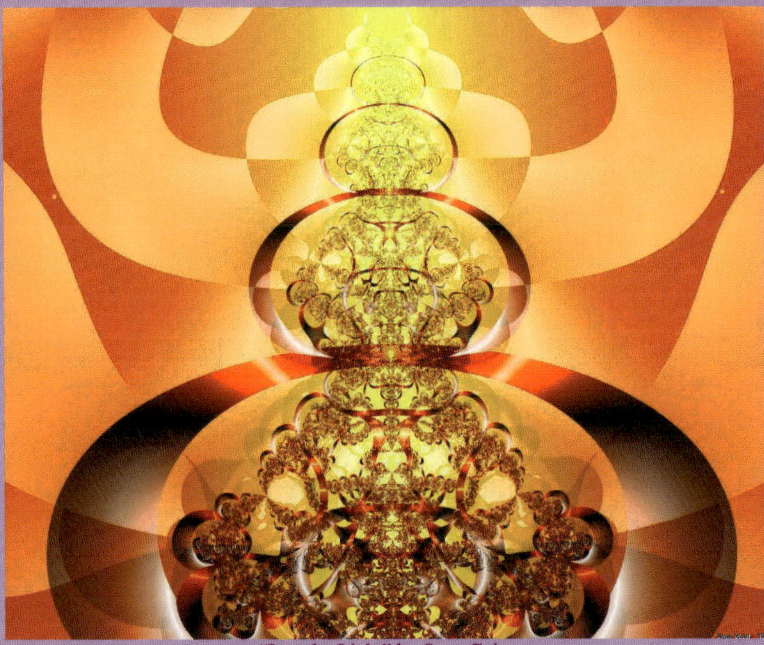

"Into the Light" by Sven Geier

Yet I am hopeful. Not hopeful that human beings will become more benign … or that evil will evaporate … or that greed will be regulated out of existence. But I am hopeful that in the New Economy people will see the power that comes from taking responsibility for their professional lives. I am hopeful that that they will also find pleasure in unleashing their instinctive curiosity and creativity that has been so effectively quashed by schools and corporations alike.

Tom Peters

The Self-Weaving Tapestry

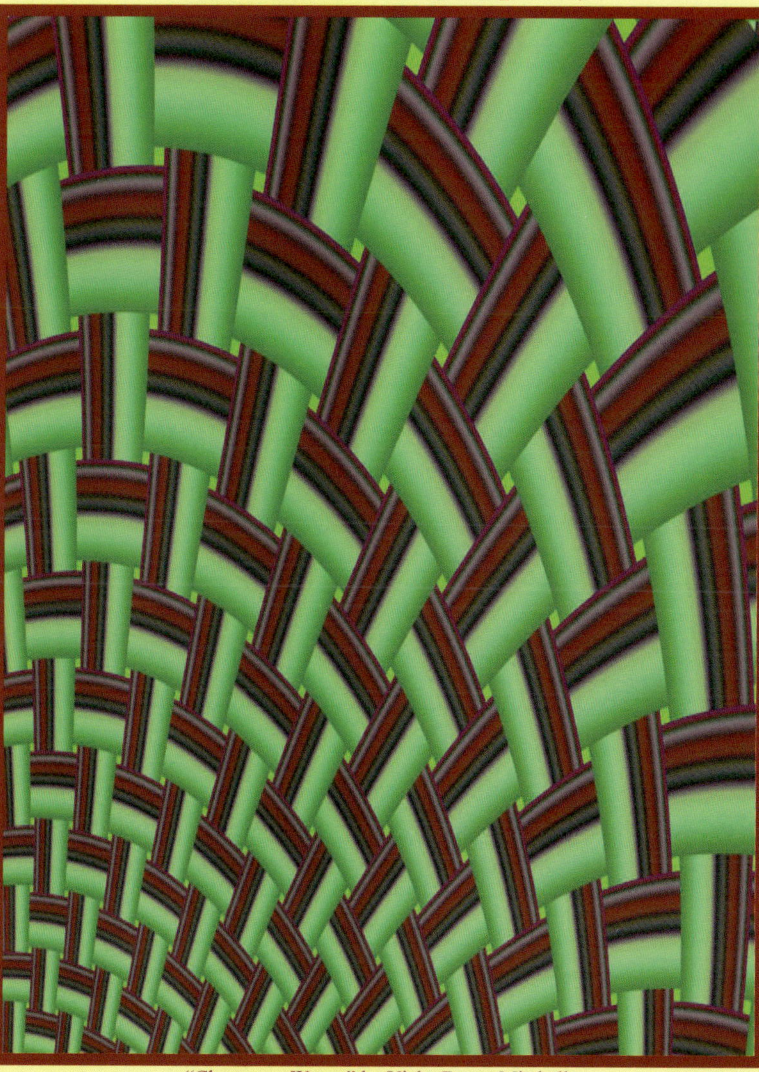

"Chartreuse Weave" by Vicky Brago-Mitchell

We are the loom.
We are the threads.
We are the weavers.
Imagine.

Judith A. Sturnick

–31–

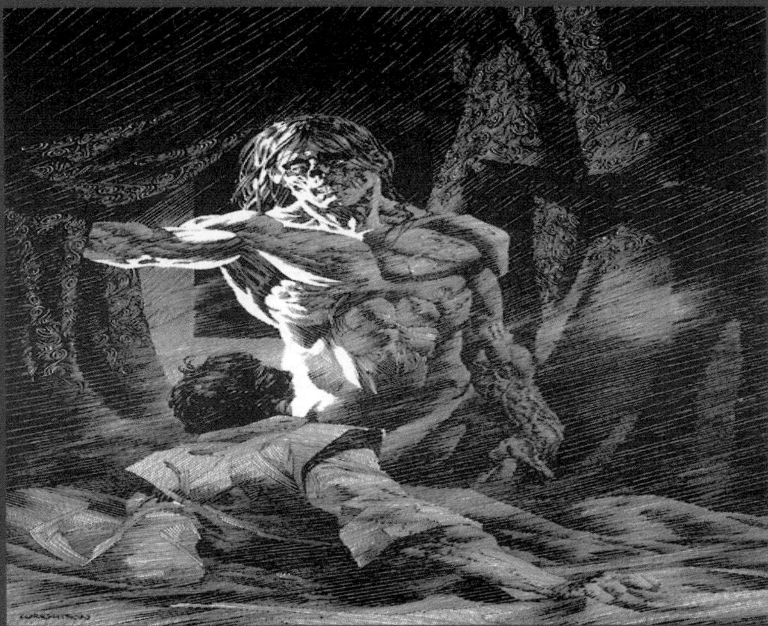

"Frankenstein" by Bernie Wrightson

The Baron Frankenstein, with full knowledge of **specialization** at his fingertips, sought to create a perfect man from the "best" parts of the "best" dead bodies; but the premise was its downfall, the brain was damaged, and with the loss of organic cohesion the result was a powerful moron.

Lawrence Blair

A primary method of top-down bureaucratic control is the notion of "best practices." The "best parts" of the process are ascertained by researchers with mental models geared to pinpointing such parts. Those best parts are then imposed on present and future practitioners. The socialistic mindset cannot comprehend that teaching is like writing; the reflective practitioner can learn from others in the field, but, in the end, success is an individual responsibility, an idiosyncratic, creative, and courageous construction.

The subtitle of Mary Shelley's *Frankenstein* is *A Modern Prometheus.* The story came to her in a dream when only nineteen. She fed the image, and it grew into the novel that has become so much a part of our cultural heritage. Shelley describes the nightmarish vision which came to her in the author's foreword to the 1831 version of her book:

> I saw the pale student of unhallowed arts kneeling beside the thing he had put together. I saw the hideous phantasm of a man stretched out, and then, on the working of some powerful engine, show signs of life and stir with an uneasy, half-vital motion.

When Baron Viktor Frankenstein realized that his machinations had succeeded in creating a monster, he ran from it. The young scientist had been so caught up in the arrogance of his reductive capabilities that he believed he could piece together a holistic reality. He was wrong, for he did not understand the magic of life, the synergy of the whole. Baron Frankenstein may have been a modern Prometheus, but the monster he created only wanted to destroy him.

Each classroom, each school, is an idiosyncratic relationship. Each is a whole beyond the measurable sum of its individual parts. Synergy defines the uniqueness of each, for good or bad. The "best parts" of other classrooms and schools stitched into the organic cohesion of different situations systemically generates disruption and dissociation. "Best practices" can inform and perhaps even inspire, but they cannot be used as rubrics to assess and control the efforts of teachers to instill life into the learning of their students. That can only result in uneasy, half-vital motions. True aliveness comes from sincere, integrous, interaction.

Each classroom and each school must discover and construct the conditions for its own individual organic cohesion; otherwise, they are leached of their uniqueness, and they lose their vitality and meaning. The "life force" of each classroom is an individual creation forged by the community of teacher and students that happen to reside there at that particular time. The initiative of both teachers and students is essential to this task—and should be treated as sacred—especially in a democracy.

Our educational system is a powerful moron because it strives to scientifically manage—through socialistic metaphors, methods, and materials—the endeavor. This requires ignoring the interactive realities of schooling and disregarding the developed intellects and accrued experience of teachers. It suppresses both teacher and student initiative in a fixation on training. With undue faith in the operating metaphor of "scientific" control, we created a Frankenstein, the monster that is a powerful moron—one capable of causing deep systemic costs, even of soul murder. The arrogance, foolishness, and blindness of Baron Frankenstein are hard at work in our schools.

The Lesson

While the professor lectures, the student experiences the severe pain of a toothache. But the professor has been trained to cover the curriculum as given; authentic interaction is not part of the rubric, so he ignores her cries of anguish until they are too disruptive—which is when he strangles her. The play ends as another student arrives for <u>his</u> lesson.

A synopsis of the play by Ionesco

—32—

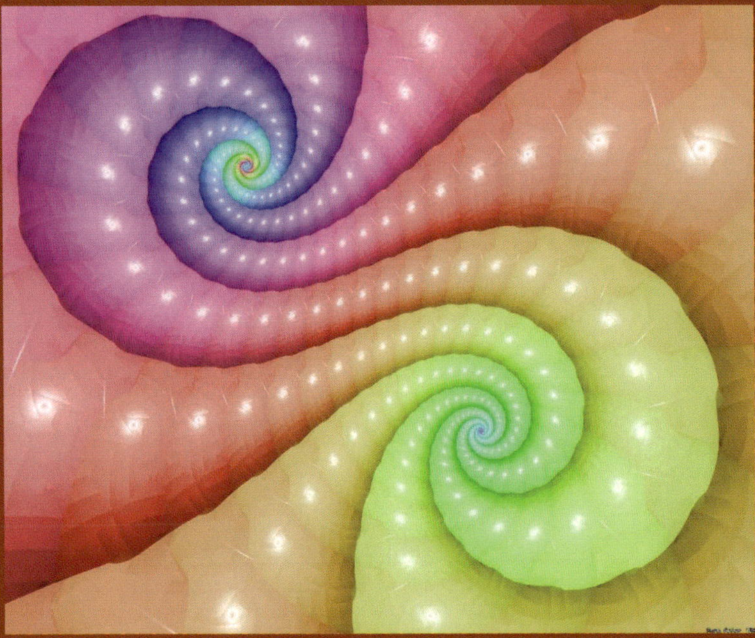

"Constipation" by Sven Geier

Don't improvise on materials . . . . Don't introduce variations of the instructions. Don't wander off into other tasks. Don't present additional exercises . . . . And above all, don't become involved in lengthy explanations. Resist the impulse to "tell" the children. Chances are they won't have the faintest idea what you are talking about; you will unfortunately demonstrate that you cannot be relied on to clarify, that you only confuse.

Excerpt from a Teacher's Guide—Science Research Associates (SRA)

The preceding quote—taken directly from a teacher's guide—illustrates the present image that defines teaching. Good teachers, by that perspective, should suppress their initiative in order to maintain the so-called integrity of the "scientifically" (note the company's name) designed curriculum materials. Teacher initiative will only derail curriculum alignment; teacher judgment is not only unnecessary but disruptive. Teachers are therefore perceived as mere "curriculum implementation specialists." No sense of symphony is necessary; "it" is all taken care of by the curriculum design. No wonder the educational process is characterized by resistance and inertia. The process itself constipates both the teaching and the learning.

The old definition of schooling once produced such absurdities as teacher-proof textbooks. Curricula were designed that discounted the interactive relevance of teachers—that were then imposed upon the "instructional cogs" in the assembly-line. The educational managers eventually backed off from the most egregiously teacher-proof materials, as well as such insulting directives as that on the preceding page, not because of any enlightened understanding of their systemic disrespect for the teaching profession, but because the implementation problems were insurmountable. However, the culture of education is still focused on taking teachers out of the pedagogical equation.

Missed Opportunities

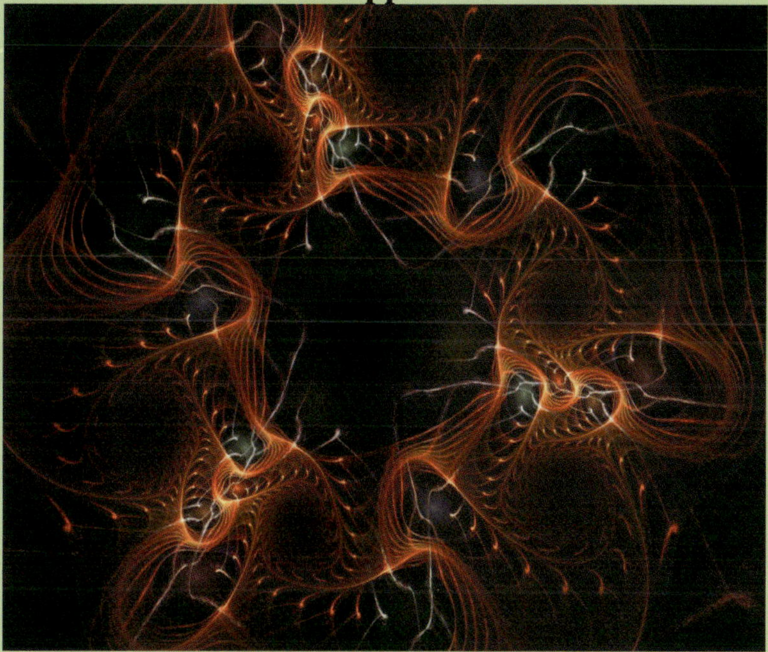

"Frankenstein Winter" by Lauren Zorn

It is a sad historical note that there has been no explosion of outrage at such pedagogy without representation—an educational equivalent of the Boston Tea Party, where teacher-proof textbooks and curriculum plans were thrown into the nearest harbor. Instead, millions of dollars were (and are) spent for their purchase and immeasurable amounts of trust and cooperation squandered as countless district offices imposed "scientifically designed" instruction programs upon classroom teachers. Hundreds of thousands of teachers and millions of students have had their initiative suppressed by such, in their very essence, un-American perspectives and materials. Teaching Redefined will make such arrogant disregard of the interactive importance of teachers impossible. **Never Again!**

A Cautionary Story

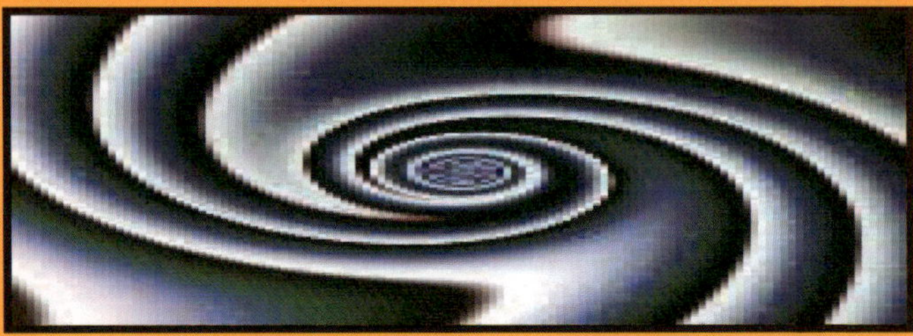

"Going Nowhere" by Tina Oloyede

When I taught reading to fourth graders, I complained to the publisher's representative that if I handed out all the ditto worksheets the teacher's manual insisted I should, we'd have no time for reading. He told me that I must not invalidate the program by skipping worksheets and not to worry so much about reading. "In this new approach," he assured me, "the actual reading isn't as important as it used to be. Decoding's the thing now." I think of the teacher who blindly passes out reams of standardized lessons and feels proud when her class is two lessons ahead of the teacher across the hall, and I am reminded of the pilot who reported from somewhere over the Pacific, "I'm lost, but I'm making record time."

Susan Ohanian

An Inspirational Story

—of a real science teacher—

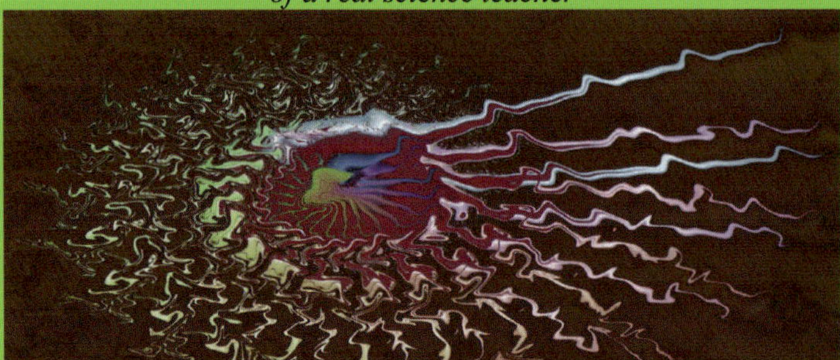

"Neuron" by Sven Geier

This reminds me of a story told by David Hawkins about another elementary school science teacher who was told she must use some fill-in-the-blank workbooks. "So," she said, "We used them. We weighed them singly and by twos and by threes. We weighed them dry and we weighed them wet."

Alfie Kohn

–33–

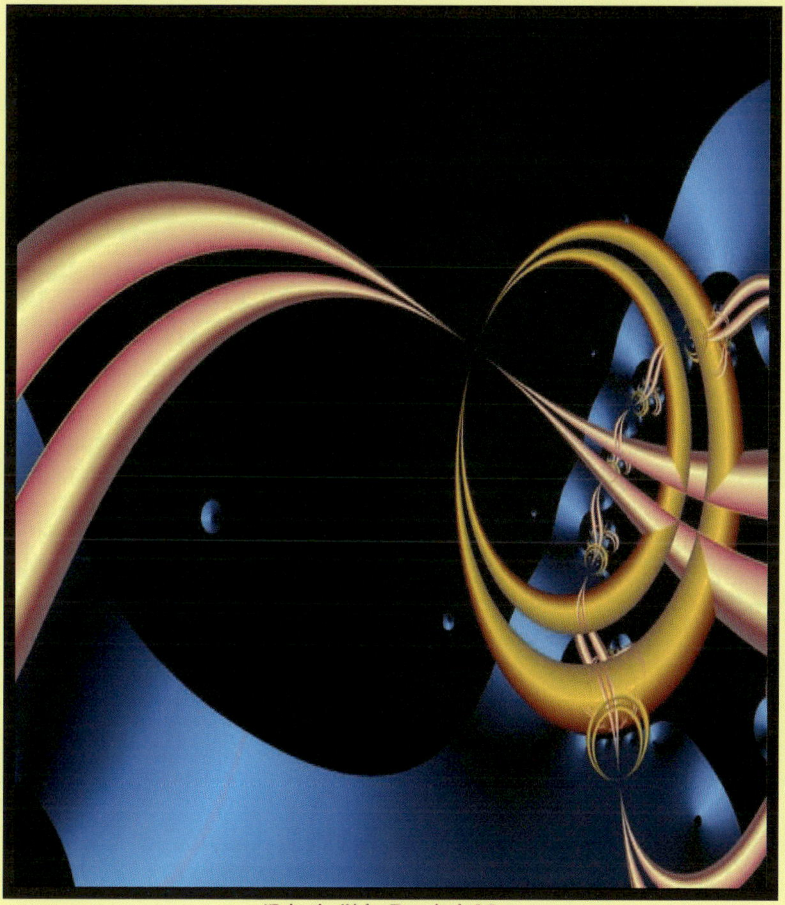

"Injective"* by Dennis de Mars

Teaching is not like building bridges between stable points, but like building flexible webs among constantly moving points—among, for example, the evanescent images of a poem and twenty-two different minds, including mine.

Joseph P. McDonald

We need to culturally recognize that the relationship between teaching and learning is complex and dynamic—not simple and static. It is not like a permanent architecture such as a bridge but by a continuously melding and unmelding web consisting of such intangibles as trust, credibility, interest, identity, meaning, judgment, and understanding.

> *"This is not as simple as going to the moon."*
>
> Robert Wycoff, President, Arco Corporation
> After one day as acting principal in a Los Angles high school

Recognition that education occurs within the momentary architectures of teacher/learner connections would dramatically increase our regard for the accrued experience and collected wisdom of our teachers. We would then give them more authority, and freedom, as well as responsibility in their efforts to forge learning relationships in their classrooms. Teaching is more of an interactive art than a solid structure of "scientifically developed" expertise, regardless of how complete and detailed the design of manipulative interconnections. Teaching is more like the art of dramatic improvisation than it is the science of engineering. The task is permeated with hard-to-grasp intangibles and constantly emerging implications. Teaching is confusion-laden interaction without end, a context-dependent process that is a source of challenge and joy for those who don't need to reduce it to a set of solidified relationships.

As Abraham Maslow commented, "People who only have hammers can only look for nails." The profession has suppressed the intellectual development of practitioners with inorganic metaphors and mechanistic methods. We have pursued "research-driven" techniques of teaching and neglected the construction of teaching webs, the collection of understandings that best image and inform educational relationships.

*The title of Dennis de Mar's fractal art fits into our focus on the importance of initiative in learning. His inventive use of the word "injective" rests upon the word inject, which means "to throw in." Injectives are the instances of provocation within the learning process, the thoughts and contributions that ***turn*** the reflection or conversation this way and that. Injectives are the bits of life, borne by the interest and imagination of learners, within individual minds or within social discourse, that give meaning and relevance to the learning. His image also fits into our image of learning redefined, as it intimates dynamic flow, surprising confluences, occasional circularity, and projection into the horizon beyond. The healthy learning process—the vital conversations—are full of injectives. The present definition of learning, however, views injectives as disruptive to the coverage-fixated curriculum. It wants nothing to be thrown into the programmed process. Injectives, such as thinking and questions, are perceived as too messy by the prevailing image, so they are systemically suppressed.

Injectives are the instances of connection that comprise "teachable moments."

—34—

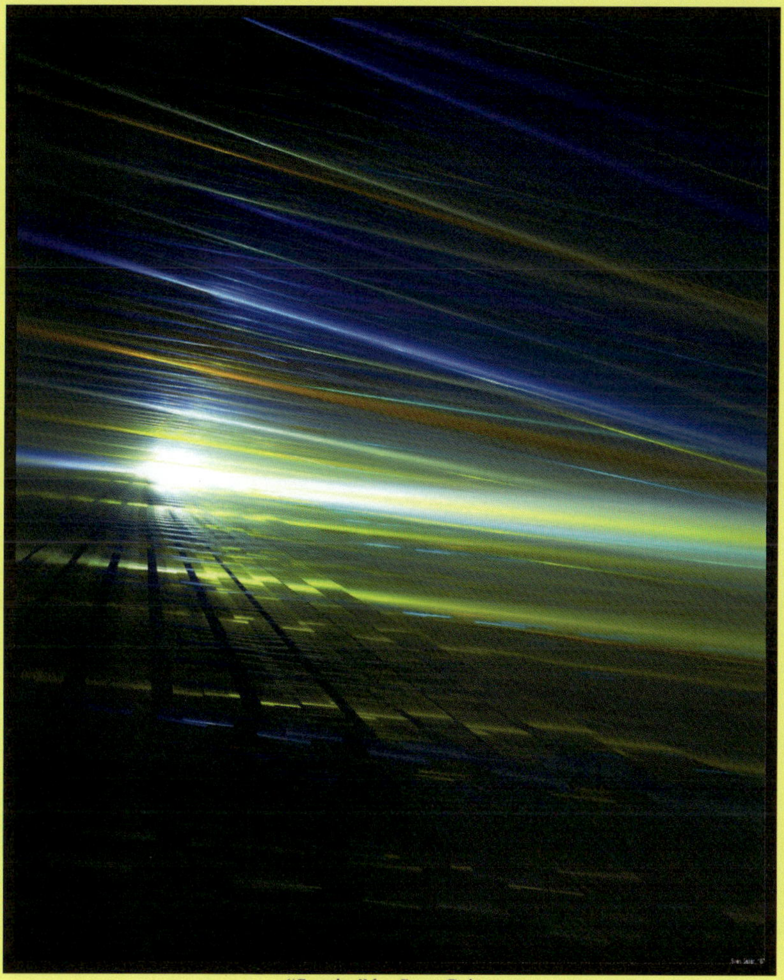

"Sunrise" by Sven Geier

The mediocre teacher tells.
The good teacher explains.
The superior teacher demonstrates.
The great teacher inspires.

William Arthur Ward

Telling, explaining, and demonstrating are important aspects of teaching, but we are really doing our jobs when we inspire our students. Inspire etymologically means to "breathe life into." It is analogous to the difference between giving someone fish and teaching them to fish. Teaching someone to fish, to harness and use their own initiative effectively, takes care of them forever.

The historian Max Lerner understands the inspirational role of teachers. As he writes, in his book, *Values in Education:*

> A good teacher—whether at home, at school, or on the job—heightens the energy field around him and makes the life force in everyone flow more strongly. Beyond biological limits, beyond the determinism of operant or aversive conditioning, the learning process is affected by the ebb and flow of the life force in the interacting organisms.

The images of teaching and leading have been, in the past several decades, melding into one another. Good leaders in organizations know that a key component of their capability is teaching. It is through teaching, not through motivational speaking and managerial pushing, that leaders breathe life into organizations. Rip-roaring presentations can occasionally be helpful, for short spurts. The real act of breathing life into organizations consists of the many and myriad conversations that teach factors such as self and inter-reliance, community, imagination, trust, hope, confidence, history, and vision.

Teachers need to understand that a key capability for them is leadership. Teaching Redefined will increasingly incorporate their roles as leaders—in their classrooms and schools. The business world has recognized that it has a crisis in leadership, too often confusing leading with managing. It is redefining leading, as illustrated by the words of Jim Autry, retired president of the Meredith Corporation:

> Becoming a manager has much to do with learning the metaphors;
> becoming a good manager has much to do with using the metaphors;
> and becoming a leader has much to do with changing the metaphors.

There is nothing more inspirational, more transforming, than changing our metaphors. When we redefine reality, and ourselves in relation to it, then we know that we are learning, and therefore growing, at our peak capacity. This breathes life into us, personally and organizationally. Thomas Merton thought that "the purpose of education is to show students how to define themselves authentically and spontaneously in relation to the world." We can add to this insight that, if teachers help students accomplish such self-knowledge, connection, and flexibility, then personal effectiveness and productivity will surely follow. How can we be authentic—and therefore effective—if ignorant of the operating metaphors guiding our behavior?

> The greatest thing by far is to be master of the metaphor.
> Aristotle

–35–

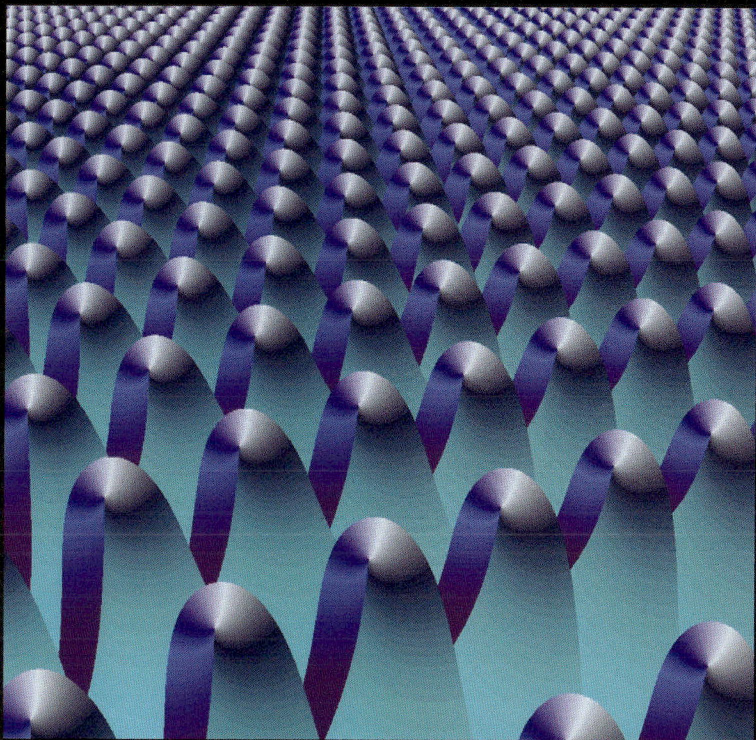

"Blue Order" by Rupert Ward

Practically all of the hundred people I interviewed in my study of very creative individuals—ninety out of a hundred—had pretty bad things to say about their formal education. They usually had one or two teachers who made a big difference in their lives and whom they remembered fondly. But the structured, mass-produced instruction that their schools generally provided was something they just couldn't take.

Mihaly Csikszentmihalyi

Do we need any more evidence than this quote that we need to redefine teaching, as well as instruction? How much creativity has not made it past the gauntlet of programmed instruction? How many creative, innovative students have had to draw a shallow and crooked breath for every minute spent in a typical classroom? For that matter, how many students have been labeled ADD and subjected to drug therapy because they were trapped in environments that suppressed their interests and potential?

We need more creative teachers. We need, as well, teachers who can recognize and foster creativity in their students, who can escape the orthodoxy of programmed instruction when necessary. The ninety percent failure rate for encouraging creativity is simply unacceptable, especially these days, because creativity is increasingly essential to our intellectual, spiritual, and economic well-being. Ray Kurzweil, inventor, entrepreneur, executive, and author of *The Age of Spiritual Machines* and *The Age of Intelligent Machines*, writes:

> The world is changing. We're entering an era in which the creation of new knowledge really constitutes the wealth and power of a nation's organizations and individuals. It's no longer just being disciplined in manufacturing or intelligent in some rote way.

Teaching and instruction that suppress the emergence and development of creativity diminish our future health and vitality, our future wealth and power. How much creativity have we lost to disengagement? How much constructive creativity have we lost because students with creativity chose a disruptive and resistive path of expression? How much creativity have we lost to Ritalin and negative labeling? How much creativity, and thus potential, will we squander before we redefine teaching?

> For the first time, research shows that American creativity is declining.
>
> "The Creativity Crisis"
> Po Bronson and Ashley Merryman

The assumption, of course, is that more creative teaching will encourage creativity. Another assumption is that initiative is essential to creativity. This makes sense logically; how can the teacher without initiative encourage it in students? How can teachers suppressed by a system of prediction and control recognize and foster creativity in their students? Another assumption we can make is that creativity is essential to the unwrapping of the gift that each student has to make to society. It takes a knowledgeable and creative teacher to be aware of and understand potential. It also takes empathy. The task is especially hampered by orthodoxy; the teacher not allowed to develop and exercise initiative will not have the perspective and judgment to see beyond the given. It is the creative teacher that images the potential gifts in students and helps them construct connections to possible futures.

Robert Freeman, Dean of the School of Fine Arts at the University of Texas, Austin, writes:

> The creative teacher—whether it was someone alive in 1800, 1900, this year, or a hundred years from now—is going to be someone who sees in each of his or her students what makes them different and can enable them to see their own futures.

Our schools of education and the professional development industry rarely foster creativity in teachers? For the most part, they are still focused on training, the installation of methods and techniques and curriculum alignment issues.

However, as the economic benefits of creativity become increasingly apparent, and the business world will see to that, schools of education and professional development will find it necessary to redefine teaching. The meeting of creativity with the bottom line will be a most interesting one. There will either be an explosion of potential as we turn the ninety percent suppression rate on its head or we will suffer economic collapse as the rest of the world finds its creative wings.

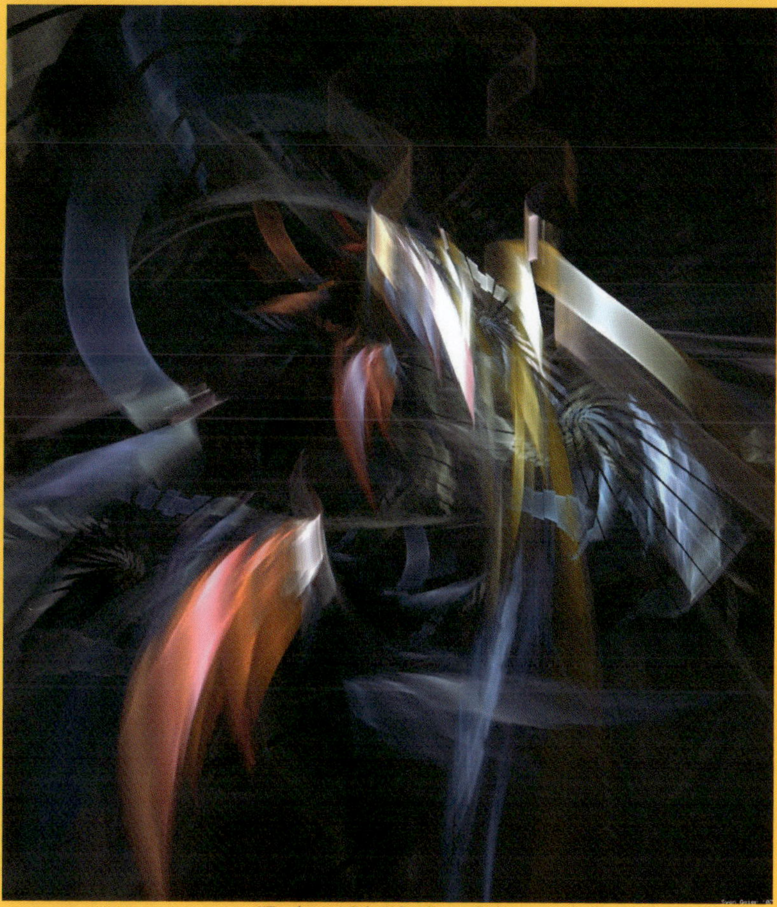

"Darkness Stirs" by Sven Geier

The graded classroom dominates, and teachers' task of bringing about learning may well be judged hopeless to begin with. There is more than a little evidence (rarely looked at) that at least a considerable share of conventional teaching has *negative* results: it inhibits, prevents, distorts, or holds back learning.

Leslie A. Hart

–36–

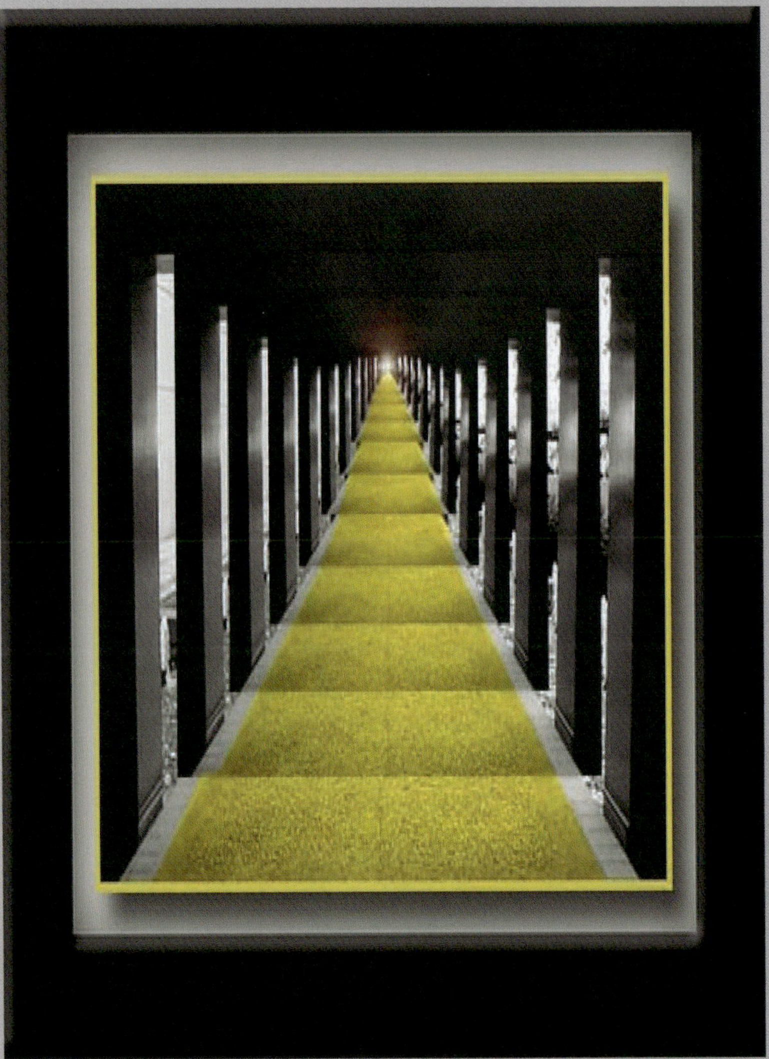

"Goodbye Yellow Brick Road" by Lynne

Wooden-headedness, the source of self-deception, is a factor that plays a remarkably large role in government. It consists in assessing a situation in terms of preconceived fixed notions while ignoring or rejecting any contrary signs.

Barbara Tuchman

Unquestioned operating metaphors blind us systemically. They impact all relationships. They color every interaction, making us believe we are on The Yellow Brick Road to The Emerald City regardless of any feedback to the contrary. We become addicted to the provided certainties, for they make every decision easier. We become woodenheaded.

The historian Barbara Tuchman, in her book, *The March of Folly*, defines wooden-headedness as the refusal to follow paths of wisdom. It is the habit of assessing rapidly developing and dynamically complex situations from a mental framework of preconceived fixed ideas. Tuchman wonders why human organizations, particularly governmental ones, so frequently ignore common sense and wisdom despite available evidence in their support. Wooden-headedness occurs whenever dogma trumps common sense. She comments:

> It is acting according to wish while not allowing oneself to be deflected by the facts. It is epitomized in a historian's statement about Philip II of Spain, the surpassing wooden-head of all sovereigns: "No experience of the failure of his policy could shake his belief in its essential excellence."

In the previous section, Csikszentmihalyi indicted our educational system with the statement that 90% of the very creative individuals he studied hated their schooling. Especially, as we move toward a right-brain world, failure to revision and redefine learning is wooden-headed. We need to look at another indictment of our educational system: the explosion of special education in the past decades. The question needs to be asked: “What is the cause of the exponentially expanding need for special education?” The short, but systemic, answer is that **the essential cause of special education is regular education.**

In his book, *Behind Special Education: A Critical Analysis of Professional Culture and School Organization*, Thomas M. Skrtic writes:

> Public education, acting through its institutional practice of special education, and under the legitimatizing effects of educational administration, is perhaps the most powerful profession in society. This is particularly true when we consider the pervasiveness and centrality of education in contemporary society and the fact that, as an institutional practice, it continues to classify more and more of its students as abnormal.
>
> As Foucault has argued, the most insightful way to understand society is to consider it from the perspective of the professions that have emerged to contain its failures. In this sense, special education can be understood as the profession that emerged in 20th-century America to contain the failure of public education to educate its youth for full political, economic, and cultural participation in democracy.

Skrtic answers our question, "Why has there been such an explosion of special education in this country?" Scientific management of education—a reductionist perspective applied to a holistic endeavor—will, in the throes of its blind pursuit of prediction and control machinations, damage many of the "materials" it is supposed to improve. Special education classifications such as ADD, ADHD, ODD, and LD are actually, for the most part, systemic protections of the central hypothesis: that the educational endeavor can be scientifically managed. Special education is exploding in correlation to the cumulative results of regular education *not* working. Increasing numbers of our children are crippled by the mechanistic design of our educational system. Sometimes, when we believe everything lined up in a pleasing order, with the categories in alignment with our operating metaphors, is when we are truly lost.

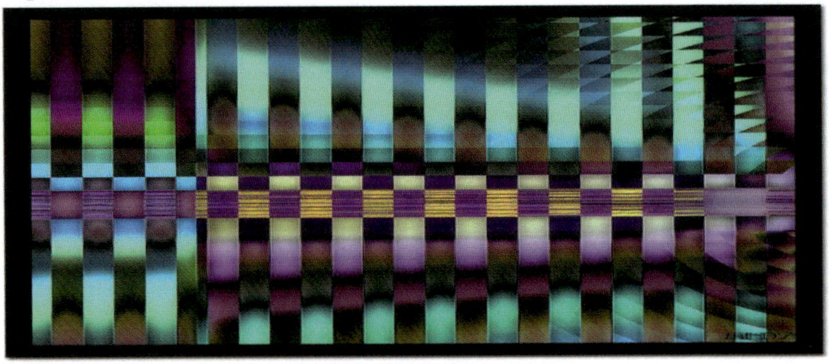

"Lost" by Mindy Sommers

The image of a fruit packaging plant comes to mind. In such a facility, the delicate fruits are thrown onto conveyor belts and sorted according to standardized criteria. Mechanical arms and metallic fingers fly about their separate tasks. Those fruits that don't fit the desired configurations—or that get too bruised by the process—are separated from the system and placed into different bins. How much more will the need for special education expand before we begin to question the manufacturing metaphors that guide the practices which frequently bruise—and sometimes squash—our children? When a process makes this many "lemons," shouldn't we seriously question the process?

Way back in 1993, U.S. News and World Report magazine published "Separate and Unequal: How Special Education Programs Are Cheating Our Children and Costing Taxpayers Billions Each Year:" The study points out some particular problems in the special education movement:

> Since implementation . . . the number of students in special education has increased every year without exception. Today, there are 5 million students in the nation's schools—10 percent of all students enrolled. One result of the growth: a bloated bureaucracy that even advocates of special education say is unnecessarily expensive. In Connecticut, for instance, a separate transportation system costs taxpayers 10 times more to bus a special ed student than one attending regular classes.
>
> Many principals have raised their schools' scores on statewide competency exams by placing low-scoring students in special education programs. [They are then exempt from the tests.]

Special education labels are so ambiguous that classifications vary from state to state—and even from school district to school district. Fifteen percent of all Massachusetts students wind up in special education programs, for instance. Yet in Hawaii, just 7 percent of all students are in special education. Classifications vary wildly from state to state, even within special education categories. In Alaska, only 3 percent of all special education students are classified as retarded; in Alabama, 28 percent.

Nothing drives the special education system like money. No state has more students classified as emotionally disturbed than Connecticut, for example. But it's not that there is more stress, paranoia, or pathology there. It's simply that the state's complex funding formula encourages school districts to send emotionally disturbed students to separate schools . . . Some cities, like New Haven, actually save money when they send students to out-of-district schools, even though these schools can cost more than $100,000 per student, because the state picks up the bulk of the cost.

. . . Black students are overrepresented in special education programs . . . [especially] when they are students in predominately white school districts . . . Critics of the special education system attribute the overrepresentation of African-American students in the system to cultural bias in testing and placement procedures—not to any inherently high level of disability.

By far the largest class of special education students, at 49.9 percent, learning-disabled pupils are the most difficult to identify properly. One reason is definition. A learning-disabled child, according to the Department of Education, is one who has "a severe discrepancy between achievement and intellectual ability." This is squishy territory.

The definitional problem is compounded by another. It is up to state education departments to suggest which tests and procedures are used to measure a learning disability, and, as a result, school practices can vary wildly.

A Memphis newspaper, *The Commercial Appeal*, adds these considerations about the expanding use of Ritalin, a drug that, in its effects, is virtually identical to cocaine:

The Drug Enforcement Administration is reporting with alarm that prescriptions for the drug are up 600 percent this decade. It's so popular, according to a new DEA report, that in some schools 20 percent of the students are medicated.

They are Generation RX. Nearly all are white, from middle and upper class families, typically with two working parents who place high value on academic performance. School bells ring, and long lines of pupils form at the nurse's stations or principal's offices for pills to slow them down and lock out distractions.

> This is a phenomenon seen in no other country. The United States consumes five times more of this drug than all the rest of the world combined. The United Nations International Narcotics Control Board has twice voiced warnings about this country's dependence on Ritalin.

We are supposedly fighting a war on drugs in this country, but are we not predisposing many of our citizens to drug dependence and abuse? Why do so many of our students need drugs in order to get through their school days? The costs to intellectual, emotional, and even physical health of children sorted into the category of exclusion from "normalcy" are beyond calculation. Why has this development occurred? And why have we not responded wisely to the situation? Why aren't we shocked and dismayed at this evidence of failure to educate and care for our young?

A more recent development is the rapidly growing need for developmental education at the university level. Special education has graduated into college. Can we soon expect it to shove its way into graduate level and even doctoral level education? Why do we keep adjusting to the situation instead of fixing it?

A bizarre item in the news is of the couple in Kansas where the woman developed a phobia about leaving the bathroom. For whatever reasons, her vision of the world, and thus her operating metaphor, necessitated a retreat into the constricted horizon of a tiny room with only a toilet to sit on. Both she and her boyfriend fell into the trap of continuously adjusting to the systemic stupidity, with him bringing her food, water, and clean clothes, and her sitting on the toilet until she became stuck to it. The only explanation for such behavior is "diminished mental capacity." Future historians may arrive at a similar diagnosis when they strive to explain our mindless adjustment to the systemic damage to our children by our educational process.

The March of Folly persists. Our operating metaphors make us wooden-headed. Dogma continuously trumps common sense. The evidence of special education is ignored. The lack of engaged, prepared, and capable students is also ignored. Such evidence as the 90% of very creative individuals who hated their schooling reported by Csikszentmihalyi is discounted. No evidence of the operating metaphor's failure is considered. The present dominating operating metaphors seem impervious to real change. Because of this wooden-headedness, we have lost sight of ourselves, our roots, values, and dreams—our essential selves. We have lost our initiative, and without initiative we have also, logically, let go of our responsibility. Our present educational process diminishes rather than develops us. Bill Moyers, in *A World of Ideas*, relates a conversation with the novelist E. L. Doctorow:

> The general crisis of the age is the loss of our identity as a democratic nation with constitutional ideals . . . Not as a sudden thunderclap kind of loss, but as a slow, almost invisible transformation of ourselves under the pressures of our history and our time and our ideologies. I'm reminded of de Tocqueville's remarks that when tyranny comes to the United States, it

will be very, very quiet. It will be the somnolence that comes over quiet and pacific industrial animals.

What are we doing? The present operating metaphor prefers quiet and pacific students—and it wants the same kind of teachers. The system wants those who comply with the curriculum as given, who do not question and disrupt the process. Our schooling is training the democratic foundation right out from under us. How wooden-headed is that?

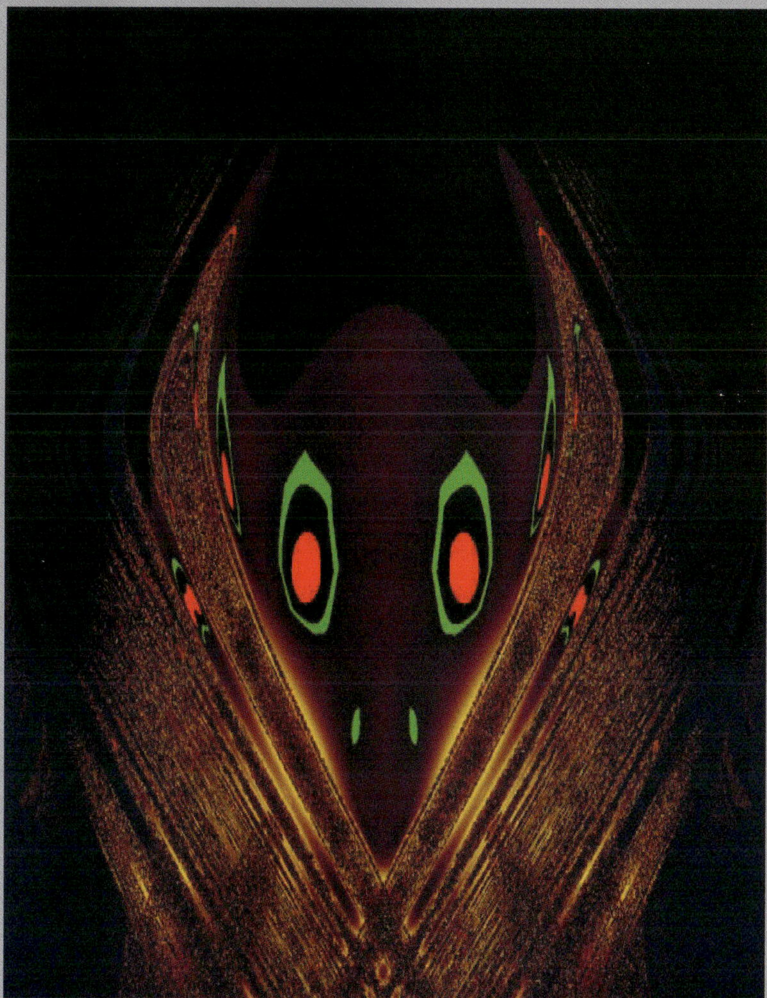

"Demon 2X" by Angela Wilczynski

The greatest menace to freedom is an inert people.

Justice Earl Warren

The Farewell Symphony

In this work by Franz Joseph Haydn, the music begins with a full orchestra but as the piece proceeds the musicians individually withdraw their contributions to the performance. As the musicians finish their parts, they blow out their candles and leave the stage. They do this, one by one, until the light of the last candle is extinguished, the stage is dark and empty; the music is over. Are we, unwittingly, disintegrating the composition of ourselves?

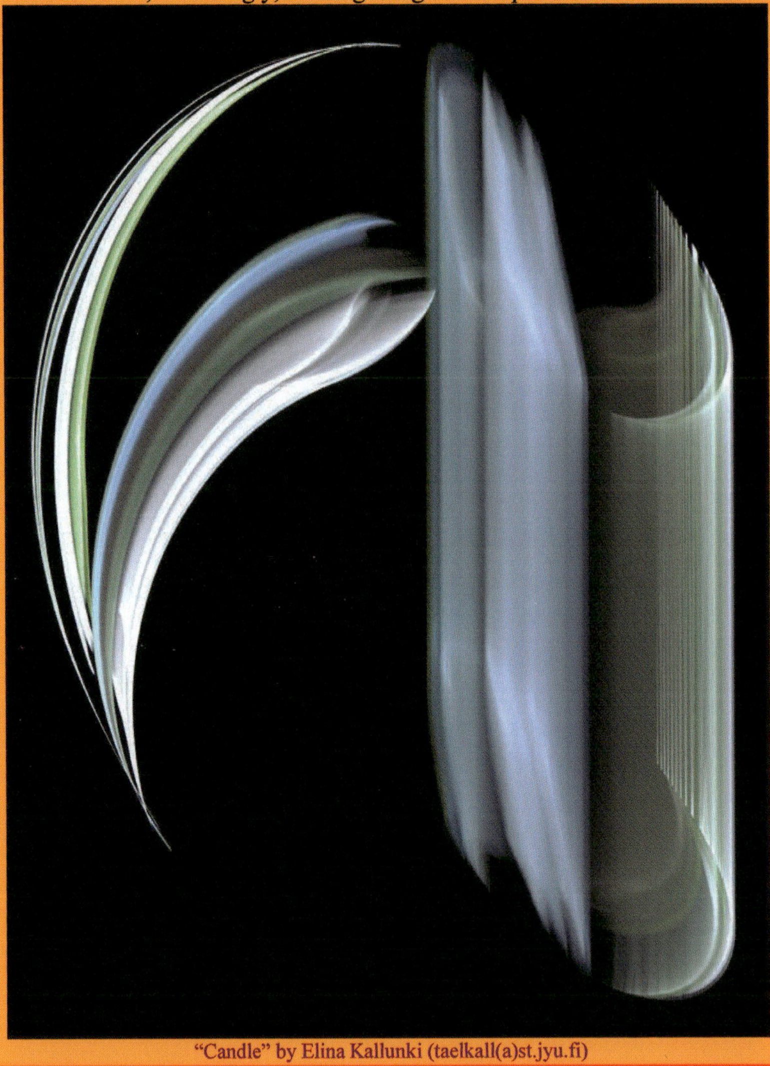

"Candle" by Elina Kallunki (taelkall(a)st.jyu.fi)

–37–

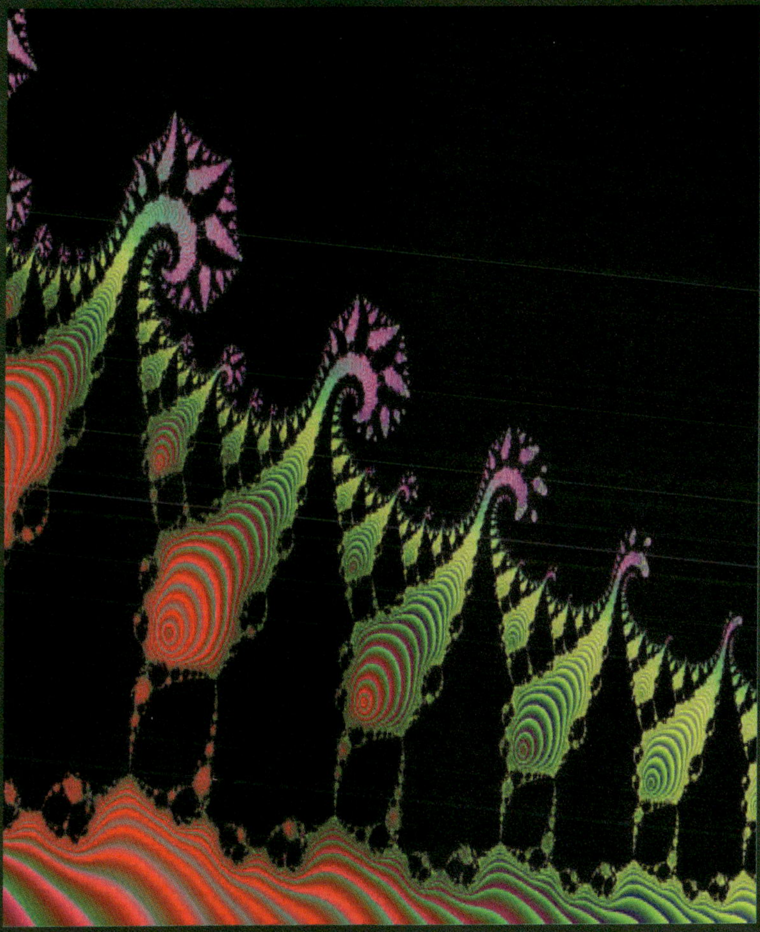

"Emus on Parade" by Karen Moore

What everyone appears to want for students—a wide array of learning opportunities that engage students in experiencing, creating, and solving real problems, using their own experiences, and working with others—is for some reason denied to teachers when they are learners.

Ann Lieberman

The redefining of learning must begin with teachers. After all, they model the image of learning ingested by students during their schooling. If what they see are teachers forced to be "on the same page," to "march in unison," then the message they get is not individual responsibility but adherence to the program-in place, whatever that may be. If students see teachers lacking initiative, or with their initiative suppressed by the educational system, then they learn the image of passive learning, or they learn begrudging compliance and maybe even sabotage. They also learn that the judgment and integrity of teachers are not to be trusted. Trust is to be placed in the system of controls, such as research-driven assessments, canned curriculum, and top-down management. (A hot new word in the educational world today is "fidelity.")

Professional development needs to move away from the "sit and git" image and recognize the need for programs that excite and nourish teacher intellect—and individual responsibility. As Aristotle said, "Teaching is the highest form of understanding." Understanding is constructed through conversation and reflection. Teachers can't sit and git understanding—they must interact and reflect and make choices of what they value and don't value. Dennis Sparks and Stephanie Hirsh (1997) write:

> Many events of the past few years bode well for the field of staff development. Reports issued by governmental bodies, business groups, and various commissions emphasize the central role staff development must play in school reform efforts. In addition, there is greater recognition today at the local, state, and national levels that sustained, high-quality staff development is essential if all students are to achieve at high levels.
>
> At the same time, however, more people are realizing that this professional development must be considerably different than that offered in the past. Soon to be gone forever, we hope, are the days when educators (usually teachers) sit relatively passively while an "expert" exposes them to new ideas or "trains" them in new practices, and the success of the effort is judged by a "happiness quotient" that measures participants' satisfaction with the experience and their off-the-cuff assessment regarding its usefulness.

The problem is that there is little support for professional development that helps teachers develop their intellects as teachers. Understanding is an emergent capability, one that must be constructed within the learner; it cannot be handed down by the traditional top-down mindset which presently dominates teacher training. Intellect cannot be developed through passive learning. Teachers need to demand teacher-training that nourishes their intellects as teachers. They, like their students, have been compelled by our educational system to be passive learners. The challenges of our cultural diversity, turbulent times, and a confusing future demand education for understanding.

Teacher development is the systemic lever that will help us redefine learning, for until teachers model and teach for active learning, passive learning will control our schooling. Teachers have the power to teach for initiative, to turn our nation toward a new, more active, definition of learning; they should be allowed the control necessary for the expression of their initiative and responsibility. That means that we develop teacher intellect and judgment, and, most importantly, teacher autonomy. This would free us from the absurdity of striving to teach democratic values through socialistic methods.

As Joe Frattaroli comments:

> It is most satisfying to demonstrate the link between professional development and student outcomes. The investment in quality teaching is the most important investment we can make. All educators need the opportunity for continuous improvement. I believe professional development will be the major educational issue of the 21st century.

Frattaroli is correct: professional development will be the major issue of this century. But it is the operating metaphors guiding that development that will be the key. Will they be socialistic or democratic in spirit? Quality teaching is not teaching from socialistic metaphors, methods, and materials—not in a democratic society. The notion of continuous improvement does not mean more stringent adherence to the old metaphors and vigorous polishing of the old methodologies. Quality and continuous improvement, like learning, will also have to be redefined. It is not improvement in quality to get better at doing what has not worked before. It is not ever tighter allegiance to socialistic metaphors and methodologies.

Continuous improvement, considering today's challenges and opportunities in light of the democratic ideal, is not more training in the old ways of seeing and doing things. It is professional development that inspires and informs teacher initiative and individual responsibility. Continuous improvement is a reconnection to our democratic roots, movement toward the ideals of individual vision and voice. Continuous improvement, from the perspective of the democratic spirit, is movement away from socialistic metaphors and methods toward individual freedom and responsibility, where initiative is encouraged and informed.

A Cautionary Consideration—The assumption here is that if we stop gavaging our student teachers and teachers then they will eventually stop gavaging our students. However, teachers have usually attained their achievements through that very process; they often harbor the mental model of correct-answer schooling—not realizing the power of and need for education for understanding. They have been led to expect programs of correct answers in professional development. Education for understanding starts with our teachers, through conversations, reflections, and projects that develop their intellects and response-ability—but can they transfer that realization to their students? Professional development has a lot to accomplish. But right-brain research, brain-based learning, and the expanding insights and evidences of neuroscience give us hope.

–38–

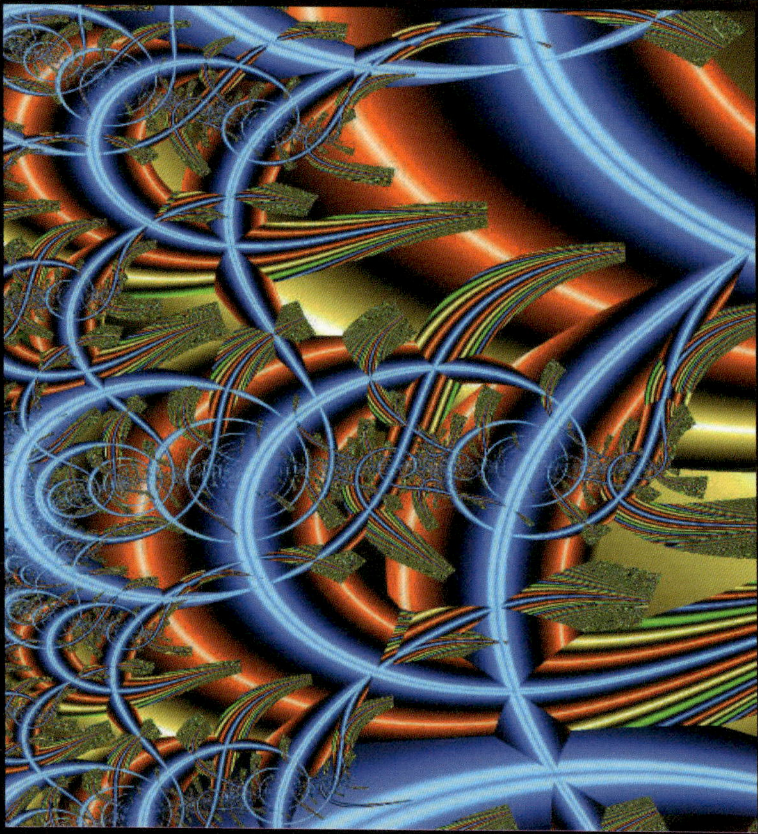

"A Vision of Music" by Ken Keller

The conductor Leopold Stokowski dispensed with the uniform bowing of the strings, knowing that the strength of each player's wrist varies, and, to achieve the richest string tone, each player should have maximum elasticity. Leopold also encouraged the wind players to breathe as they wished. He didn't care, he said, how they made music as long as it was beautiful.

Marilyn Ferguson

If we can develop the wisdom and courage to give up on our prediction and control machinations, and stop demanding everyone to be on the same page, then we could unleash the power of our individuality. We need to learn from Stokowski: it is not the uniform bowing of the strings but the beautiful music that matters.

The business guru Steven Covey, in *The 8th Habit: From Effectiveness to Greatness*, talks about the challenge for organizations to understand and redesign in response to the power of choice. Will organizations have the emotional intelligence necessary for engaging constructive rather than destructive or disruptive choices? He writes:

> At the core, there is one simple, overarching reason why so many people remain unsatisfied in their work and why most organizations fail to draw out the greatest talent, ingenuity, and creativity of their people and never become truly great, enduring organizations. It stems from *an incomplete paradigm of who we are—our fundamental view of human nature*. . . The fundamental reality is, human beings are not *things* needing to be motivated and controlled; they are four dimensional—body, mind, heart, and spirit. . . So what's the direct connection between the controlling "thing" (part-person) paradigm that dominates today's workplace and the inability of managers and organizations to inspire their people to volunteer their highest talents and contributions? The answer is simple. People make choices. Consciously or subconsciously, people decide how much of themselves they will give to their work depending on how they are treated and on their opportunities to use *all* four parts of their nature.

The New Productivity demands the engagement of choice from workers. Simply doing the job is no longer sufficient. Organizations that cannot design, establish, and maintain the conditions conducive to the engagement of commitment will lack the emotional intelligence for dealing with tomorrow's problems and products. Covey sees that the fundamental problem facing organizations today is figuring out how to adjust to this need for engaging the constructive choices of the workforce. He quotes Peter Drucker:

> In a few hundred years, when the history of our time is written from a long-term perspective, it is likely that the most important event those historians will see is not technology; not the Internet, not e-commerce. It is an unprecedented change in the human condition. For the first time—literally—substantial and rapidly growing numbers of people have choices. For the first time, they will have to manage themselves.
>
> And society is totally unprepared for it.

Covey believes that leaders should develop not only their own voice but that of others as well. Leadership increases organizational intelligence, which means removing the factors that impede growth and contribution. Democratic leaders, unlike those who are bureaucratic or totalitarian, change conditions within organizations to more often encourage and nourish personal vision and individual voice. Covey writes:

> Despite all our gains in technology, product innovation and world markets, most people are not thriving in the organizations they work for. They are neither fulfilled nor excited. They are frustrated. They are

> not clear about where the organization is headed or what its highest priories are. They are bogged down and distracted. Most of all, they don't feel they can change much. Can you imagine the personal and organizational cost of failing to engage the passion, talent and intelligence of the workforce? It is far greater than all taxes, interest charges and labor costs put together!

Learning how to learn, and how to teach, are key ingredients in leadership that **develops voice in self and others** (the 8th habit of effective leadership). Voice, defined by Covey as "unique personal significance," is essential to our health and vitality because the "new productivity" demands **unique personal contribution.** Organizations will increasingly depend on the power of voice to marshal the emotional intelligence necessary for solving tomorrow's problems and fashioning tomorrow's products. Unique personal contribution is, after all, the hallmark of Social Mental Health in democratic organizations. This means that we must learn to unleash the initiative of teachers, so that they can teach their students to unleash their initiative.

Covey's thinking strongly influences the business world. We need to give him similar attention in the education world. If we provide the business world with passive and disengaged learners, they will be unable to provide the "unique personal contribution" necessary to fuel tomorrow's productivity—or fulfill themselves spiritually, emotionally, and intellectually.

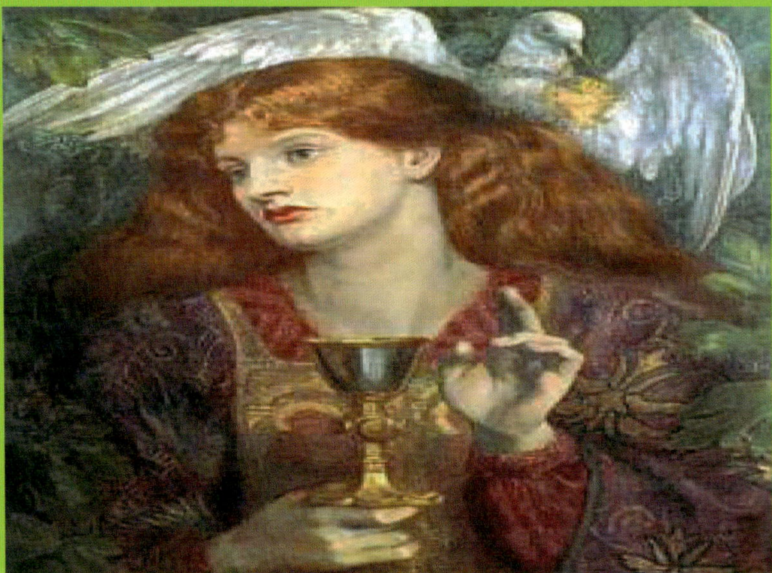

"The Holy Grail" by Dante Gabriel Rossetti

Unique personal contribution is the new Holy Grail in today's business world. It should also become the new Holy Grail in the educational world.

–39–

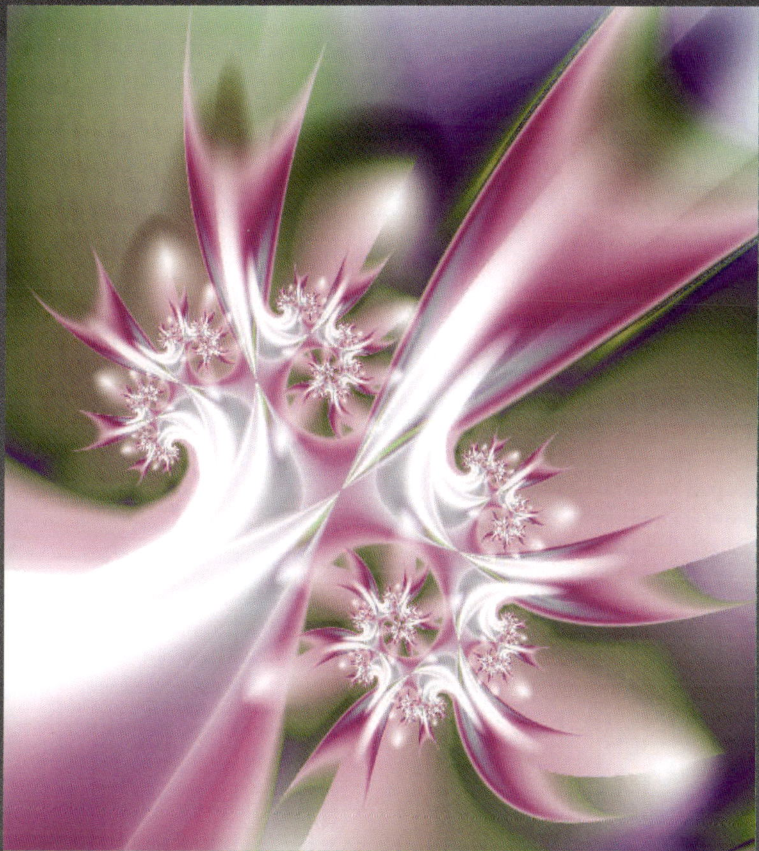

"Bursting into Bud" by Anna Laurie

It is essential for the heart's coronation
For the pawn to realize
There is nothing but divine movement
In this World.

Hafiz

But fundamentalism wants pawns; it wants individuals chained, unable to move on their own, without initiative, easily trained.

Lack of knowledge is rarely the biggest impediment to intelligence. Ignorance, after all, is easily remedied: just stir in a little appropriate knowledge and voila! —a changed perspective. Intentional ignorance, on the other hand, is hell to eradicate. It digs in roots and resists the pressure of insights and understandings to enlighten.

When I was sixteen, my father said something apropos of nothing in the context of any prior discussion:

> "You are going to find, Dennis, that bad people will rarely hurt you."
>
> "Say what?"
>
> "There are two reasons for that: One, truly bad people are extremely rare. You will almost never run across them. Two, if you are at all smart, you will sense their presence and get away from them."
>
> "Uh, okay."
>
> "The people who are going to hurt you are good people—who are weak."
>
> I made no response to this comment other than look at him curiously. I had an inkling of what this meant, but no real understanding.

Ears grow slowly. I wasn't able to fully hear what my father said until exactly sixteen years later. Driving across country, my mind revisited that conversation so many years before. I heard him then, having been hurt by weak people, and, sad to say, having hurt people because of my own weakness.

Our biggest problem is not ignorance but weakness. It is weakness that compels intentional ignorance. It is weakness that fouls up so many political processes, that compels knee-jerk partisanship. It is weakness that prevents cooperation and productivity in the business world. It is weakness that perpetuates and fuels sexism, racism, and all the other prejudgments that suppress intelligence as well as potential. It is weakness that degrades community.

> It is weakness that underlies what will probably be the biggest threat to growth, peace, and survival in this century, fundamentalism—of any kind: Christian, Muslim, Atheist, Buddhist, Republican or Democrat, whatever doctrine that insists on some form of dogmatic intentional ignorance.

Fundamentalism is an arch-enemy of learning; it closes off curiosity, intellect, and investigation—and, most importantly, understanding and empathy. Fundamentalism is essentially a philosophical disorder, in that the quest for wisdom is forsaken for the clarity of a conviction. Fundamentalism is a form of intentional weakness, a weakness of mind, of intellect, of spiritual health, of perspective, of connection with others. Fundamentalism rejects any learning not fixated on its tightly controlled box.

What does education do?

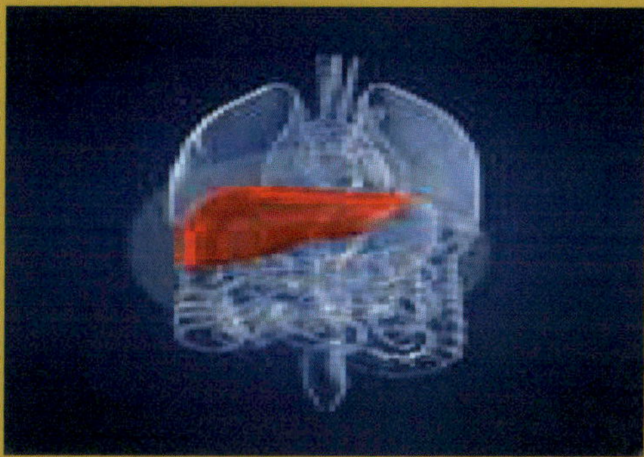

The educational process is analogous to the body's liver. It cleanses personal and social poisons from our systems—poisons such as ignorance, misunderstanding, prejudice, incapability, and immorality. It also prevents addiction to the simplistic clarities of totalitarian beliefs. What we cannot forget is that if we look closely enough, weakness underlies all of those poisons, making it ironic indeed if the educational process is itself weak. If the liver is to do its job, then it needs to be aware of its systemic problems. It has to be especially careful of its operating metaphors and the resulting methods and materials. It has to be particularly mindful of its assessment strategies, for the dynamically complex, interactive, and fuzzy hard-to-measure factors are essential to its health and vitality. Without a strong liver, the social body will weaken and die.

To the question, "what does education do?" we can add that, ultimately, it expands our awareness and intelligence in order to help us poor disconnected humans make integrity, to forge a moral as well as a capable soundness within ourselves, and to connect ourselves to the world. Knowledge is essential to the expansion of intelligence, but it is only one of many factors. What good is knowledge without capabilities such as imagination and empathy and the strength to use them courageously and wisely?

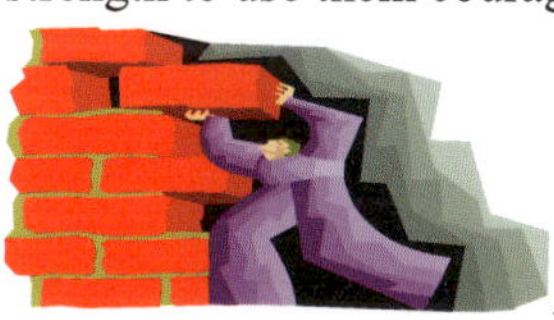

As we learned from the story of *The Three Little Pigs,* we should build our houses (identities) out of bricks, not sticks or straw. Sooner or later, and in one form or another, the wolf (bad circumstances) is going to come along. Houses made of straw or sticks will soon disintegrate. But do you remember what happened when the wolf tried to blow down the house made of bricks? The house actually settled more firmly on its foundation. And when the wolf, in its exasperation, tried to sneak down the chimney, the third little pig was not the kind to panic:

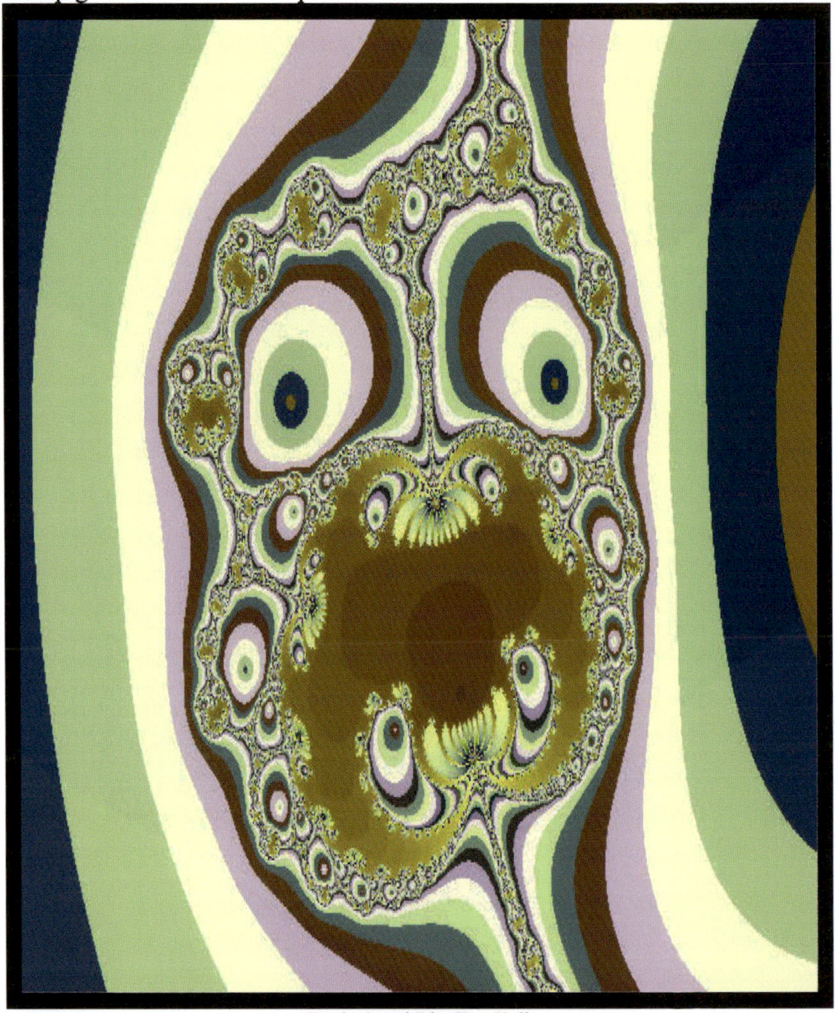

"Panic Attack" by Ken Keller

She had a cauldron of boiling water waiting for him. The bad old wolf was turned into a hearty stew, proving that if you build your house out of bricks and keep your wits about you—and don't let panic raise its ugly head—you can make nourishment out of whatever happens to you.

> *Educare*, the root of the word *education*, means "to lead forth the hidden wholeness," the innate integrity that is in every person.
>
> Rachel Naomi Remen, M.D.

—40—

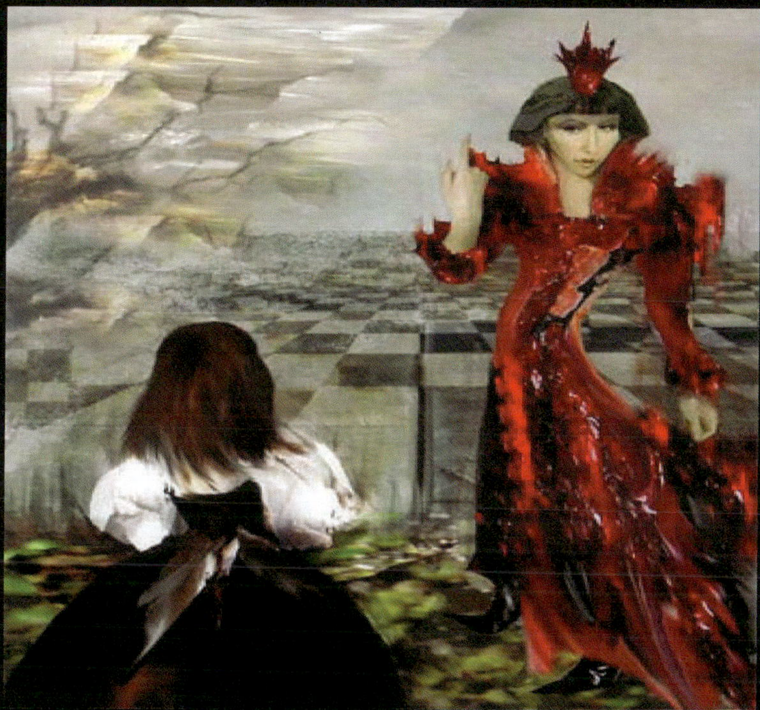

"Alice and the Red Queen" by Marina Valuiska

The future is not what it used to be.

Paul Valery
[backed up by the Red Queen]

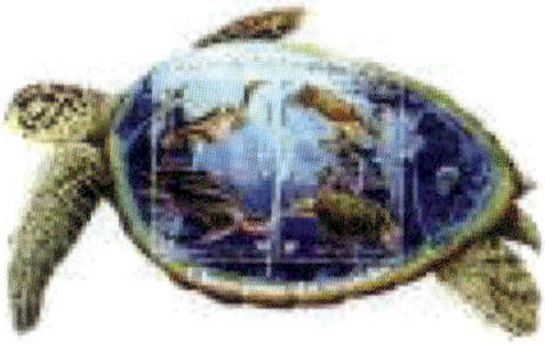

The world used to progress in a stately, slowly moving manner. Sometimes, it didn't seem to move at all; decades, even centuries, would roll by with everything staying pretty much the same. After all, the world rested on the back of a giant turtle. But now we dance in rubbery terrain. The world heaves and flexes beneath our feet. Relationships of every kind have lost their previous solidity. Though that solidity was often cheap and benighted, it still gave the comfort of the known and given. Things pretty much stayed in their places; people pretty much stayed in their stations. There was occasional static, even flare-ups, but the world pretty much kept its moorings.

But then the ropes holding the world in place started giving way. Many of them were rotten and we should celebrate their unraveling. But the good frayed with the bad, and the world was cast adrift. And now we strive for balance and direction in a haphazardly contingent, constantly twisting, topsy-turvy world. The solid, dependable shell of the slow moving turtle is gone, replaced by a trampoline held up by a huge herd of rampaging elephants. (Or would the reader feel more secure on the wings of flippantly flapping butterflies?) Education has therefore become more important—exponentially so.

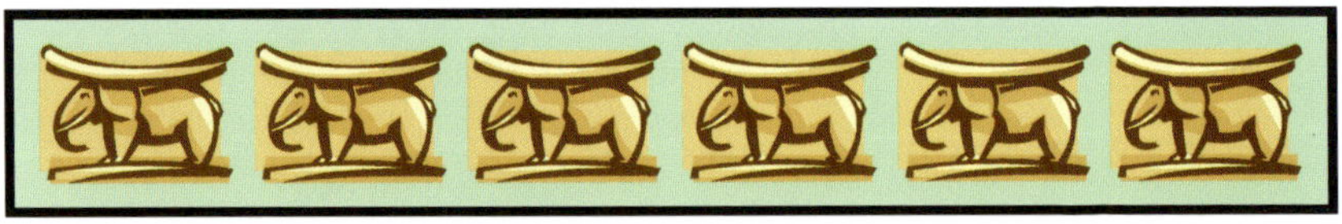

After all, we are now in the land of the Red Queen. When Alice encountered the Red Queen, she had to run at a fast pace to even have a conversation with her because the landscape constantly roared past them. If they didn't run, they fell behind. Education is the way we run in this slippery, rapidly sliding-by trampoline terrain resting upon the backs of agitated elephants. Education is the feet we grow in response to the challenges and opportunities of our worlds, to give us direction and traction in our ever-changing terrains.

> Education is the process through which we transform ourselves. The Red Queen World has us by the metaphors—so we better grow new ones.

We must adjust to the new reality—or fall increasingly behind the changing landscape. If we fail to meet our challenges and opportunities, then we will diminish and eventually perish. The postmodern, Red Queen World, calls for a redefinition of and resurgent concern for the educational process. We either continuously revision and reform the process—or fall off the bucking trampoline.

> One thing needs to be made clear: schooling is only part of the educational process. Literature, movies, and even music have important roles in the process. The worlds of religion, community, business, and especially family affect the process.
>
> **Education is a culture-wide endeavor.**

We can bemoan the passing of the comfortable, slowly changing world resting on the solid, stately back of the giant turtle, but we must also be pragmatic and find a way to get to our feet and learn how to progress while on top of a heaving bouncing trampoline supported by a herd of rampaging elephants. Ready or not, this is our new reality. Training is insufficient for the postmodern world. It could carry individuals, and societies, in the mechanistic, simple (relatively speaking) modern times. But now we need more imagination, more creativity, more ownership, more individual contribution, and more personal integrity if we are going to muster the intelligence to master the problems coming our way and fashion the products necessary for meeting our challenges and opportunities.

> Initiative is the magic in the educational mix. It carries the life-force. It is at the core of the Democratic Promise.

The good old turtle is dead and gone; long live the rampaging elephants. The world of the Red Queen is a bouncy, rubbery trampoline. Live with it.

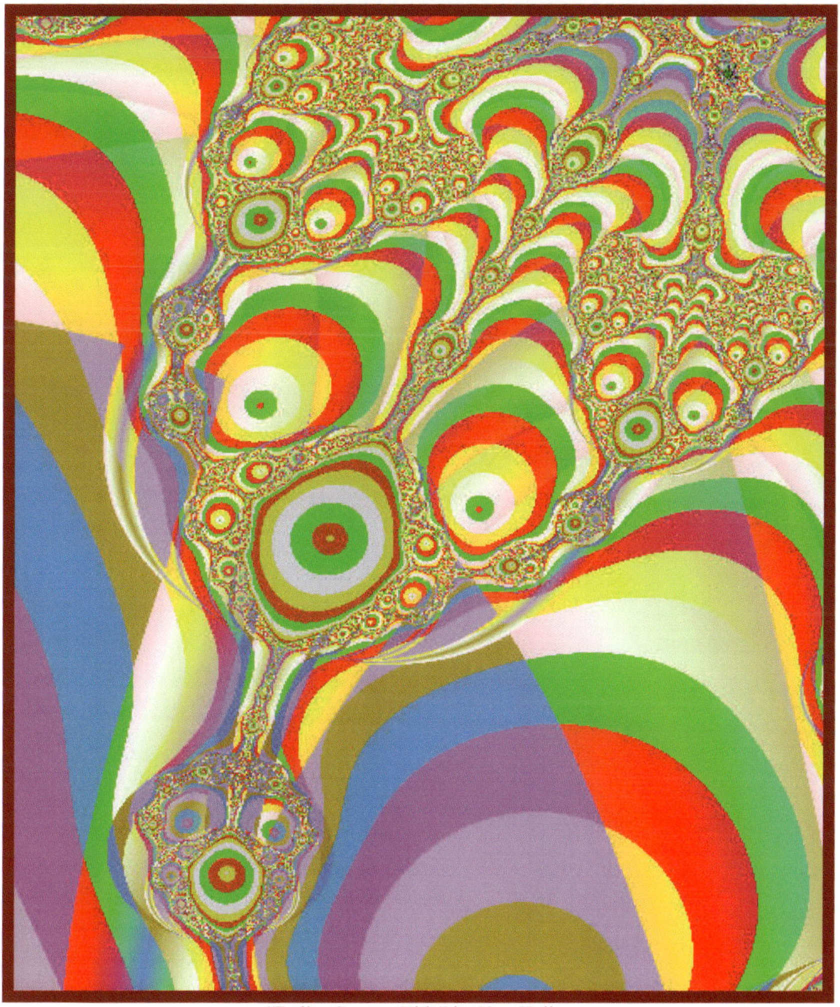

"Roller Coaster Ride" by Ken Keller

—41—

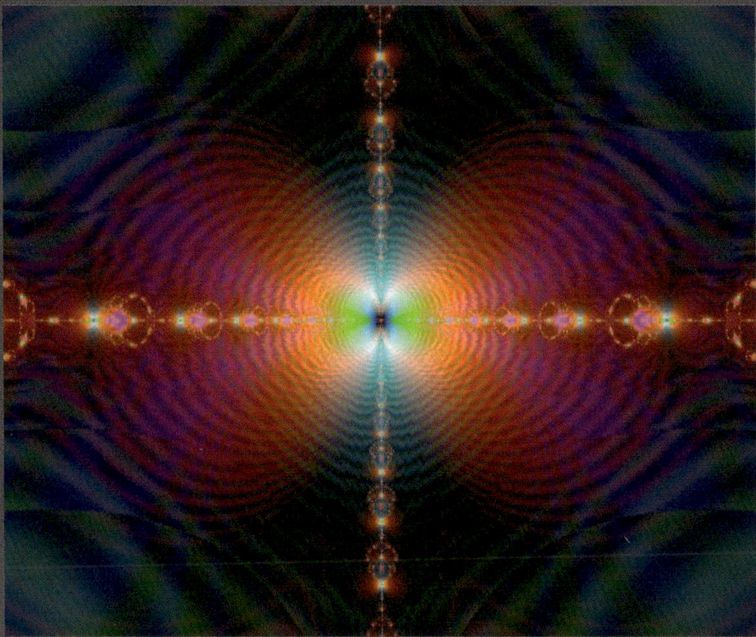

"The Splendor Kingdom of Harmony and Oneness" by Jack Haas

Wisdom is the right use of knowledge. To know is not to be wise. Many men know a great deal, and are all the greater fools for it. There is no fool so great a fool as a knowing fool. But to know how to use knowledge is to have wisdom.

Charles H. Spurgeon

We rarely aim for the development of wisdom in our educational system, though we culturally understand its importance. The curriculum ignores the notion of adulthood, though we disrespect immaturity. Learning Redefined will return to a focus on both wisdom and adulthood, concerns that are especially relevant in these confusing and challenging times. John Dewey, in *How We Think*, warned us about the trap of confusing knowledge with wisdom:

> The distinction between information and wisdom is old, and yet requires constantly to be redrawn. Information is knowledge which is merely acquired and stored up; wisdom is knowledge operating in the direction of powers to the better living of life. Information, merely as information, implies no special training of intellectual capacity; wisdom is the finest fruit of that training.

> Because their knowledge has been achieved in connection with the needs of specific situations, men of little book-learning are often able to put to effective use every ounce of knowledge they possess; while men of vast erudition are often swamped by the mere bulk of their learning, because memory, rather than thinking, has been operative in obtaining it.

We can think of wisdom as the capacity to perceive and escape traps. It is wisdom that perceives our predicaments and forges pathways of escape. Especially when the trap is of our own making, wisdom is called for, though it is then much harder to imagine and construct. Our operating metaphors can not only lead us into our predicaments, but also keep us from envisioning the pathways of action that could help us escape them. Geoffrey Vickers, in his book, *Freedom in a Rocking Boat: Changing Values in an Unstable Society,* provides a helpful analogy:

> Lobster pots are designed to catch lobsters. A man entering a man-sized lobster pot would become suspicious of the narrowing tunnel, he would shrink from the drop at the end; and if he fell in, he would recognize the entrance as a possible exit and climb out again—even if he were the shape of a lobster. A trap is a trap only for creatures which cannot solve the problem that it sets. Man-traps are dangerous only in relation to the limitations on what men can see and value and do. The nature of the trap is a function of the nature of the trapped. To describe either is to imply the other. . . . We the trapped tend to take our own state of mind for granted—which is partly why we are trapped. With the shape of the trap in our minds, we shall be better able to see the relevance of our limitations and to question those assumptions about ourselves that are most inept to the activity and the experience of being human now.

The socialistic operating metaphor (and its constellating methods and materials) guiding our educational process has funneled us into an increasingly narrow tunnel. We have locked onto presentation, memorization, and measurement, because you can't objectively scale a conversation, predict and control thinking, or metric understanding and wisdom.

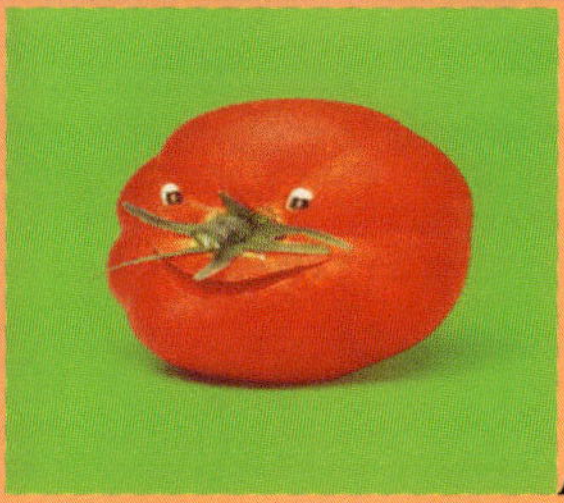

A humorous illustration of the difference between knowledge and wisdom is the following: Knowledge is knowing that tomatoes are a fruit. Wisdom is not putting them into a fruit salad.

The relationship between wisdom and maturation is an essential one. The trap of a left-brain fixated school system, because of the easy measurability of left-brain capabilities, is one of our own making. We have taken our own state of mind for granted, in particular our definition of learning. Can we muster the maturity to develop the wisdom to escape our traps, whether circumstantial or self-constructed?

A Cautionary Image

Mature antelope have learned how to spot and avoid lions.

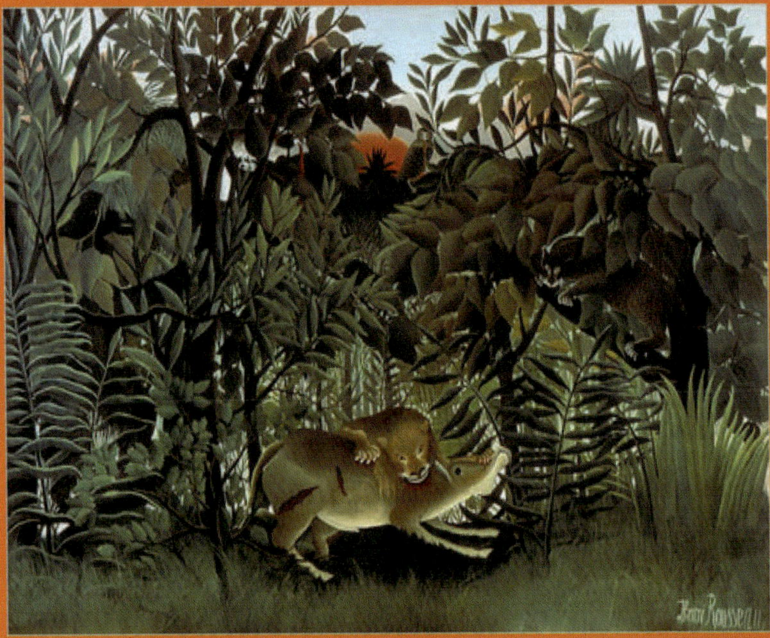

Art by Henri Rousseau

The Pluto Test

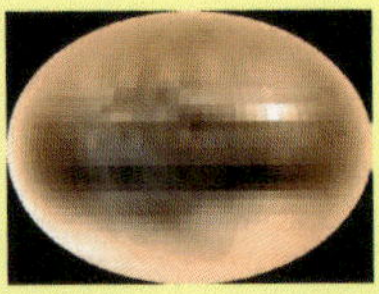

Poor Pluto is no longer considered a planet. It has been redefined out of that rare category. Planethood is now defined as a body of material with sufficient gravity to cleanse debris from its orbit. When you think about it—the same can be said for adulthood.

The fuzzy picture is the best we have of the former planet.

Is there a better definition of an adult than one who cleanses debris from his or her orbit? Adulthood is achieved through the successful avoidance of becoming lost in the maze, through overcoming any obstacle, whether external or internal. This requires an increased focus on emotional intelligence, the capacity to solve relational problems and fashion relationship-dependent products. And emotional intelligence addresses both intrapersonal and interpersonal issues, with cleansing the debris from our inner orbits the most difficult and the most important.

The stone in your path must
become a brick in your house.

Wisdom and adulthood call for education with the right side of the brain in mind. Capabilities such as courage, imagination, initiative, and empathy are essential for the development of either. The debris caused by the present operating metaphors guiding our schooling is the explosion of special education, disengaged students, resentment and resistance, undeveloped intellects, suppressed initiative, and passive learners. The worst debris is students disconnected by their schooling from the capability and responsibility necessary for democratic citizens. Our educational system will transform itself to a more comprehensive and effective maturity or it will fail us. Can we, as a profession, mature beyond our present weaknesses? Can we cleanse the educational system of the debris that presently pollutes it, especially that of our own making?

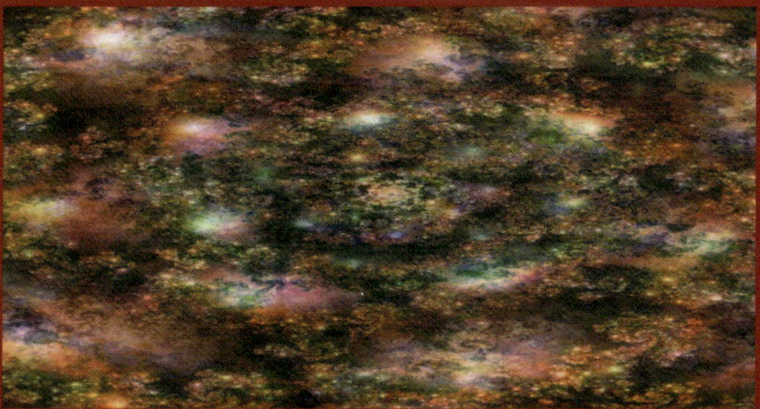

"Finding the Center" by Keith Mackay

My will shall shape the future. Whether I fail or succeed shall be no man's doing but my own. I am the force; I can clear any obstacle before me or I can be lost in the maze. My choice; my responsibility; win or lose, only I hold the key to my destiny.

Elaine Maxwell

—42—

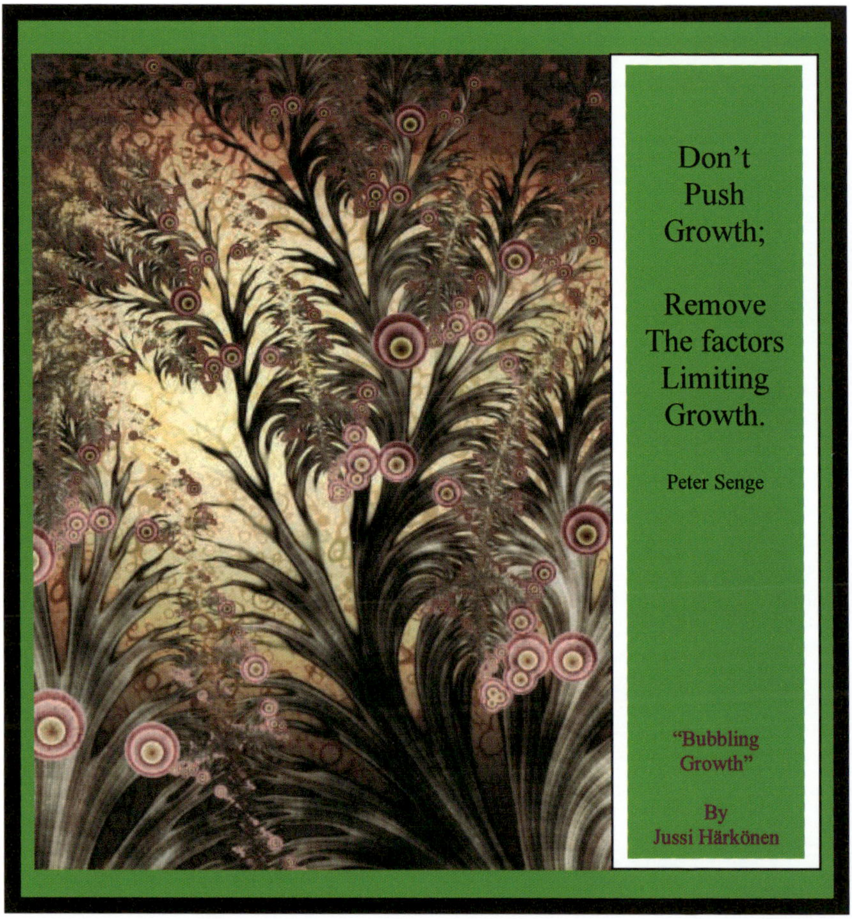
Don't
Push
Growth;

Remove
The factors
Limiting
Growth.

Peter Senge

"Bubbling
Growth"

By
Jussi Härkönen

In recent conversations with public school teachers, some in rural areas, others in inner cities, and from various social-economic situations, a frequent complaint is the growing prevalence of discipline issues and the lack of learning. (Even some of my university colleagues voice both of these concerns.) The teachers also find that their administrators don't seem to know what to do. The situation is getting worse, despite numerous plans and the continuous expansion of special education programs.

The question is why: Perhaps the youth of this country are spoiled; they don't know what it means to work; achievement is not necessary, for they will still never be deprived of anything. Perhaps the breakdown of family structure is generating a nation of dysfunctional youth. Perhaps the culture itself generates the problem, with gangs, drugs, and a general attitude of disrespect. Perhaps the times are simply too crazy. But perhaps the systemic problem is that our educational system, by pushing a benighted definition of growth, has developed factors that suppress it.

It makes systemic sense for educators to focus on the last possibility, for we lack the power to change any of the other possibilities. What we can change is how we perceive and practice our endeavor. We can hope that down the road those changes will alleviate the other factors. But we can definitely address and remedy our contribution to the overall problem. We can remove the factors, within ourselves, that prevent growth.

The challenge is to think systemically. Where are the levers within the system to increase both its stability and its effectiveness? In order to find them, we need to go back to those operating metaphors, those images harbored in our individual and social minds that guide our perceptions and behaviors. The problem is, ultimately, philosophical. It can only be fixed by changing the operating metaphors that govern teacher education and the everyday practice of schooling.

Mrs. Moore's Price of Admission

My tenth-grade English teacher, Mrs. Moore, always demanded a price of admission to her classroom. That ticket was the homework given the day before. (Good behavior during class was so assumed it wasn't even mentioned.) Failure to have the price of admission: "My dog ate it;" "The house burnt down, killed my dog and my sister and, really tragically, burned up the just finished assignment;" or "I suddenly came down with bubonic plague," was met with a calm directive to see the principal. The kind principal would look at you sadly and send you directly to Mrs. Clobber, the giant and bitter study hall teacher. Just being within a hundred feet of that woman dried up even teenage hormones and stopped all neurogenesis in its tracks. You just didn't want to go there.

On the other hand, Mrs. Moore's class was where the action was. She was funny and she had a way of making even Shakespeare understandable and entertaining. She also invited conversation, and had set up conditions in her classroom where students felt free to contribute. Not only that, it was a guaranteed period of time when I could be in close proximity to Diane, Tootie, Donna, and a few others of considerable charms, and I had a few male friends in there to boot. I consistently, and even sometimes enthusiastically, paid her damned price of admission.

School is where the action is, or at least where it could be. It certainly should be. Schools are social centers where intellectual, emotional, athletic, and romantic connections are made. When they are also places of real learning, they will become so desirable that prices of admission can be asked, and they will be paid.

Learning, real learning, after all, and we tend to forget this—is deeply pleasurable. Lehrer writes:

> . . . Scientists have discovered that antidepressants work by stimulating neurogenesis (at least in rodents), implying that depression is ultimately caused by a decrease in the amount of new neurons, and not by a lack of serotonin. A new class of anti-depressants is being developed that targets the neurogenesis pathway. For some reason, newborn brain cells make us happy.

Both my hormones and my neocortex were happy in Mrs. Moore's class. That is why I paid her price of admission. The principal also supported her approach, and Mrs. Clobber did her part. Other teachers didn't demand a price of admission, and couldn't have, even if Diane, Tootie, and Donna were sitting right in front of me, because they excited my resentment or resistance instead of my desire to learn. Theirs were not neurogenic classrooms, usually because they were curriculum-fixated, lecture-driven, and test-focused gavagers—where the individuality, initiative, and ownership of the teachers were not present. Mrs. Moore was a successful teacher not only because of Diane and Tootie and Donna, but because "for some reason, newborn brain cells make us happy."

Build a [real] field of learning—they will come.

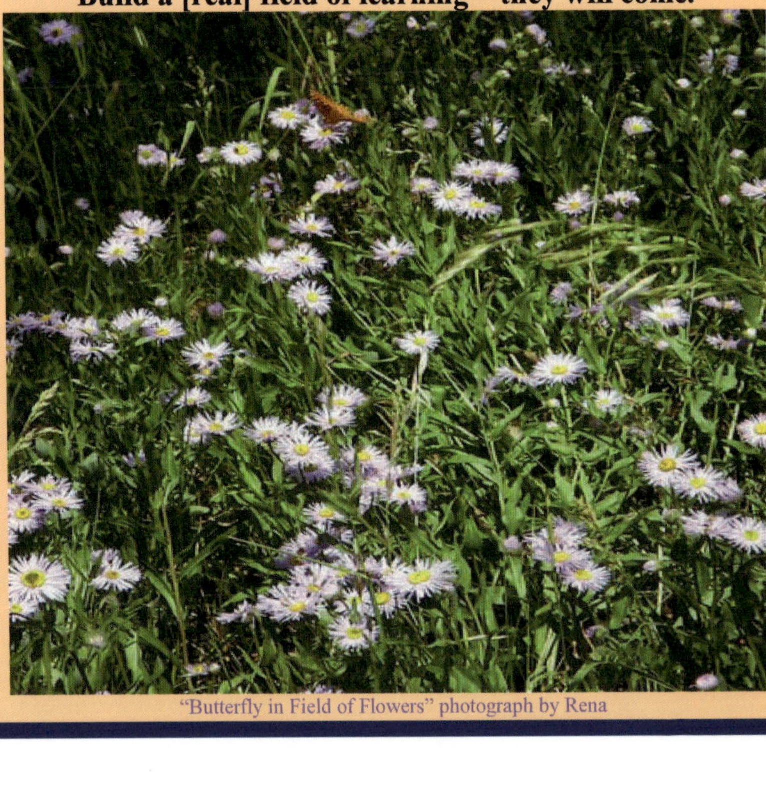

"Butterfly in Field of Flowers" photograph by Rena

Teachers have the power to build the fields of learning, but they must be built anew in each classroom with each new community of students. Too often, however, their efforts are impeded by prediction and control machinations emanating from top-down bureaucracies. They are not able to establish either a price of admission or classrooms that students will pay to attend. Teachers have the responsibility to build fields of learning, but must must fight against the power of the educational system to disrupt and suppress their efforts.

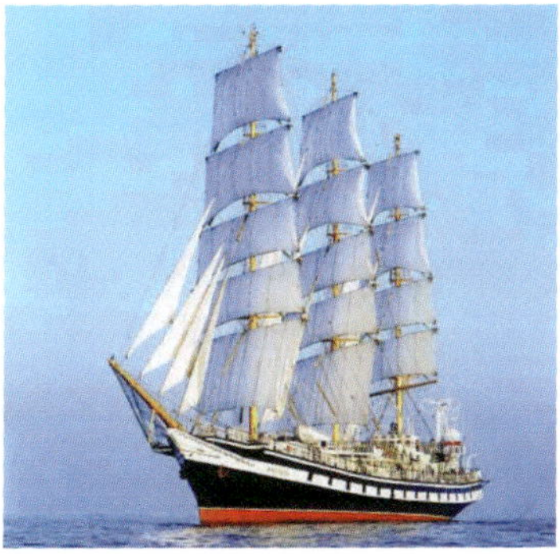

Today, our teachers are not captains of their own ships, the operating metaphor regarding the role of a teacher that Mrs. Moore held firmly in her mind and heart, one very much supported by the principal. In democratic schooling, this would be increasingly the case. Teachers should captain their own ships. How can a democracy, a system of government dependent upon the principles of individuality and personal responsibility, not image its teachers as captains of their ships?

There will be systemic costs in such a shift in operating metaphors. The present image of top-down management will have to be turned on its head. The primary function of administrators will be to support their teachers. Regrettably, some teachers will not be fit captains; they will be pugnacious bullies producing either victims or static, or weak incompetents inviting either boredom or mutiny. But then, and only then, can we truly call for teacher accountability. A democracy must depend upon the capability and integrity of its teachers to teach the principles that constitute its foundation.

What do teachers do?

What was the texture of his [Shakespeare's] imagination? Would mapping his brain have told us? If he were alive today, could scientists begin to explore the mountains of his mind? What would they find? A rare bounty of connections among neurons, which makes it easier to link unrelated images from different parts of the brain, the stuff of metaphors?

Diane Ackerman

In her book, *An Alchemy of Mind,* Ackerman talks about "the natural brain process of 'spreading activation.'" And right there, in a biological context, is our task as teachers: to spread activation, to excite the neurons in growing brains—which in turn excite other neurons. What we do is make possible futures more real for others, and we do that through establishing neurogenic relationships. We spread activation in the brain—if we are teachers. Ackerman writes: . . . "As the neurologist Martha Denckla wryly observes: 'Every teacher is a brain surgeon, a scary thought . . . every teacher is making little dendrites sprout and connect up neurons.'"

A Cautionary Rule

If we are to think systemically about our problems and opportunities, then we must always bear in Peter Senge's

Take Two Aspirin and Wait Rule.

Headaches are usually a systemic problem. Something is wrong within the body system, dehydration or whatever, that is the underlying cause of the pain. Aspirin is a systemic medicine, an analgesic that affects the whole body. It also takes time to have effect, to percolate throughout the body system. You don't take two aspirin, declare the headache still there and pounding, and immediately take two more tablets; you wait, giving the medicine time to take effect. Failure to follow this rule can result in the medicine becoming itself toxic.

We must be careful in removing the factors preventing growth in our schooling. It will require considerable reflection and genuine conversation to ascertain the systemic levers and decide which ones to apply and how to assess their effectiveness. Neuroscience supports Senge's intuition that growth cannot be pushed, for that is not only counterproductive but destructive—but it can be encouraged and informed. Most importantly, conditions can be created and established that excite rather than suppress it. We only have to ascertain what those conditions are and remove the ones that limit growth.

We can assume that everyone wants to learn, grow, and contribute. A theory of human development that fits in with learning redefined will hold this belief as fundamental to the human experience. The present definition of learning, and thus teaching and schooling, assumes just the opposite.

In the words of Joseph Featherstone, an astute observer of the educational process,

"Our schools assume the worst of teachers —as well as children."

That negative assumption is itself a factor limiting growth. It represents the absence of belief in both teacher and student desire to develop and produce. A new theory of human development will understand that we can generally assume the natural desire to learn, grow, and contribute. The growing capability of neuroscience will support that assumption, as well as help us discover the factors limiting growth and remove them.

Education change depends on what teachers think and do. It's as simple and as complicated as that.

Seymour Sarason

Systemic Stupidity

*80 percent of CEO's and CFO's said they would not spend money to make their factories more efficient and save money in the long run if it hurt their next quarter bottom line. That is functionally insane.**[2]

Al Gore

Growth, real growth, in either business or education, is suppressed by such mindsets. Addiction to the easily measured is one of our most profound cultural weaknesses. Even most of our CEO's and CFO's, supposedly our best and brightest, suffer from such systemic stupidity. This inability to look ahead to the greater but harder to measure gain is a weakness we must address and eradicate. Otherwise, we are functionally insane.

We will also fall behind other cultures that do not share that systemic stupidity. Witness the decline of our auto industry, which, through its addiction to the bottom line, measured assiduously every quarter, neglected quality and development. Years ago, Hyundai, a South Korean ship builder, decided to expand into the automotive industry. After five years, the head engineer of the new division went to the president of the company with the resignations of himself as well as those of his entire division. After five years of intense effort, they had failed to make a decent car, and they had spent millions of dollars in the attempt. They were ashamed of their failure. The president, however, refused to accept the resignations, informing the division head to go back and work another five years, then the company would take another look at the situation. That is an example of systemic wisdom, as their later success bears out.

Our cultural addiction to the easily measured explains Yong Zhao's puzzlement in his book, *Catching Up or Leading the Way*. He cannot understand why we are increasingly fixated on test scores, in order to catch up with those of other countries, when those countries desire our culture of creativity and innovation. Those countries have perhaps mastered education for the easily measured, but they want to remove the factors that limit the growth of creative and innovative people. As he states: ". . . While the United States is moving toward more standardization and centralization, the Asian countries are working hard to allow more flexibility and autonomy at the local level."

Zhao warns us: "American education is at a crossroads. There are two paths in front of us: one in which we destroy our strengths in order to 'catch up' with others in test scores and one in which we build on our strengths so we can keep the lead in innovation and creativity."

*How can we define functional insanity? I image individuals or organizations so habitually self-defeating, so fixated on short-term gains or simplistic momentary pleasures, that they are incapable of either perspective or understanding of how their mindsets and behavior are eroding the very substance of themselves.

—43—

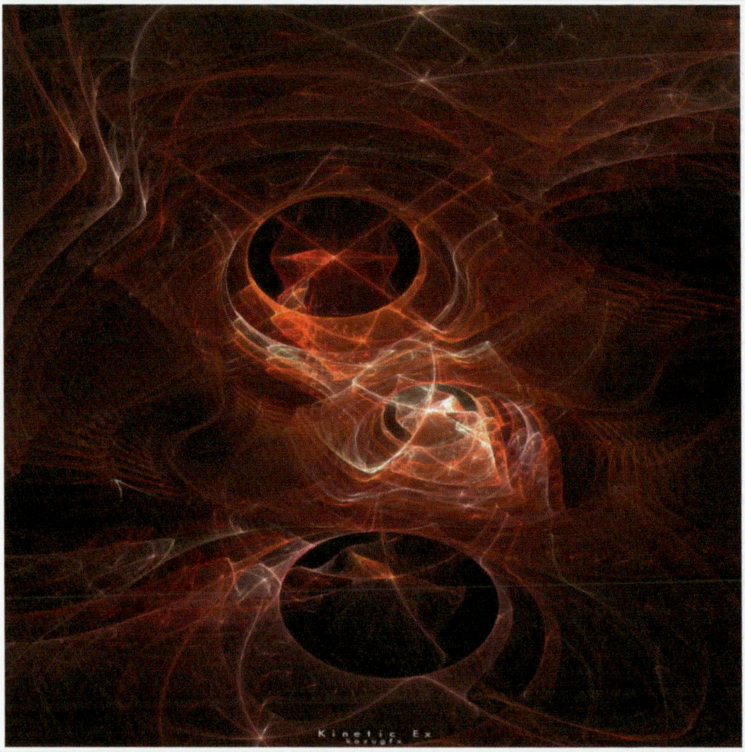

"Kinetic ex" by Phil Marsh

If you can keep your wits about you while all others are losing theirs, and blaming you, the world will be yours and everything in it. What's more, you'll be a man, my son.

Rudyard Kipling

In a topsy-turvy Red Queen World, the task is to keep our wits about us despite the increasing turbulence and confusion. This calls for the capacity to redefine and redesign ourselves while on the move—to not only keep ourselves glued together while on the fly—but to revision and remake ourselves even when our feet are not firmly on the ground. If we do not dramatically improve our capacity for creating and hanging onto our wits, then the world will whittle us down, and become too much for us.

We have to dream more, as well as develop the responsibilities to those dreams. This is one reason Pink calls for the development of right-brain capabilities. The strength we will increasingly need in the Red Queen World is **kinetic stability.**

Kinetic Stability is the personal or organizational ability to maintain, repair, and even develop one's gyroscope in the midst of dynamically complex situations and life's assaults upon balance and direction—to keep moving with purpose and effectiveness despite disruptive influences.

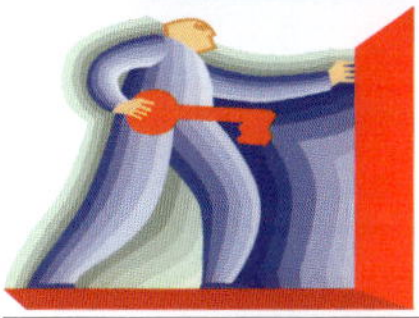

KEY POINTS

- **Kinetic Stability is the best indicator of possible intelligent action. Problems are consistently faced and solved; products are consistently imagined and produced.**
- **Those individuals and organizations that lack Kinetic Stability will more easily wobble, weaken, and fall to the wolves. They will lack the wisdom to forge strength and effectiveness.**
- **Individuals and organizations that have Kinetic Stability are more likely to establish and maintain the psychological state of flow, the momentum of effectiveness. They continuously learn.**
- **Good learners, whether individual or organizational, increasingly move with purpose and effectiveness despite disruptive influences—because they learn from those influences. (Influence means "to change the flow.")**
- **Change is mandatory—Growth is not. Individuals and organizations with Kinetic Stability consistently find ways to choose and forge growth—to move constructively.**
- **Kinetic Stability indicates the "flexible soundness" of an identity—its true integrity.**

When the psychologist Mihalyi Csikszentmihalyi discusses the phenomenon of flow, he is referring to kinetic stability. The term indicates both movement and balance—action guided by an inner gyroscope. Individuals, or systems, with kinetic stability are dynamic, changing, effective, and, at the same time, hard to knock out of kilter. They maintain purposeful direction despite disruptive and derailing influences.

The athlete in the zone, the philosopher or poet lost in thought, the musician at one with the music, the child enraptured by the placing of colored beads on a string, all exhibit kinetic stability. The kinetically stable have focus but not fixation, attention but not dysfunction. Distractions may surround them and occasionally burst through the intensity of their focus, but their confident passion soon reasserts itself. They find a way to stay true to the call of their endeavors.

Witness Michael Jordan

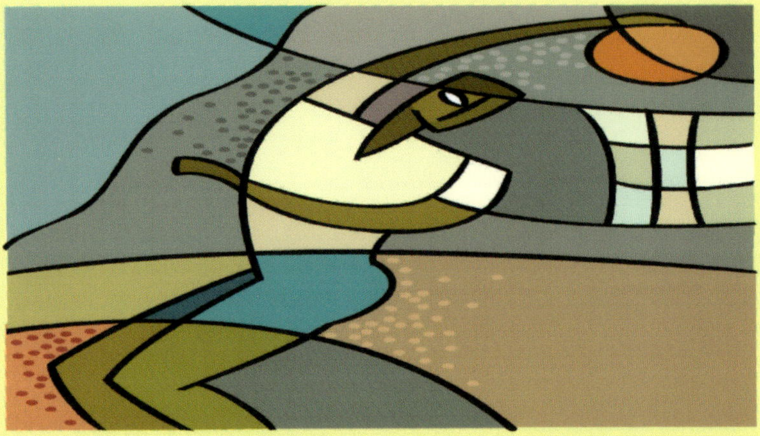

Jordan's poised confidence on the basketball court emerged from years of effort and success at his chosen endeavor. He has reflected deeply and consistently about the challenges, both internal and external, of the art and science of his sport. He found the factors, whether internal or external, holding him back—and got rid of them. It is extremely difficult, and unusual, as his opponents will attest, to either shake his confidence or disrupt his focus. Jordan is a reflective practitioner of the game of basketball, who knows how to achieve and maintain a state of flow while playing, with tremendous kinetic stability at his chosen endeavor.

Adjustments to ever-changing surroundings are continuously created. Initiatives are developed and implemented as learners, through reflective, predictive, and spontaneous thinking, make the endeavors their own. The focused commitment is deep and satisfying—indicating the seamless melding of identity with endeavor. When one is doing what one is supposed to do, failure is unlikely. Such individuals or groups are in the zone, so-to-speak, highly resistant to distraction or disruption. They are dynamically entwined with the ongoing effort and purpose necessary for successful completion of their tasks. The kinetically stable not only succeed where others fail, but evolve their capability for future endeavors. They are increasingly effective and dedicated. The energy of their initiative and the wisdom of their judgment grow in strength and breadth.

The present definition of learning cannot encourage and inform the phenomenon of kinetic stability. It is so addicted to illusions of order that hints of disorder throw it into cognitive dissonance and then intentional ignorance, a truly witless response to turbulent times. The present definition fosters kinetic instability. But change will happen in our commotional world, whether we are ready for it or not, whether we can grow in response to its challenges—or not. We will either learn to deal with the increasing commotion, or become stupefied by it.

The Kinetic Stability of the Brain

The human brain grows continuously in an interactive complexity but, somehow, maintains a coherent sense of identity through the mystery of mind. It has a kinetic stability which gives it coherence but also flexibility—a dog never too old to learn new tricks. Some neurons grow only a few connections while others grow thousands in an ever developing web of interacting relationships with other neurons. The kinetic stability of Michael Jordan's basketball prowess may be traceable to the jungle of connections of certain dendrites and axons. Diane Ackerman writes, in *Alchemy of Mind:*

"Neurons grow like quaking aspens in the forests of the mind . . . Unlike other cells, they don't move or divide. They assume branching shapes from pyramid to star. Best of all, they talk among themselves, eavesdrop, dash off messages. For that purpose, they have two kinds of limbs, dendrites and axons; the former to listen, the latter to speak. Dangling from a neuron's pouchy trunk, dendrites hear what neighboring neurons signal through their axons. Like elegant ladies air-kissing so as not to muss their makeup, dendrites and axons don't quite touch. The contact happens in less than one thousandth of a second, a spell of microtime as powerful as fate."

Perhaps this explains our immense variability: as we choose to pay attention to certain aspects of reality we come to understand them better—and we sprout dendrites and axons accordingly. The evolution of seeing—and intellectual/emotional/spiritual development—resides in the dynamic rhythm between attention and interpretation. We attend to what we understand and attention expands as understanding increases—thus choosing the evolution of our kinetic stability.

For increased KINETIC STABILITY we need education that:

Helps us recognize the power of operating metaphors, and how to change them when necessary.

Encourages the imagination, interest, and initiative of both teachers and students—as well as the understanding and judgment that guide those factors.

Recognizes that learning has a dynamic ecology—and that making ground-up, not top-down, adjustments to the process in mid-flow is essential.

Redefines learning toward a balance between educating both left and right-brain capabilities.

The art of progress is to preserve order amid change
and to preserve change amid order.

Alfred North Whitehead

—44—

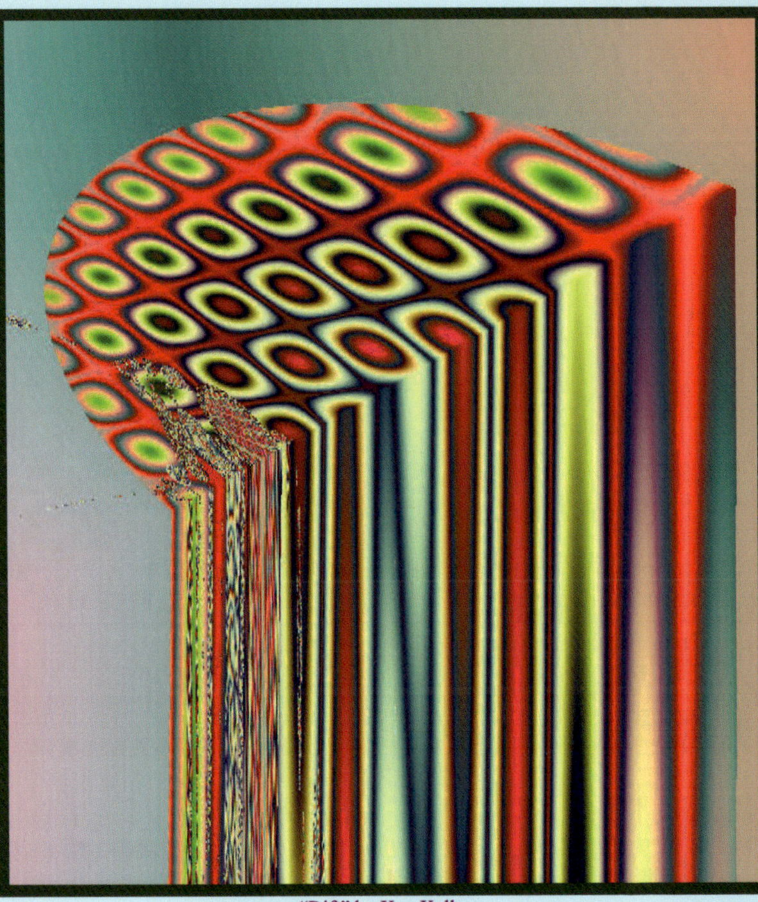

"Rift" by Ken Keller

Education can be a cohesive force in a society, as it was in an earlier America, or it can be a dissolvent force, as it has been in the past half century.

Max Lerner

The imbalance between initiative and training not only degrades individual potential but the integrity of our country as well. Each mindless suppression of initiative in either teachers or students by a training-poisoned system diminishes our strength as a nation. In a world of dynamic complexity and entwined economic and political realities, the commitment and contribution of a nation's citizens are more important than ever before in human history.

We ignore student resistance and resentment to the educational process at our peril. There may be wisdom in their feelings, borne of their perhaps inarticulate and inchoate knowledge that their individuality, and therefore their uniqueness and responsibility, is being attacked by the philosophy, methods, and even the materials of schooling. As the historian Max Lerner's warning points out, we have developed a system that dissolves rather than coheres the structure of ourselves. We need to redefine learning to where initiative, commitment, and, ultimately, responsibility are inspired and informed.

The phenomenon of **ressentiment** is little understood, researched, or even heard of, but it has powerful consequences in our school environments. **Ressentiment is the feeling of free-floating resentment and resistance.** Like "free-floating anxiety," ressentiment is a systemic disorder because the sufferer doesn't know where to direct a response to the stress. Ressentiment tears at the cohesion of ourselves individually and socially—a condition that corrodes community, degrades engagement, dissolves commitment, and prevents productivity.

In *Society's Children: A Study of Ressentiment in the Secondary School*, published way back in 1967 but neglected by the temper of the times, the authors Carl Nordstom, Edgar Z. Friedenberg, and Hilary A. Gold, voiced their concerns:

> We seek to determine whether there might be an unrecognized process by which schools actually do something to students, and in the doing, seriously interfere with the development of what used to be called a strong and forceful character . . . In our preliminary judgment ressentiment operated to stifle enthusiasm, to undermine fortitude, and to discourage the development of self-mastery; and to the degree that this is true we saw ressentiment as insidious when endured, difficult to fight, and stultifying in its consequences.
>
> We also thought that this process was not only unrecognized, but, in a formal sense, unintended. And, to the degree that this is true, we felt that it should be brought to the attention of responsible persons.

Ressentiment in American schools has two primary sources:

> The reductive perspective applied to a holistic endeavor produces procedures that are ignorant of interactive factors and therefore systemically disruptive to the educational process. Friction is both caused and exacerbated.
>
> Many of the practices of American schooling are not aligned with the values dear to our democratic hearts. They corrode against initiative and ownership, wearing and tearing at both teacher and student individual autonomy.

Students in our schools are beginning to recognize how they are being governed by atmospheres of manipulation and coercion without hope of personal representation in what happens to them. An academic Boston Tea Party, of sorts, occurred in a suburb of Los Angeles, Torrance, California, in 1989. The Los Angeles Times reported:

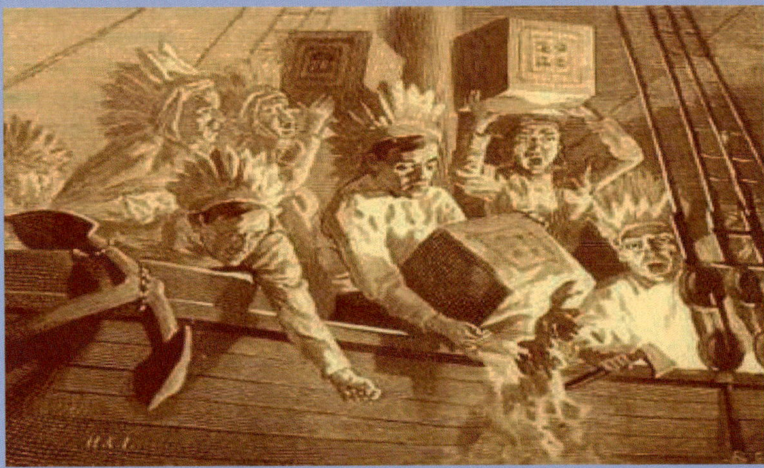

Picture of Boston Tea Party Copyright 1996-2008 Early America

A group of seniors at Torrance's academically rigorous West High School intentionally flunked the latest California Assessment Program test in an attempt to send a message to administrators who they believe place too much emphasis on the exam . . . some seniors became disgruntled when some teachers interrupted classes to prepare them for the state tests . . . students also believed that administrators who visited classes to stress the importance of doing well were too concerned with maintaining the school's image . . . The principal blamed the state Department of Education and the press which does not publish other indicators of school performance . . . The head of the Torrance Teacher's Association blamed it on a trickle-down effect, saying the pressure starts with the state Department . . . and works its way down through the local school districts, principals, teachers and eventually students. And he added, "I think students are feeling like pawns in a game that is much bigger than they are."

This example of directed resentment indicates the possibility of how much directionless resentment is floating around in our schools. (And this was over twenty years ago; we can assume conditions have not improved.) Students intuitively recognize, or at least suspect, that their integrities are not being respected by the educational process. They sense that the shapes and substances of their identities are suffering from forced immersion into a manipulative environment. Within the conventional educational atmospheres generated by a culture of scientific management, the wonder is that more students, and teachers, don't understand and express their resentment.

No wonder the educational process tears at our sense of cohesion.

—45—

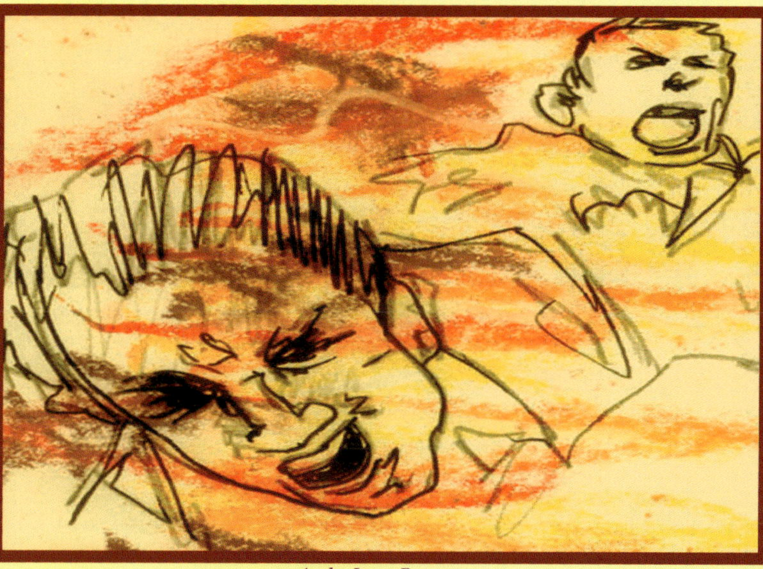

Art by Irene Pereyra

When one considers in its length and breadth the importance of this question of the education of the nation's young, the broken lives, the defeated hopes, the national failures, which result from the frivolous inertia with which it is treated, it is difficult to restrain within oneself a savage rage.

Alfred North Whitehead

Whitehead is talking about soul murder, the destruction of the enjoyment of learning. The result of suppressed constructive learning is not only the impediment of intelligence, but the squelching of the human spirit. It is through the increasing capacity of intelligence, we must remember, that individuals actualize the potential of personhood. Thus, education, as it is culturally framed and practiced, results all-too-frequently in soul murder—because it suppresses growth.

In his essay, "Whitehead on Soul Murder in Education: The Continuing Problem for Teachers," Foster N. Walker talks about Whitehead's notion of inert ideas:

> Ideas are inert only if the student's mind is inert, and if the student's mind is *characteristically* inert in school, the consequences may be life-long and the teachers and administrators are guilty of an irresponsibility of immense ethical proportions.

Inert minds are the haunt of toads. Bitter feelings emerge from the swamp. Disruptions, even sabotage, become perceived as avenues of constructive response. The suppression of initiative, in both teachers and students, generates conditions inviting resentment and resistance. Teachers and students feel disrespected, discounted, and trapped in an insincere situation. The mind not engaged productively will find alternative avenues of expression. The mind cannot be truly inert, but it can be trapped in situations of make-work designed to take care of the "managers' needs for control."

In an interactive endeavor, insincerity is one of the worst sins, as indicated by Jacques Barzun's admonition that manipulation in place of teaching is cruel and harmful. Falseness is not only immoral, it is ultimately ineffective. It generates resistance and resentment within teachers to the educational system that manipulates them and within students who frequently suffer from ressentiment. Students therefore lash out at the nearest representatives of authority—their teachers—when they feel trapped in an insincere, inauthentic situation.

In his book, *A Different Kind of Teacher: Solving the Crisis of American Schooling,* John Taylor Gatto describes the ressentiment of our students:

> Children are condemned to hours of desperation in schools, pretending to do work that doesn't exist. School is a liar's world, it cannot deliver on its promises; at the end of each day children are full of aggression which they take out on their families. School children are sad and desperate people, they recognize they are dying but don't understand how the execution is being managed. They are the developmental stages of a proletariat in the making, without heart, without initiative, without knowledge of their own families or histories and without any abiding loyalties. Their spirits are broken on a government dole which in a short time becomes addictive. Even when they are offered real work to do, most drift back to the secure meaninglessness of busy work. Anyone who has ever tried to lead public school students into generating lines of meaning in their own lives will have felt the hostility with which broken children fight to be left alone. "Just tell me what to do," they say through gritted teeth.

Suppression of initiative always generates hostility and insincerity. Whenever teachers are forced or cajoled onto district, state, or federally approved bandwagons, the result is insincerity, sabotage, or, at minimum, distraction from the real task of teaching, figuring out the best way for individual teachers to forge working relationships with students, given their unique strengths, abilities, and temperaments. As Barzun pointed out in his book, *Begin Here: The Forgotten Conditions of Teaching and Learning*, the lack of sincere relations is the cause of an appalling amount of nonsense. The resulting distrust chokes every interaction. It pushes teachers and students into inauthenticity. Compulsion to be insincere, to be inauthentic, to be divorced from one's true self, is a force that pushes toward schizophrenia. Thinkers such as R. D. Laing and Lionel Trilling believe that pressures against the individual's essential sense of self generate schizophrenic responses. Training, as it crowds out initiative, prevents a fundamental way our identities establish and express themselves. Teachers often respond to such pressures upon their sense of self by going underground or burning-out.

Students respond by either developing a habit of false compliance or dropping out. Every instance of manipulation instead of teaching is a choke point in the flow of schooling. Hesitations, confusions, fears, and angers develop. Enthusiasm is suppressed. In a top-down, bureaucratic system of schooling, curriculum and polices become toxic to the psychic and even physical health of students.

> Imagine yourself trapped within a work environment that made you feel dumb and inadequate frequently and systematically. How long would you put up with it? What if you had no choice—that the situation compelled you to bite your tongue and stay within the toxic environment? How would you deal with the stress? Drinking? Kicking the dog? Lashing out at convenient targets? Is it any wonder that many teachers and students feel ressentiment?

The cultural lack of empathy for the lives of so many of our students in our school system is a puzzle. To a great degree, the lack of anger at the damages generated by the system is explained by our cultural fixation on the easily measured. The soul murder going on is hard to either envision or measure. The loss of potential is likewise hard to comprehend and put a handle on. But how much of our failure of empathy is because of an intentional ignorance? Why are we not listening to our students and teachers like Gatto?

Jane M. Healy writes, in *Endangered Minds: Why Children Don't Think and What We Can Do About It:*

> The day's worksheets were distributed. Each day brought a new lesson, whether or not the students had understood the last one. This lesson consisted of a long list of complex analogies calling heavily on abstract verbal categorization skills. They were phrased in high school to college level vocabulary. . . . It soon became clear that most of the kids, whose tested reading abilities ranged mainly between third- and eighth-grade level, could not understand this assignment at all. Indeed, as I puzzled over some of the problems, I decided they would make challenging work for a group of graduate students.
>
> . . . . Soon the bell rang, the teacher unlocked her door, and the students left, convinced once again by their loving school system that learning was a mystery and they were all inadequate. I found myself admiring them for hanging in there for so long—and feeling within myself the rage that must impel violent acts.

Dr. Healy was in the classroom at the invitation of one of her graduate students, inner-city reading teachers, who were compelled to teach "thinking skills" to students who lacked ability to comprehend the assignments. They complained about being forced to install the program into the heads of students because of decisions made by absentee decision-makers. Healy: "Their major beef was that the program consisted of an extensive (and expensive) series of workbooks and worksheets that the students often did not understand—but that they were required to cover."

Here is an illustration of methods and materials emanating from an inaccurate operating metaphor. The best way to teach thinking is through a culture of inquiry and classroom conditions conducive to the emergence of conversation and reflection, one that utilizes projects of different kinds. A gavage mindset cannot coerce thinking into existence. It will, in fact, suppress thinking, as undoubtedly happened in the class observed by Healy. But the present definition of learning is blind to this truth about education for thinking:

> The emergence and habit of, and thus capability for, thinking requires a culture of self-governance, in both teachers and students—not a culture of gavage and regurgitation.

Thinking is what gives life to ideas, but the way we school makes ideas inert. Ideas are powerful motivators; it takes a systematic and systemic approach to drain the life out of them. But our educational system has done so because it has forgotten a fundamental reality about human development:

Growth

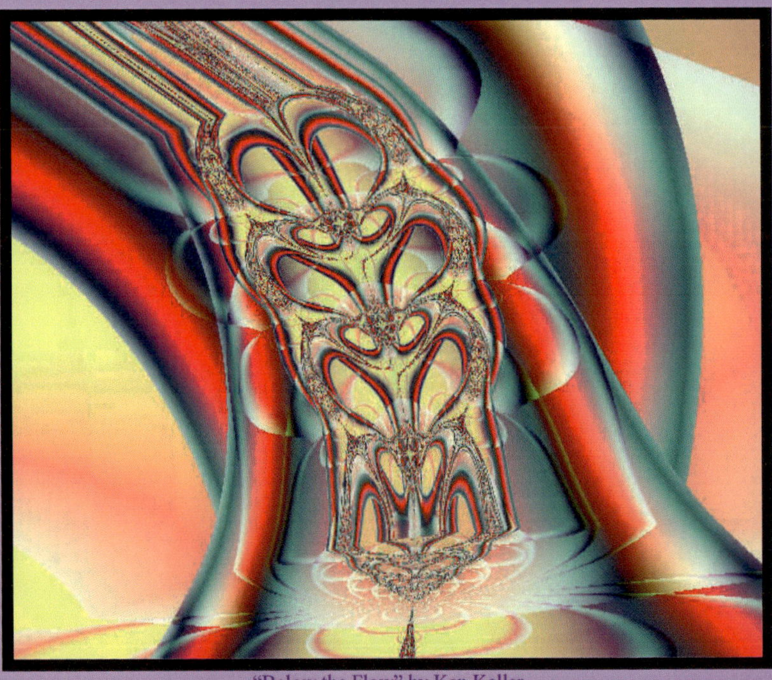

"Below the Flow" by Ken Keller

Emerges from the confluence of

Knowing—Thinking—Doing

Keller's fractal was inspired by the following poem:

***Below the Flow**

**Below the flow
Is where I know
I must go**

**Below the flow
Is where I know
I have seeds to sow**

**Below the flow
Is where I know
I must go**

**Below the flow
Is where I know
Life is not so shallow**

by savannah skye

The poem by Skye is a statement of protest against the superficiality of our times—which includes the sciolistic nature of our educational process. Keller's image captures that dynamic of going beneath the surface, getting below the flow, into the depths where things matter, where life is real.

Our present educational system has forgotten about the fundamental reality of growth emerging from the confluence of Knowing/Thinking/Doing because of an intentional ignorance about the human condition:

> The soul cares enough about only one thing to take note of its presence or absence. It measures nothing else: not success, not fame, not money, not even love. The only thing that matters to the soul is growth.

Success without—and especially at the cost of—growth hurts the soul. Fame is empty without it. Money is without value. Is even love, whether of self, another, or God, truly love if it is not growing? Even learning is harmful, if it is not entwined with growth. People know when they are not growing, when they are squandering their spiritual health and developmental potential—or having it squandered.

When Whitehead talks about soul murder, we should take him seriously. It is not hyperbole. What are we doing to our children? When we lock them into a system of learning without thinking and doing, we trap them on the surface of what learning is supposed to accomplish. We prevent growth, and in so doing murder souls.

Knowing is essential to growing—unless distilled to a toxic level—then it suppresses growth. Growing depends not just on knowing but also thinking and doing. Whenever one crowds out the other, growing is crippled. Real growth, not the delusion of growth resulting from the temporary memorization of data and the passing of tests, depends upon the thinking that establishes personal ownership of the knowledge and the doing that establishes personal capability and a sense of effectiveness, the using of knowledge.

Students know their souls are being disregarded, malnourished, and even murdered, as the phenomenon of ressentiment indicates, along with the explosion of special education needs in this country. They may not fully realize the problem and they may not be able to articulate their anger and anguish, but they resist and resent the process, and wish it were different. Mary Poplin and Joseph Weeres, in their book, *Voices from the Inside: A Report on Schooling from Inside the Classroom*, report the anguish of students at their school lives. One student succinctly answered a fundamentally important question asked by Poplin and Weeres in their study of life inside schools and classrooms:

> "What is the problem of schooling?"
>
> "This place hurts my spirit."

This student knew that his or her soul was in trouble. The student sensed that the schooling process was whittling away at his or her significance and potential. The student felt trapped, unable to effectively rebel. The odds are even high that this student was considered "successful" by teachers and administrators. Poplin and Weeres comment:

> Most students, particularly after fifth grade feel that many of their classes require them to learn or memorize irrelevant things they perceive are not connected to their lives. Even students who do well in school do so with little effort. They learn what they are told because it is easy for them to memorize and they are obedient. Other students actively resist attempts to get them to learn what they see as boring or irrelevant facts. Students who do not do well in school or for whom schools hold low expectations often experience even more routine and boring activities in remedial or basic classes.

Theodore R. Sizer, in *Horace's Compromise: The Dilemma of the American High School,* discusses Charles Silberman's *Crisis in the Classroom*:

> He argued that the students quickly learn what it takes to survive in school, and that it is to conform to what the system and its teachers want. "The most important strategy for survival is docility and conformity," Silberman asserted. "Docility is not only encouraged but frequently demanded, for teachers and administrators seem unable to distinguish between authority and power." The students accept the power. "The tragedy is that the great majority of students do not rebel; they accept the stultifying rules, the lack of privacy, the authoritarianism, the abuse of power—as The Way Things Are.

> A colleague, Peter Holland, recently told me [Sizer] that, if anything, the situation has worsened since the 1960s. "The schools may be anaesthetizing the students . . . There's not enough stimulus."
>
> Many schools are quiet, apparently happy, orderly, but intellectually dull. They are not provoking, stimulating places, and their students are not hungry. A Hamilton, Ohio, athletic coach is quoted to the effect that schools allow students "to practice stupidity as long as they don't become discipline problems. They get good at dumbness." David Seeley sadly sums up his view: "Education has become a massive process for producing passive minds."

A passive mind will not, cannot, grow, thus the soul dependent upon that mind is slowly suffocated and finally murdered by an educational system responsible for its growth. Passive learning, a fundamental characteristic of the present definition of learning, makes ideas inert and souls stymied. This is The Way Things Are in our schools.*

One parent who did not want his child suffocated in an inert atmosphere is Yong Zhao, who writes in *Catching Up or Leading the Way:*

> What really pushed me to abandon my original writing plan [about Chinese education] is what I've witnessed over the last few years: broad damage inflicted by NCLB as well as the growing enthusiasm for more standardization and centralization. Frankly, when NCLB was passed, I did not expect it to have much impact on what goes on in American schools, given my experience with past reform movements. Apparently, I was wrong.
>
> I was proven wrong by my son about five years ago. One day at breakfast he told me that he had figured out how to get a better score for his writing on the MEAP, the standardized testing Michigan uses to satisfy NCLB requirements. . . . My heart sank as he was explaining to me how he would improve his score. The essence of his strategy was to stop being creative and imaginative. Instead he would follow the scoring rubric, which was analyzed and taught by his teacher. Indeed his score improved the next round. Because of this experience and many others, we decided that it was best to move him to a school that was not governed by NCLB.

Most of the time, in too many classrooms, in too many schools, the conditions are stultifying, in the etymological sense of the word, "to make stupid." Stupidity is the absence of intelligence. When we suppress student—and teacher—initiative, we also suppress the heart of intelligence, for without initiative, problems have to be solved by others, and the passive mind has to be directed regarding what products to fashion.

*If the reader doubts any of these assertions, visit any public school, from kindergarten to university, and walk down the hallways. Glance in at the classrooms, take a moment to listen to the proceedings, and make a record of any indications of student initiative versus those of trainer-centered coverage. Alternatively, talk to some students known to you about their school days.

Is this what we want to accomplish in our schools? Do we want to perpetuate our fixation on the easily measured, even at the cost of hurting the democratic spirit and the souls of our children? What is the ultimate stupidity?

> In fact, the more inventive and creative capacity of students is "brutalized," the more they are simply being conditioned to accept "answers" to questions which have not been asked. The more students adapt to such a procedure, the more, ironically, it is reckoned that this is "productive" education.
>
> Paulo Friere

A Cautionary Voice

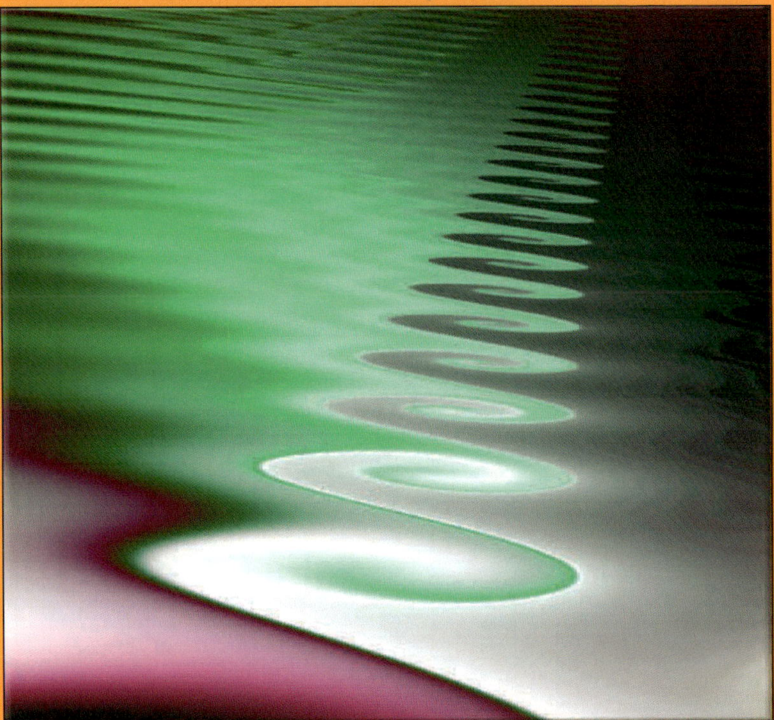

Fractal from www.matrixandmeaning.com/reviews/

What avail is it to win prescribed amounts of information about geography and history, to win ability to read and write, if in the process the individual loses his soul; loses his appreciation of things worthwhile, of the values to which these things are relative; if he loses desire to apply what he has learned and, above all, loses the ability to extract meaning from his future experiences as they occur.

John Dewey

Consider

On April 22, 1999—two days after two students attacked their high school in Littleton, Colorado, killing twelve students and staff, and, finally, themselves—the entire staff and student body of the Open School [five miles away in Lakewood] marched to Columbine High School to pay their respects and show their support. No other school in Jefferson County joined them.

One month after the Columbine murders, a group of Jefferson County principals and administrators met to discuss strategies to prevent such tragedies in the future. The questions of the day: How could this have happened in one of the most affluent school districts in Colorado? Why didn't we see this coming?

Columbine was a large high school. It was easy for students to get lost or hide out. Then there were the cliques: the Jocks, the Goths, the Stoners, and others. Some kids felt they were outcasts. Many felt that there was no sense of school community except for the pep rallies for the sports teams, which only about twenty percent of the school participated in.

How could these kids have gone so far? After all, they were not bad students. Perhaps they were ignored because they got good grades and performed well on the standardized tests. Did anyone really get to know these boys?

At the principal's meeting, the question was raised: do we have a model for some kind of counseling program that can reach all kinds of kids? Only one of the principals offered a response. The director of the Open School stated that her school had been conducting an effective advising program for thirty years. She added that every student had an advisor whose job was to get to know him on a deep, personal level. No one at the meeting took much interest in the advisor program, and the discussion went on to consider some packaged, formulaic counseling programs, It was as if to say that the Open School was an anomaly that had nothing to offer the real world of conventional schools and education.

The aftershock of the Columbine shootings rocked the foundations of the education system across the country. Most of the talk was about metal detectors and searches. Some debate involved parental responsibility. Little of the discussion involved the idea of personalizing the educational system and getting to know kids. In fact, if anything, there was a retrenchment to a back-to-basics, impersonal approach to education and schools. The social and personal domains were, once again, given little attention. The importance of relationships and community responsibility was pushed back into the closet.

In the days after Columbine, many parents were afraid to send their kids to school. High school students, fearing a copycat incident, stayed home in huge numbers. Tensions were high. Meanwhile, the Open School went on with its business of building a safe, nurturing community in which to learn. Students actually used the school as a haven. Kelly, class of 1999, wrote:

"I remember, the day after Columbine, I couldn't wait to go to school. I felt so safe and supported there. It felt like walking into my own living room with my family around a table. I don't think a Columbine could ever happen there. At the very least, we would have known something was coming because everyone gets to know each other so well."

Excerpt from *Lives of Passion: School of Hope: How one Public School Ignites a Lifelone Love of Learning*, by Rick Posner, PhD.

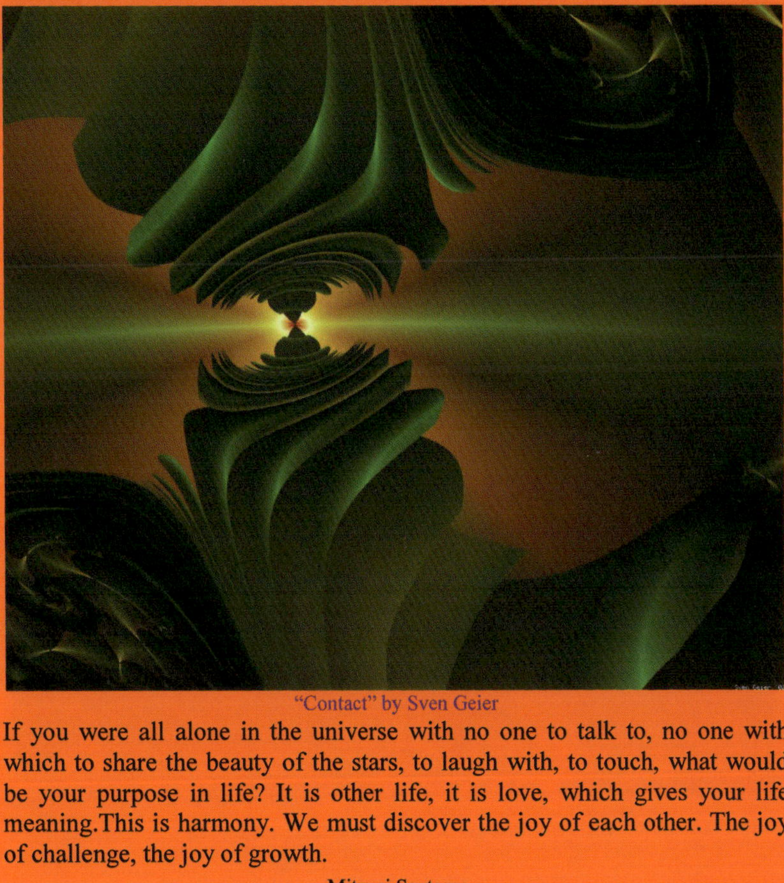

"Contact" by Sven Geier

If you were all alone in the universe with no one to talk to, no one with which to share the beauty of the stars, to laugh with, to touch, what would be your purpose in life? It is other life, it is love, which gives your life meaning.This is harmony. We must discover the joy of each other. The joy of challenge, the joy of growth.

Mitsugi Saotome

—46—

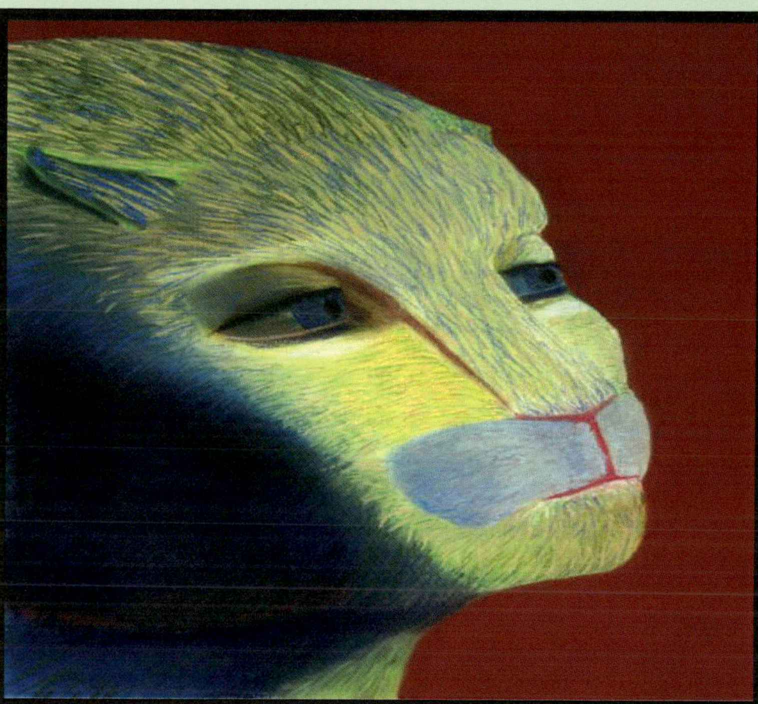

"Understanding" by James Williams

I believe that the United States could lead the world in achieving an entirely new educational aim: the design and implementation of an education that yields understanding.

Howard Gardner

Our schools are busy places. A lot goes on; much of it is meaningless noise and the wasted heat of resentment and resistance, but a lot is happening. Curriculum is applied frenetically. Students acquire, even if temporarily, the transmitted knowledge—or they busy themselves disrupting instruction. Much of what is happening is not learning related, at least not in a developmental, intellectual sense. Teachers and administrators assume that learning is occurring in classrooms where students are listening and teachers are talking. But understanding comes from a more contemplative space. Understanding more often comes from reflection and solitude, or through quiet discourse. Activity, no matter how furious or tightly regimented, is no substitute for the development of understanding.

In *The Unschooled Mind: How Children Think and How Schools Should Teach,* Howard Gardner writes about how schooling compels teachers and students to constantly make right-answer compromises to the cost of education for understanding:

> Teachers require students to answer preset kinds of problems, to master lists of terms, and to memorize and then feed back definitions upon request. They do not ask students to try to reconcile their earlier, partial forms of understanding with the notations and concepts of school; instead they deal only with the latter forms of knowing, hoping that students can later develop the reconciliation's on their own. Nor do teachers pose challenging problems that will force their students to stretch in new ways and that will risk failures that might make both teachers and students look bad.
>
> Neither teachers nor students are willing to undertake "risks for understanding"; instead, they content themselves with safer "correct answer compromises." Under such compromises, both teachers and students consider the education to be a success if students are able to provide answers that have been sanctioned as correct. Of course, in the long run, such a compromise is not a happy one, for genuine understandings cannot come about so long as one accepts ritualized, rote, or conventionalized performances.

Teachers who dedicate class time to encouraging "risks for understanding" get reprimanded when they fail to cover the required material. When students fail to (temporarily) memorize enough data, both they and their teachers are penalized. Teachers are always fearful of hurting their students. They know how the game is played. If they teach their students to make the necessary "right answer compromises," students will then pass the tests and proceed on down the pedagogical pipeline. If teachers instead teach for understanding, they may impede the academic careers of their students, for understanding is not easily measured. Virtually all tests are geared to measure correct answers, and both teachers and students suffer the systemic consequences of "diversions" into searches for understanding.

Teaching for understanding is therefore crowded out by focus on correct-answer schooling. The systemic result of this dynamic is the corrosion of the learning environment because teachers adopt the attitude of "defensive teaching" while students respond with "defensive learning." Constructivist teaching and learning become increasingly rare. Both teachers and students respond to a schooling environment that crowds out education for understanding with resentment and resistance. They withhold their commitment because the learning environment lacks, in Gardner's phrase, "educational inspiration." It therefore suppresses initiative, and then we puzzle over the lack of commitment and self-directed learners.

Reflection is a form of internal conversation, where parts of the self become alive in striving to puzzle together, to construct, an instance of learning that produces understanding. Reflection, as well as conversation, is a characteristic of engaged, self-directed learners. Reflection, however, is a habit and capability rarely supported by the present definition of learning. A personal story illustrates the role of reflection and engagement in constructive learning:

> Some years after finishing my doctorate, I had the opportunity to audit a class taught by the historian Max Lerner. Max was not only an esteemed historian but a good teacher. However, I was not really learning. I attended the classes, enjoyed the lectures and discussions, and took the occasional note. I had no problem with the subject, social transformation; I was certainly interested. I had no problem with the teacher; he was doing his job well. The problem was me; I simply was not really learning.
>
> Then one night Max delivered a particularly interesting insight. I don't even remember what it was, and that is not really relevant. What I do remember is my response to his insight. My reflection, curiosity, and desire to construct an understanding suddenly engaged, and I left the lecture, in spirit if not in actuality.
>
> For the next forty-five minutes, I did not hear a word uttered by Professor Lerner or anyone else. I was engaged with furious thinking and writing as I strived to pull together the fleeting, flitting insights drifting around in my mind into a new comprehension of this dynamic complexity called social transformation. Finally, feeling like I had managed to nail something to the wall (possibly jello but regardless, it was my construction), I closed my notebook and listened to Max end that evening's class. For the past forty-five minutes, I had really been learning.

The questions are: Can I allow this kind of learning with my students? If I can't, I should. Can I set up conditions in the classroom that generate such fierce engagement? Can I encourage reflection and conversation? And those personal questions can be transferred to our schooling in general. Can we school in such a way that fierce reflection and conversation is encouraged and informed?

The business world says that it needs people capable of such reflection and conversation. The future demands such capabilities. The issue is whether our schooling can provide them, bearing in mind that we must turn the present system on its head, forgetting top-down management, and not only allowing but encouraging and supporting the responsibility of teachers to establish learning communities in their classrooms.

Only through the capability and integrity of individual teachers, with their unique visions and voices, can we reconnect to our democratic principles. Only the teacher in the interactive maelstrom of a classroom, supported by trust and respect for their judgment and principles, can forge the necessary working relationships with their students to reach the critical mass of a learning community. Then we can have the conditions for the emergence of reflection and conversation, and for the individuality and responsibility necessary for a democracy.

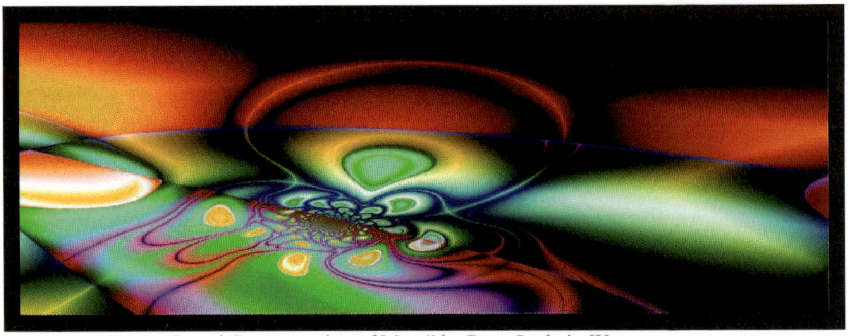

"Local Concentration of Mass" by Peter Ludwig Wegener

We become what we think—and talk—about. We build ourselves, or we fail to build ourselves. A redefinition of learning could help us take that leadership role suggested by Gardner, schooling that produces understanding. Learning redefined will have powerful and systemic impacts upon the methods and materials of our schooling. The process would cleanse itself of the poisons that now generate passive and bulimic learning and curriculum-damaged learners. As we bring concern for initiative back into the process, the development of understanding will naturally follow.

Understanding is a different kind of knowing, one more aware of the whole and its interactive variables. It comprehends that reality is not static but dynamically complex. With learning redefined away from the bulimic, static, and easily-measured image that now defines it, we could not only do more, we could become more, and we would be not only more excited but more responsible in the process. Conversations can turn us toward different definitions and different pathways—by helping us look at complicated matters from different perspectives as we turn them this way and that while striving to construct a new understanding. The redefinition of learning deserves a **National Conversation.**

The United States could lead the world in achieving an entirely new educational aim: the design and implementation of an educational system that yields understanding. Such an undertaking would be a huge systemic endeavor. However, since the task will be aligned with our democratic roots, there should be little philosophical resistance. There is a human need to think and behave in accordance with our most cherished values. The real problem will be the entrenched top-down power structures that unwittingly harbor socialistic operating metaphors regarding the educational process.

> For information to become knowledge, and knowledge to become wisdom, it has to integrate with what we know, has to become part of our personal "big picture." And that's not happening. The integrating process is "right brain," traditional schooling is "left brain." The left reasons, fragments, analyzes. The right intuits, combines, synthesizes.
>
> Marion Brady

—47—

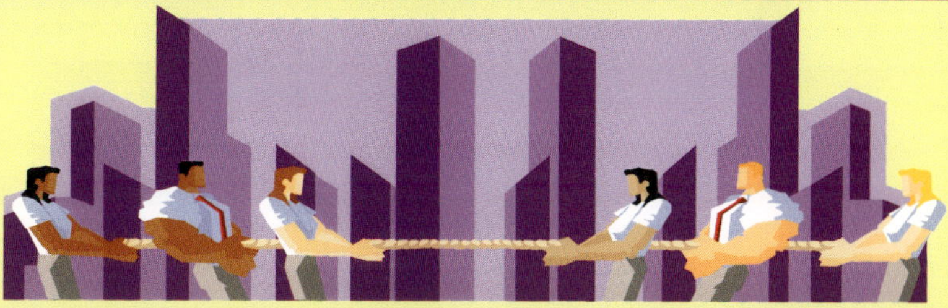

All the good-to-great companies had a penchant for intense dialogue. Phrases like "loud debate," "heated discussions," and "healthy conflict" peppered the articles and interview transcripts from all the companies. They didn't use discussion as a sham process to let people "have their say" so that they could "buy in" to a predetermined decision. The process was more like a heated scientific debate, with people engaged in a search for the best answers.

Jim Collins

Conversation—true conversation—is the way we cleanse poisons, such as false assumptions, prejudices, ignorance, misinformation, confusion, lack of perspective, lack of imagination, and stubbornness from the system. Conversation is how organizations self-correct themselves. Collins, in his extensive study of companies that transformed themselves from merely good to great were all characterized by robust conversations.

Susan Scott, in her book, *Fierce Conversations: Achieving Success at Work and in Life, One Conversation at a Time,* provides the insight that our lives succeed or fail one conversation at a time, courtesy of poet David Whyte. She then defines what she means by fierce conversation:

> But a fierce conversation? Doesn't "fierce" suggest menacing, cruel, barbarous, threatening? Sounds like raised voices, frowns, blood on the floor, no fun at all. In *Roget's Thesaurus,* however, the word *fierce* has the following synonyms: robust, intense, strong, powerful, passionate, eager, unbridled, uncurbed, untamed. In its simplest form, *a fierce conversation is one in which we come out from behind ourselves into the conversation and make it real.*
>
> While many are afraid of "real," it is the unreal conversation that should scare us to death. Whoever said talk is cheap was mistaken. Unreal conversations are incredibly expensive for organizations and for individuals. Every organization wants to feel it's having a real conversation with its employees, its customers, its territory, and with the unknown future that is emerging around it. Each individual wants to

have conversations that are somehow building his or her world of meaning.

Are we preparing our students to engage in the fierce conversations the work world is realizing is increasingly necessary for the production of accurate, imaginative, and comprehensive information? Passive learners will be at a serious disadvantage in the postmodern world. As we redefine learning and teaching, we will move from the image of presentation toward that of conversation in our schooling. Presentation generates memorization and regurgitation. Conversation generates engagement and contribution. Lecture will increasingly give way to genuine dialogue and real-world projects that demand conversation for successful completion.

The business world is increasingly aware of the importance of conversation. The education world will, ironically, considering that teaching and learning is its business, have to follow that developing awareness. After all, as the capacity for genuine conversation becomes increasingly necessary, the business world will pressure for graduates who have the initiative, responsibility, and emotional intelligence to effectively participate and contribute.

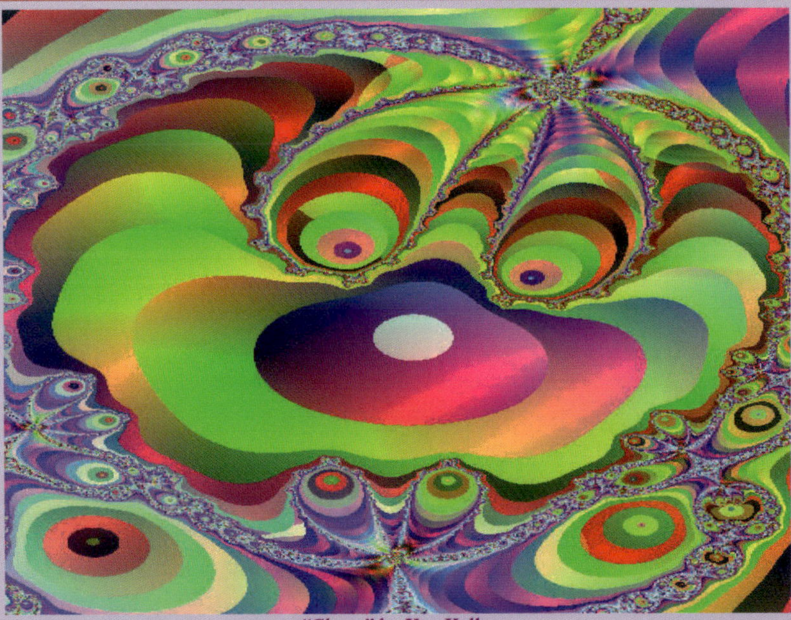

"Clown" by Ken Keller

Last year I gave a workshop to a large gathering of educators. In the evaluations, one participant thought it contained too much conversation and not enough presentation of facts. That evaluator, guided by the old image of learning, did not get my desire to encourage conversation. Where I thought I had succeeded, he or she thought I had failed and wasted his or her time.

When the poet Robert Frost taught at Dartmouth College, he once asked his students if anyone had written anything in their first assignment they could defend with passion. No one responded and Frost tossed all the papers into a wastebasket and left the room. We can imagine that this threw the students for a loop; after all, they had completed the assignment. But Frost applied a different standard; he did not want compliance and coverage but an intense conversation about things that matter.

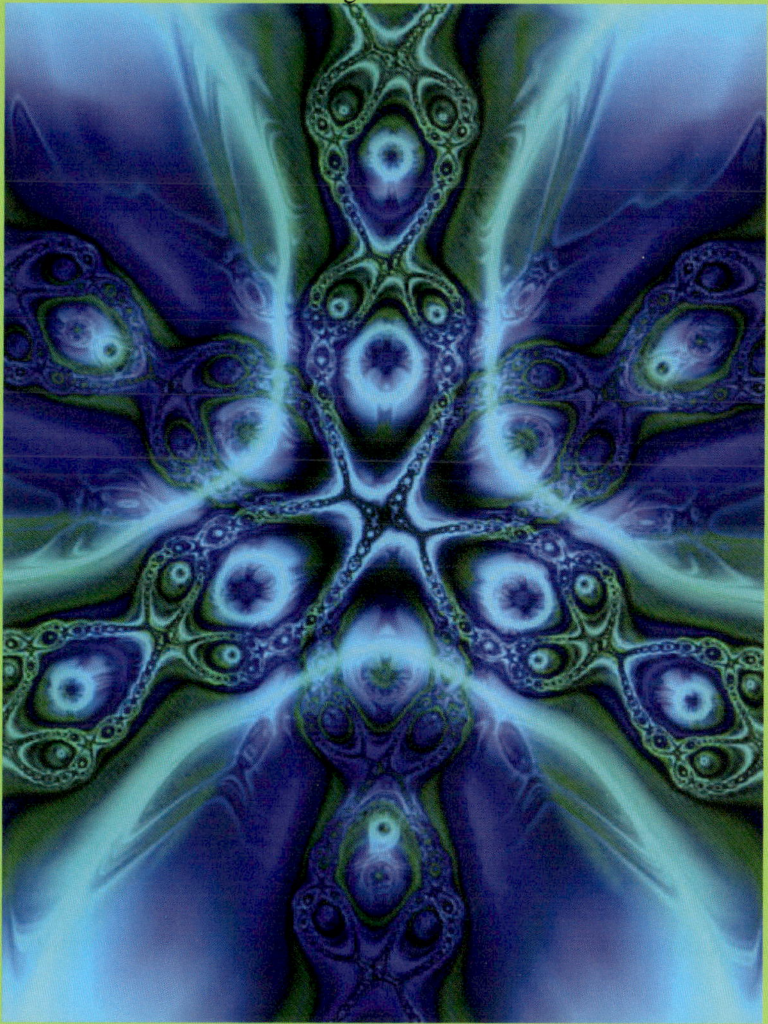

"Intersecting Paths" by Lori Ann Basile

Just as a picture is worth a thousand words, one thought is worth a thousand memorizations, and one conversation is worth a thousand coverages.

–48–

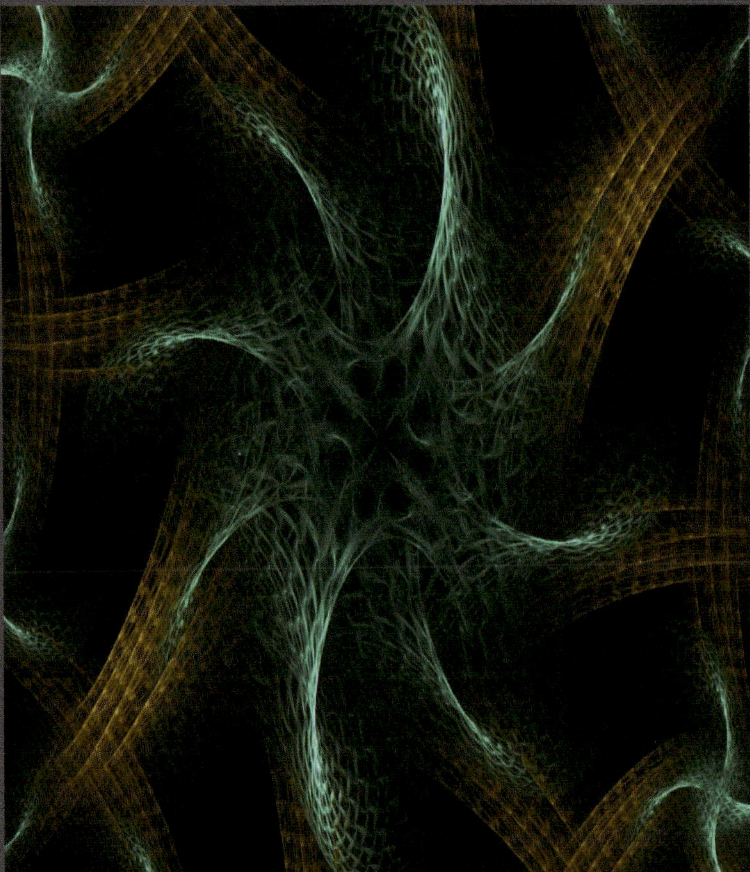

"Gordian Knot" by Lauren Zorn

I would not give a fig for the simplicity this side of complexity, but I would give my life for the simplicity on the other side of complexity.

Oliver Wendell Holmes

American education has increasingly channeled its capabilities into simplistic (even if detailed) answers to its predicaments. We have consistently placed our resources, and our hopes, in rigid manipulation schemes based on uncomplicated cause to effect connections. We chased after the conciseness and clarity of Occam's Razor, which in classical science is commendable, but in an interactive endeavor amounts to simplism, the reduction of problems to false simplicities by the ignoring of complicating factors.

It is a weakness to buy the simplicity on this side of complexity. It is the weakness that underlies ineffectiveness. It is the weakness that avoids responsibility. It is the weakness of intentional ignorance. It is the ultimate weakness, the weakness of intentional weakness: "I am confused and befuddled, so will somebody please take charge." Life is messy; denying that truth only results in worse messes, such as dysfunctional schools, and, eventually, fundamentalism and totalitarianism. But there is a simplicity on the other side of complexity. The economist William Brian Arthur comments:

> People [finally] realized that logic and philosophy are messy, that language is messy, that chemical kinetics is messy, that physics is messy, and finally that the economy is naturally messy. And it's not that this is a mess created by the dirt that's on the microscope glass. It's that the mess is inherent in the systems themselves. You can't capture any of them and confine them to a neat box of logic . . . The result has been the revolution in complexity. In a sense it's the opposite of reductionism. The complexity revolution began the first time someone said, "Hey, I can start with this amazingly simple system, and look—it gives rise to these immensely complicated and unpredictable consequences." Instead of relying on the Newtonian metaphor of clockwork predictability, complexity seems to be based on metaphors more closely akin to the growth of a plant from a tiny seed, or the unfolding of a computer program from a few lines of code, or perhaps even the organic, self-organized flocking of simpleminded birds . . . Complex, lifelike behavior is the result of simple rules unfolding from the bottom up.

Complexity Science, which can be thought of as the science of emergence, investigates those simple underlying rules that result in complex, lifelike behavior as they unfold. The trick is finding those underlying dynamics and understanding them. This is called systems thinking. Systems thinking can be thought of as the choice to not kill and cut up the elephant, to instead leave it alive and whole and moving. Peter Senge writes:

> Sometimes people go ahead and divide an elephant in half anyway. You don't have two small elephants then; you have a mess. By a mess, I mean a complicated problem where there is no leverage to be found because the leverage lies in interactions that cannot be seen from looking only at the piece you are holding.

In a curious irony, the mess of our educational system is the result of our seduction into simplistic, supposedly unmessy, reductive answers. The simplicities are seductive because they avoid the messiness of developing understanding. Ignorance of reality, however, does not protect people from the messiness of reality; it only makes them less effective and more vulnerable. But messiness in the educational process, a messy situation if there ever was one, has been systematically ignored. Here, we need to remember Aristotle's comment that "Teaching is the highest form of understanding." The understanding he was referring to is systemic wisdom, the simplicity on the other side of complexity.

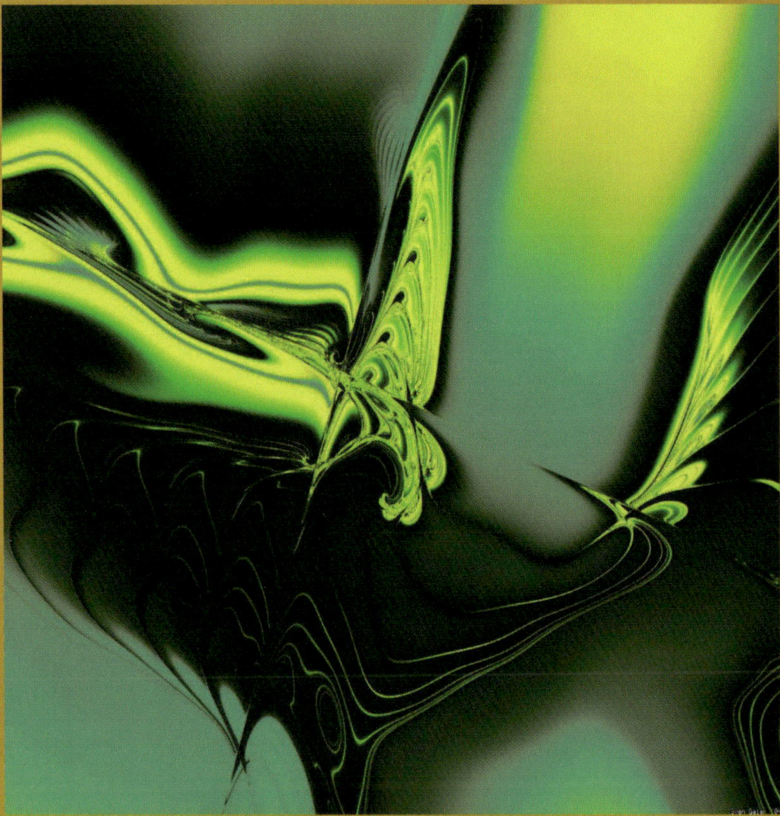

"Release" by Sven Geier

An Example of Systemic Wisdom: One fourth-grade teacher created a simple tradition in her classroom that will give rise to immensely complicated and essentially unpredictable consequences. If a student impresses her enough with a unique observation or an original thought to get her to say, "Now, <u>that</u> is interesting!" he or she gets a special prize. This is an example of the simplicity on the other side of complexity. The teacher's systemic wisdom in rewarding originality instead of only correct answers is a condition for encouraging inquiry, initiative, and individuality.

A colleague related an experience in her doctoral work which illustrates a reductionist-based allergy to the complexities of classroom realities. Her grade for a course in Change Theory was lowered by the professor because she did her project in an "unsimulated" format; that is, in a real high school. Actual situations, as we well know, have a bad habit of disrupting the "appropriate" sequence of change activities. Instead of rewarding my colleague for diving into an actual situation, however, the professor dinged her grade.

My idealistic colleague ran afoul of a cultural mindset which did not respect, much less cherish, her desire to investigate the actual confusion of real-life teaching and learning. The professor wanted the simplicity on this side of complexity, because it is so much easier to measure. The cultural message to stay focused on approved elephant parts is clear and constant to students in most graduate programs, "Keep your head down and don't look around, you'll only get confused."

Our problems are not simple, they are interactive, complex, and systemic—so the answers will not be simple. However, when we forge a way through the complexity instead of avoiding the chaos points, we will find leverage points that make us more effective. Our solutions must emerge from understanding the system—or they will only compound the problems. We need to find the simplicities on the other side of the complexities, for then a renewed respect for the art of teaching will develop.

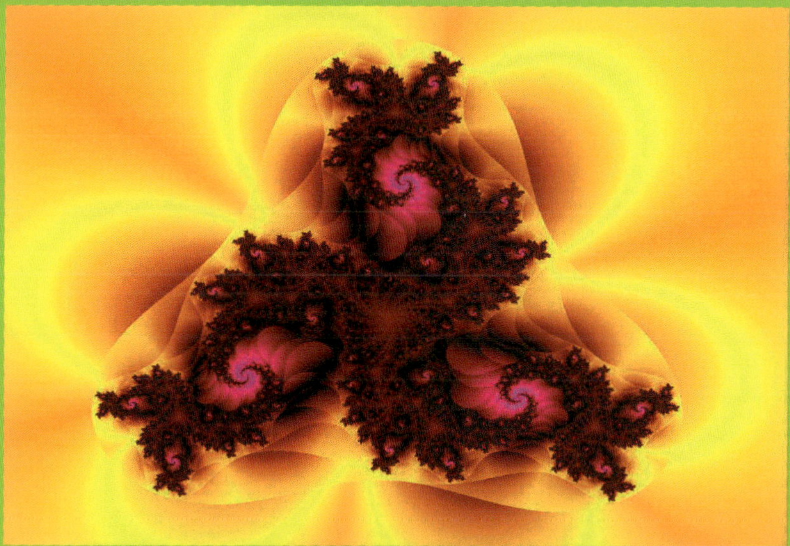

"Elusive" by Kerry Mitchell

Complicating factors are best uncovered by conversation; only then can they be dealt with. Research, even if reductive in nature, can be helpful in that endeavor, but not if it is constantly presented as the answer. **Conversation, the metaphorical equivalent of the corpus callosum, uncovers truths and develops understanding.** It weaves together the evidences and insights of the left and right brains in order to get through the complexity to find the simplicity on the other side. We need to become more scientific in our educational process. While the education world is fixated on knowing and knowledge regurgitation, the scientific world focuses on a better dynamic:

Conversation—Self-correction—Contribution.

The Quarterback Problem

Malcolm Gladwell, in his article "Most Likely to Succeed" writes about the quarterback problem in the NFL. The issue is recruitment from all of the outstanding candidates. The problem is that competence at the spread offense common at college-level play does not transfer well to the much faster, more dynamic professional level. The NFL is simply much more cognitively demanding. All potential candidates are given an IQ test, but the test is useless as a predictor. Low scorers frequently go on to The Hall of Fame. Professional teams pay seriously big money to scouts and consultants to help them make their multi-million dollar decisions. But they run up against this truth, as Gladwell states: "A prediction, in a field where prediction is not possible, is no more than a prejudice."

The NFL has a quarterback problem—it cannot figure out who will succeed.

Teachers are the quarterbacks in their classrooms. They determine whether learning and thinking and contribution occur—or not. They establish winning teams, with the emergence of learning communities, that effectively deal with disruptive factors—or fail to do so. A good teacher, even in a poor school, is the most important variable in the educational dynamic. However, teaching certificates, graduate degrees, or any other time and energy consuming credentials are useless for predicting success. Gladwell writes:

"After years of worrying about issues like school funding levels, class size, and curriculum design, many reformers have come to the conclusion that nothing matters more than finding people with the potential to be great teachers. But there's a hitch: no one knows what a person with the potential to be a great teacher looks like. The school system has a quarterback problem.

". . . . In teaching, the implications are even more profound [than in financial advising and professional football]. They suggest that we shouldn't be raising standards. We should be lowering them, because there is no point in raising standards if standards don't track with what we care about. Teaching should be open to anyone with a pulse and a college degree—and teachers should be judged after they have started their jobs, not before."

What endeavor is more pressure upon the capacity to deal with dynamic complexity than teaching? Perhaps a football game can hold a candle to it, for sixty minutes. Perhaps a general is comparable to a teacher, during the confusion and fog of a major battle. Teacher education should be an apprenticeship program, and the only coursework should be The Predicaments of Teaching—the search for the simplicities on the other side of the complexities.

Teaching is like writing;
each teacher must find his or her own way of being successful.

—49—

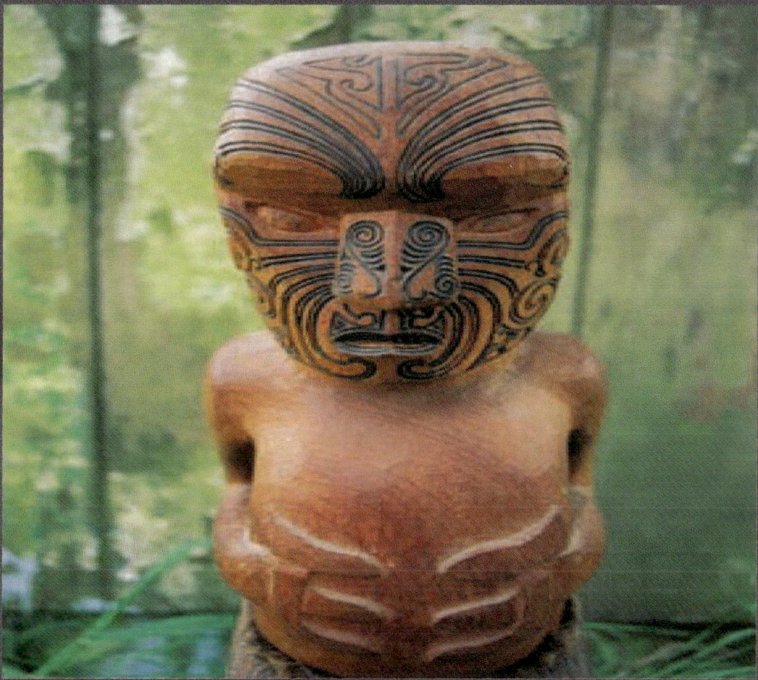

Cultures are defensive constructions against chaos, designed to reduce the impact of randomness on experience. They are adaptive responses, just as feathers are for birds and fur is for mammals. Cultures prescribe norms, evolve goals, build beliefs that help us tackle the challenges of existence.

Mihaly Csikszentmihalyi

Cultures are necessary. Otherwise, there would be too much confusion.. They provide us with structures for living. They teach us what to value—and what not to value. Cultures can be helpful. They can also be bad for us. They can suppress necessary innovation by a knee-jerk insistance on the status quo. They can blind people to potential by controlling the parameters of perception. We can become blinded by the rays of yesterday's light. This is especially dangerous in the world of The Red Queen, as Winston Churchill warned us over sixty years ago:

> We are shaping the world faster than we can change ourselves, and we are applying to the present the habits of the past.

The present culture of schooling:

—images learning as the passive acquisition of transferred curriculum.

—sees teachers as "curriculum implementation specialists" or "knowledge transmission technicians."

—envisions students as products of the educational assembly line.

—perceives the successfully taught student as one sufficiently crammed with easily-measured knowledge bits.

—assesses only a minor part of the learning dynamic, memorization of knowledge bits (even if temporary).

—defines intelligence as that which can be evidenced by IQ tests.

—suffers from scientism, the undue worship of science, that compels it to formulate prediction and control machinations based on supposedly scientific investigations.

—is socialistic in metaphor and methodology; the process therefore suppresses democratic principles.

We need new norms, different goals, and revised beliefs in our schooling. A new definition of learning will be the cornerstone of an educational culture that is an adaptive response to our challenges and opportunities.

We need a culture of schooling:

—that defines learning as constructive rather than acquisitive, as active rather than passive.

—that perceives a balance between initiative and training as necessary for a healthy educational process.

—that understands the importance of imagination to the learning process, and reinvigorates the arts back into our schools.

—that sees teachers who too often stand in front of class lecturing as probably not good teachers.

—that recognizes disorder instead of order in students sitting quietly and taking notes.

—that understands the systemic evils of the pernicious, ubiquitous, and pervasive tests.

—that weans itself from distribution of correct answers to education for understanding.

—that replaces the image of presentation with that of conversation.

—that comprehends teaching as an interactive art dependent upon initiative, emotional intelligence, and professional responsibility rather than the mechanistic application of prediction and control methodologies.

—that envisions teachers as professional practitioners who should be supported in their development and autonomy, and held responsible for their judgment and initiative.

—that images intelligence as the capacity to solve problems and fashion products, period, with all the dynamic complexity such a definition entails.

—that realizes democratic principles must be modeled instead of just preached.

Learning that is not symphogenetic, that fails to fuse ideas as they are born into developing intellects, is not neurogenic. It can be worse than wasted effort when it is a condition counterproductive to our aims, when it perpetuates a mistaken definition of learning, when it excites resentment and resistance to the learning process. Nourishment designed only for the left brain, no matter how strenuously gavaged, will not become fused into the whole. Symphogenetic education requires both sides of the brain acting in concert—a strengthened corpus callosum, the place where training and initiative weave and dance.

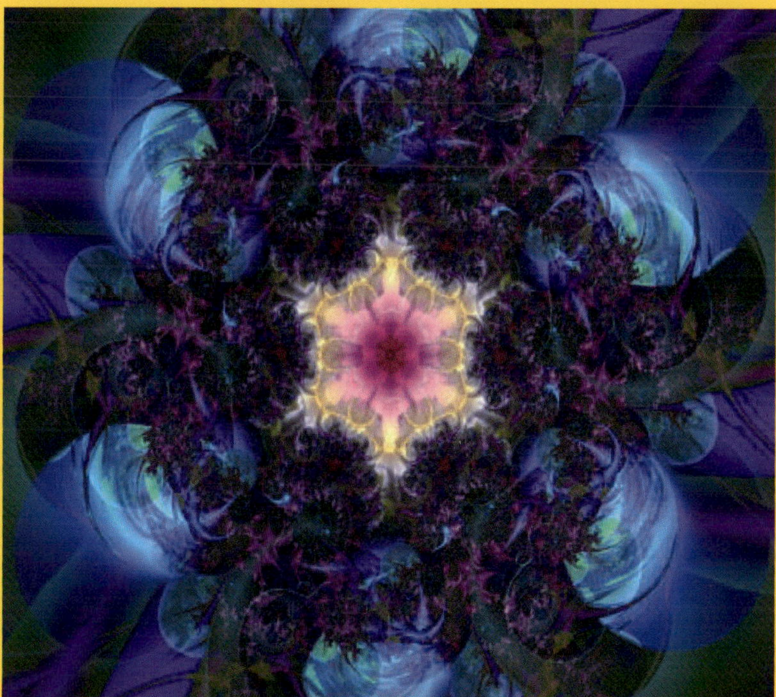

"Essence of Light" by Lori Ann Basile

Education's best claim is that it teaches a person to value what deserves to be valued.

William James

—50—

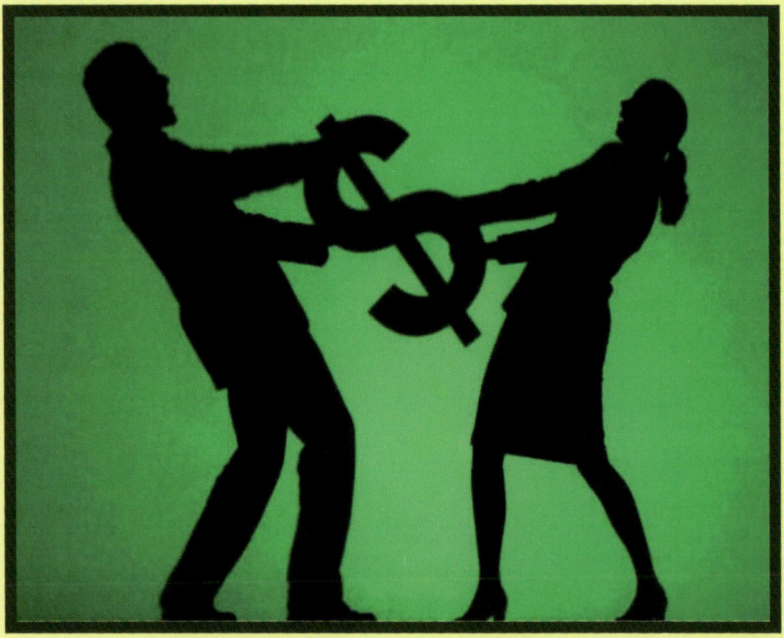

Every budget is a moral statement.

Assessment drives instruction, and defines learning and governs teaching. Schooling is geared to assessment. It's as simple as that. What we care enough about to measure, and through the measuring, judge, determines the process. The systemic questions are: what are we measuring and why, and is this truly what we value? Every budget is a moral decision, whether it is the budgeting of money, time, or effort. Every budget rests on a matrix of philosophical underpinnings. Assessment determines policies, the delivery plans developed to produce the results we aim for. But there is danger in assessment: the pressure is to see comprehensively and clearly. An immature assessment can easily generate immature policies. It is analogous to parents, feeling frustrated, barking at their children, who, after reassessing the situation, realize that their frustration was misdirected (for it was caused by conditions at work) and they owe their children an apology.

This nation was challenged to respond with maturity to the 911 situation. We failed. Our assessment settled on an inappropriate target, Iraq, a nation that had nothing to do with the attack. As a result of that immature assessment, we developed policies—delivery plans—that embroiled us in a costly, misdirected war. We expended our budgets of money, effort, time, as well as credibility in a delivery plan based on a faulty assessment.

So we need to examine our budgets, whether they consist of money, time, or effort. Are we accomplishing what we truly wish to accomplish? Are we solving the real problems confronting and diminishing us? How can we best meet the challenges and opportunities before us? Most importantly, what about the clarity and comprehensiveness of the assessments guiding the budgets? Is it not immature of us to fixate on the easily measured? Isn't that analogous to kicking the dog when we are mad at the boss? The easy target is rarely the most appropriate.

We need to reassess our assessment strategies.

In what ways are we ignorant of systemic realities in our present assessments? How can we best measure the not so easily measured? How can we assess an increase—or decrease—in interest, initiative, or imagination? What about factors such as courage, ownership, and responsibility? What about intellect, integrity, and judgment? Should all these factors be ignored since they are so hard to assess? How can we best determine the effectiveness of education for right-brain capabilities? Or should we continue the present course, one fixated on the assessment of left-brain capabilities—and the ignoring of essential but hard to measure factors—regardless of the consequences? Isn't assessment of the easily measured short-sighted and immature, analogous to the proverbial Smiths considering themselves successful because they have obtained all the biggest and best status symbols?

These are not fairly asked questions. They are biased in structure and intent. But we have systemically ignored the hard-to-measure for too long. If we are to muster the intelligence to meet the challenges and opportunities of the future, then we better get our budgets in order. Educators and politicians frequently talk about the importance of factors such as imagination, character, and integrity. So what? Do our schools reflect those values? Is money, time, or energy allotted to their instruction? The true values and principles of individuals and organizations are always accurately reflected in their budgets. Therefore, those factors are not valued, regardless of words to the contrary.

The systemic problem preventing allegiance to our democratic principles is our addiction to the easily measured. Standardized assessment strategies compel socialistic methods and materials. This is how training crowds out initiative, for it is so easily assessed (and its transmission supervised). This also explains why we ignore educating for the right-brain and fixate on the left-brain. We need to look carefully at the effectiveness of the educational process. In what ways are we systemically ineffective, and even wrong-headed? We are dumbing ourselves down—through our assessment strategies.

Are we truly winning the war against ignorance, incapability, and prejudice? Are we cleansing such poisons from the social body? The tests say so, but we should be suspicious of their assertions. The tests are addicted to the easily measured, the congelated knowledge bits that align so comfortably with curriculum and assessment. What can be easily quantified are rarely the truly important variables.Andrea Batista Schlesinger, author of *The Death of Why: The Decline of Questioning and the Future of Democracy*, writes in the Fall 2009 issue of *Yes* magazine:

> Schools increasingly focus more on the answer than the question. Teachers are deemed successful if their students answer exam questions correctly, not if they can think critically. Science, civics, art, and other inquiry-based subjects get pushed aside in favor of subjects that are more quantifiable. This is a profound irony, considering that what society needs from citizens, and what business needs from workers, is the ability to inquire, analyze, and discern.

Because questions disrupt coverage and therefore test-taking, they are budgeted out of the curriculum. But, as Schlesinger reminds us, “We’re not just teaching content, we’re not even just teaching skills. We’re teaching habits of mind.” Right there is where we are killing the geese that lay the golden eggs: the capacity to question, for critical thinking, is essential for productivity and democracy in a dynamically complex world. And our schooling considers educating that capacity disruptive to its definition of assessment.

Robert McNamara, as the Secretary of Defense for much of the Vietnam War, was the high priest of perceiving only numbered aspects of reality. For him and his minions, we were winning the war. The numbers proved it. And much of America believed them. Such factors as the tonnage of bombs dropped supposedly outweighed the dedication of North Vietnam, and the lack of belief of our allies, the South Vietnamese. How could such spiritual factors overcome our overwhelming numerical superiority? The issue is—they did. The real question is why we would think otherwise. McNamara belatedly realized that while numbers give us power, they demand a heavy price. They disconnect us from ecological realities. They separate us from the world of actual experience. In what has come to be known as The McNamara Fallacy, years later he wrote:

The McNamara Fallacy

The first step is to measure whatever can be easily measured. This is OK as far as it goes. The second step is to disregard that which can't be easily measured or to give it an arbitrary quantitative value. This is artificial and misleading. The third step is to presume that what can't be measured easily really isn't important. This is blindness. The fourth step is to say that what can't be easily measured really doesn't exist. This is suicide.

One of the reasons our educational system is so ineffective is that our understanding of human development is simplistic. Psychology decided, over a century ago, to focus its energies and capabilities on only what could be assessed, and therefore predicted and controlled. This necessitated a simplification of what it meant to be human. Anything that couldn't be easily defined and measured was simply excluded from the calculations. Jonah Lehrer, in *Proust was a Neuroscientist*, writes:

> . . . Modern psychology turned its back on William James' view of the mind. A "New Psychology" had been born, and this rigorous science had no need for Jamesian vagueness. Measurement was now in vogue. Psychologists were busy trying to calculate all sorts of inane things, such as the time it takes for a single sensation to travel from your finger to your head. By quantifying consciousness, they hoped to make the mind fit for science.
>
> William James didn't think much of this New Psychology. He believed that its reductionist approach had lost touch with what reality *felt* like, privileging the mechanics of the brain over the "infinite inward iridescences" of the conscious mind. The fashionable obsession with measuring sensations neglected the fact that every sensation was perceived as part of a whole process of thinking.
>
> . . . The New Psychology that William James fiercely resisted didn't last very long. The brain failed to disclose its subtle secrets, and psychology grew bored with measuring the speed of the nervous system. By the 1920's, scientists were busy trying to empirically explain the mind from the *outside*; the brain had become a black box. This new approach was called behaviorism. According to the behaviorists, behavior was everything. There was no idea, belief, or emotion that couldn't be restated in terms of our actions. The world consisted of stimuli to which we responded, like animatronic machines.

The mind was too dynamically complex, too full of "infinite inward iridescences" for psychologists to deal with scientifically, so it had to be excluded from study. It became a black box, analogous to ancient maps where cartographers categorized unknown, and perhaps unknowable, territories with the caution "There be dragons." The mind, since it was beyond easy measurement, had to be ignored. Don't go there, practitioners were constantly warned, at the peril of professional suicide, because they will only become lost and confused, and destroyed by the dragons of the impossible to measure.

The McNamara Fallacy explains why Tony Wagner, in *The Global Achievement Gap: Why Even Our Best Schools Don't Teach the New Survival Skills—and What We Can Do About It,* writes:

The skills needed to be a successful knowledge worker today continue to evolve and grow in importance everywhere—except in our schools.

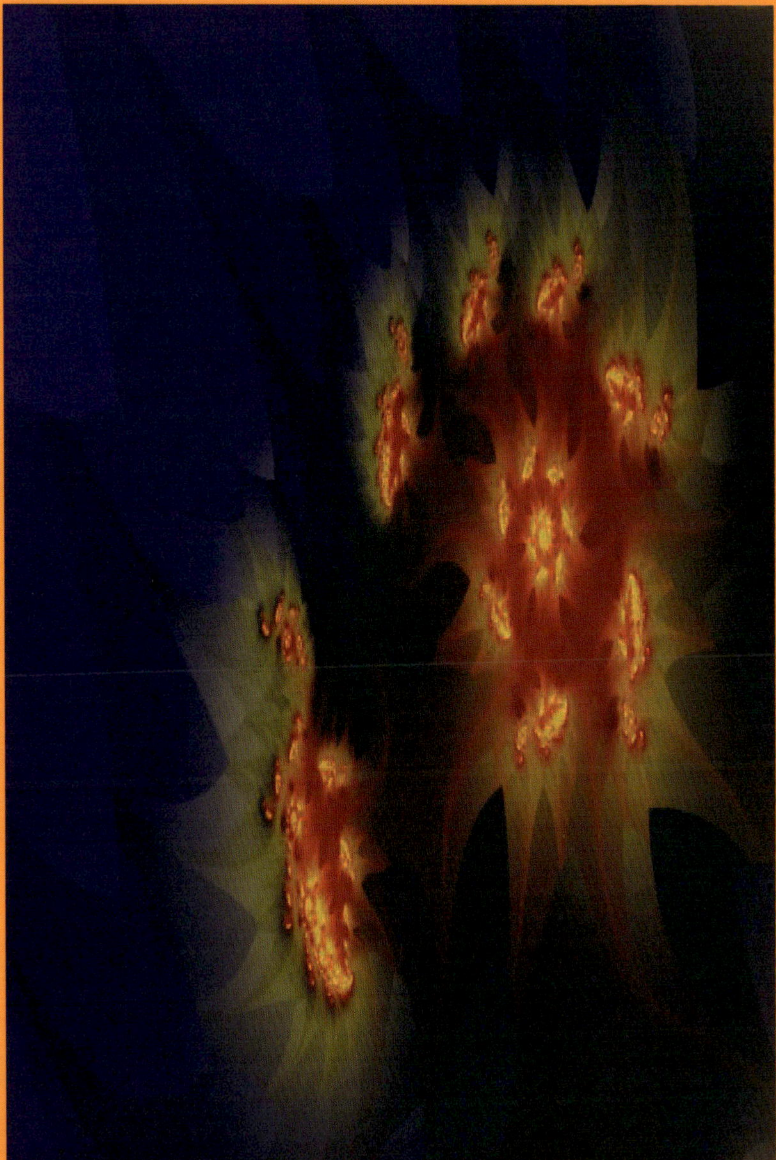

"Dousing the Embers" by Brett Szymik

If we keep treating our most important values as meaningless relics, that's exactly what they'll become.

Michael Josephson

–51–

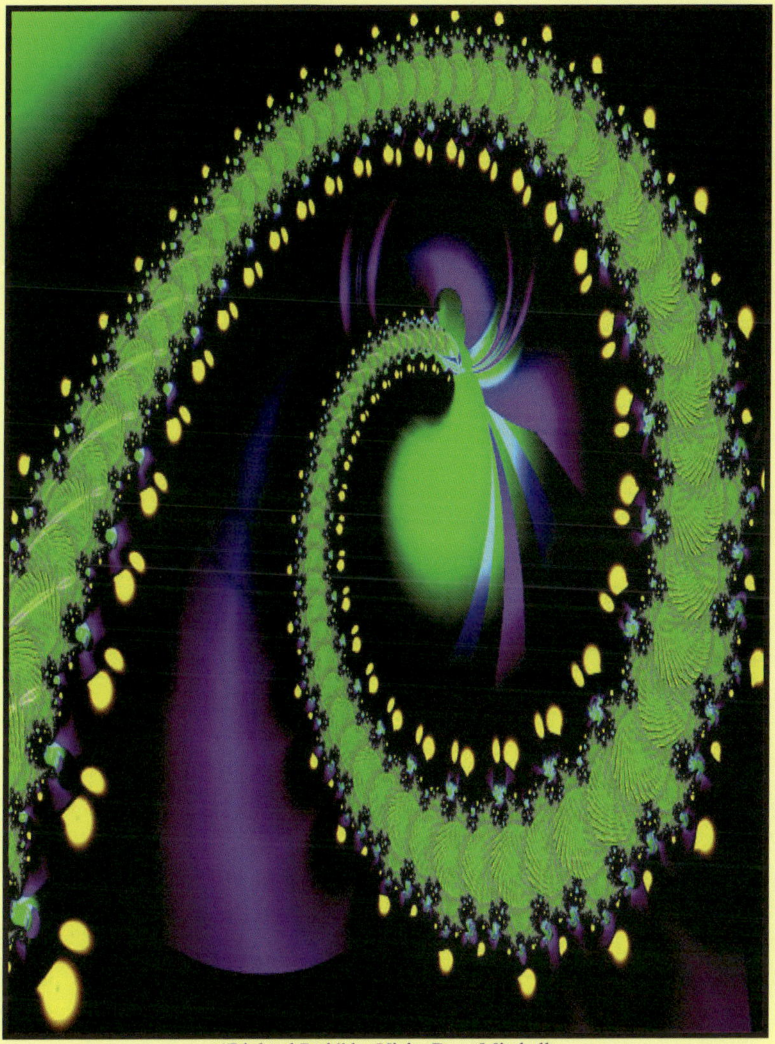

"Lighted Path" by Vicky Brag-Mitchell

We are at the very beginning of time for the human race. It is not unreasonable that we grapple with problems. But there are tens of thousands of years in the future. Our responsibility is to do what we can, learn what we can, improve the solutions, and pass them on.

Richard Feynman

We can reasonably hope that Feynman is correct, that our time does stretch far into the future, but that is not necessarily so. A lot depends upon that race between education and catastrophe pointed out by H. G. Wells. Will we succeed in effectively responding to the problems and possibilities of the future? We are presently busy educating for capabilities needed for the Industrial Age. Is that wise at this point? The real questions are these:

- **Can education educate itself out of its blindnesses?**
- **Can the educational process correct itself like science?**
- **If not, what then?**
- **How would it be redesigned?**

We are often blinded by the rays of yesterday's light. We see things as they were. It is so much harder to see things as they are—and even harder yet to see things as they will be. Michael Maccoby, in his book, *The Leader: A New Face for American Management,* investigated the values on knowing between Harvard doctoral graduates in the natural sciences and literature. He writes:

> One of the questions we asked was "What do you think it is necessary to know in order to get a Harvard Ph.D.?" We found a dramatic difference between the answers of natural sciences and doctors in literature. The natural scientists all said, "There is nothing special one needs to know in order to get a Ph.D. in physics, biology, or chemistry. Rather, a Ph.D. needs to prove that he can contribute to knowledge. The fewer requirements [of congelated knowledge bits] the better." In contrast, the Ph.D. in English literature or languages all said, "Yes, no one should get a Ph.D. from Harvard who does not know . . . ." However, each of them put in a different requirement. One said that everyone should know Chaucer, another said that everyone should know Shakespeare, the Romantic poets, or James Joyce. The humanities have become bureaucratized, interest groups defending their turf, rather than a force for deepening our understanding of human values.

This habit of orthodoxy construction permeates the educational endeavor. It percolates down from the universities to federal and state departments of education, and from there down to school districts. A body of "best practices" is determined and a bureaucracy is developed to govern its implementation. A knowledge base is also developed and prescribed, full of easily-measured knowledge bits. Turf battles, the striving for position rather than either understanding or contribution, characterize the educational process.

Science is itself more careful in not letting knowledge production crowd out the possibility and potential of understanding. It prevents the pursuit of disconnected facts and the construction of knowledge silos from crowding out holistic wisdom. Education, however, is, in its current design, not a self-correcting process but the opposite, a self-embedding process. It digs deeper into its assumptions.

Delta Willis, in *The Sand Dollar and the Slide Rule: Drawing Blueprints from Nature,* quotes the geologist Dolf Seilacher, winner of the Crafoord prize, which is given by the Swedish Academy of Sciences to honor research in areas not covered by the Nobel Prize:

> Science is not about being right or wrong. It is about understanding more, and we learn much more if we put our heads together in the field.

Seilacher not only preached but practiced this principle. With the prize money, he further investigated one of his pet theories in a trip to Australia, Namibia, and the Andes. He invited another scientist to accompany him, all expenses paid, even though he held an opposing view of his pet theory. Such metaphoric inclusiveness is not unusual in the scientific world. It is often customary to invite scientists from different disciplines to important meetings. The "included others" help generate out-of-the-box thinking. Such practice not only encourages the emergence of creative perspectives and approaches, it discourages the rigidity of orthodoxies.

The embedded value of developing concretized knowledge beds results in an infestation of academic tribalism in our universities, especially in the so-called schools of social sciences. Orthodoxy, one of the strongest enemies of the scientific spirit—and that of the artistic spirit as well—dominates our schooling. A systemic disorder of progressive intellectual parochialism takes root and crowds out holistic perspectives and ecological considerations. Orthodoxy is especially distrustful of the right brain, for it is too nonlinear, intuitive, and out-of-the-box. The tendency to self-embed rather than self-correct is why neuroscience has trouble educating the profession about the nature of learning. Common sense has never been able to break through—but it is now buttressed by neuroscience.

Feynman, a Nobel Prize winning scientist, has the optimism borne of a lifetime of involvement in a self-correcting process when he says "our responsibility is to do what we can, learn what we can, improve the solutions, and pass them on."

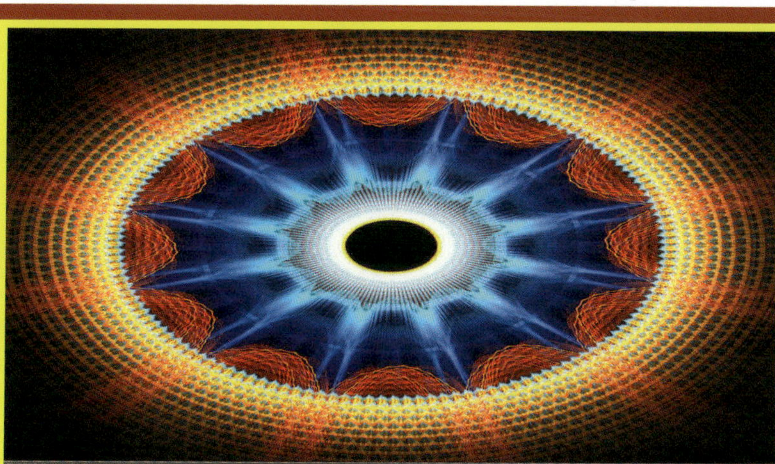

"Round and Round" by Exper Giovanni Rubaltelli

Science discards operating metaphors that prove either inaccurate or ineffective. But, can education?

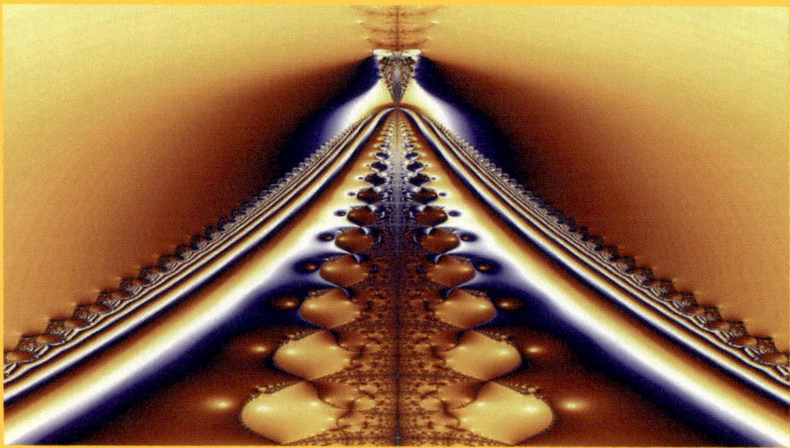

"Tower of Babel" by Lauren Zorn

We pursue preservation. But the old order is doomed. We value permanence. But "permanence" is the last refuge of those with shriveled imaginations.

Tom Peters—*Re-imagine: Business Excellence in a Disruptive Age*

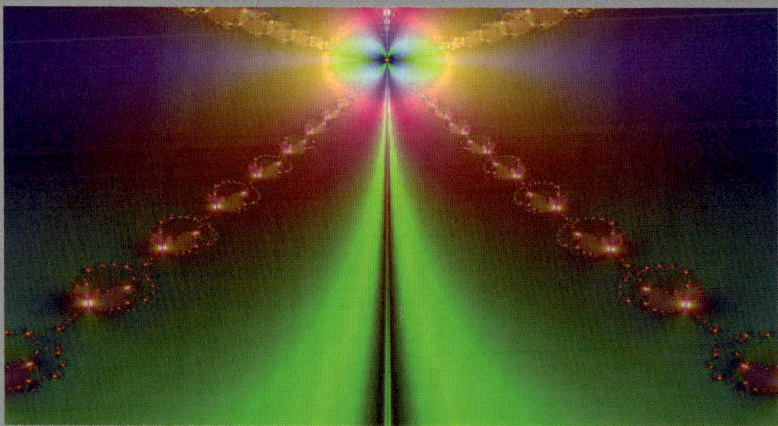

"The Way to the Higher Consciousness"from realeoni's photostream

Across many different realms, there's a growing recognition that spirituality—not religion necessarily, but the more broadly defined concern for the meaning and purpose of life—is a fundamental part of the human condition. Indeed, our capacity for faith—again, not religion per se, but the belief in something larger than ourselves—may be wired into our brains. Perhaps not surprisingly, this wiring seems to run through the brain's right hemisphere.

Daniel H. Pink

If we can escape our orthodoxies and refrain from falling back into our previous addiction to them, then education can become a self-correcting process like that of science. We can learn to pay attention to the possibilities and problems of our operating metaphors. We must, if we are to outrun catastrophe, if we are to deal with the dancing, rubbery terrain of The Red Queen World.

One thing is clear, we need to educate for the right-brain, not to the exclusion of the left-brain, but in addition to, for we need both sides of our brain if we are to attain a holistic approach to our problems and potential. Pink recognizes that we will need more right-brain capabilities for the Conceptual Age:

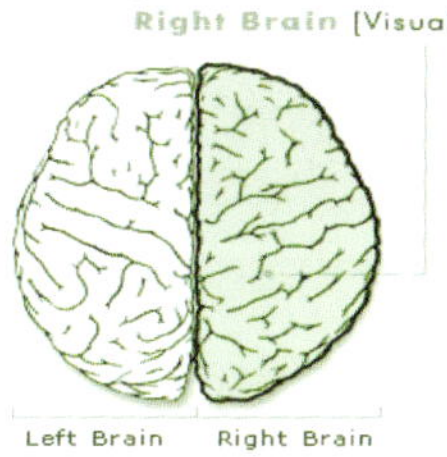

> Scientists have long known that a neurological Mason-Dixon Line cleaves our brains into two regions–the left and right hemispheres. But in the last 10 years, thanks in part to advances in functional magnetic resonance imaging, researchers have begun to identify more precisely how the two sides divide responsibilities. The left hemisphere handles sequence, literalness, and analysis. The right hemisphere, meanwhile, takes care of context, emotional expression, and synthesis. Of course, the human brain, with its 100 billion cells forging 1 quadrillion connections, is breathtakingly complex. The two hemispheres work in concert, and we enlist both sides for nearly everything we do. But the structure of our brains can help explain the contours of our times.
>
> Until recently, the abilities that led to success in school, work, and business were characteristic of the left hemisphere. They were the sorts of linear, logical, analytical talents measured by SATs and deployed by CPAs. Today, those capabilities are still necessary. But they're no longer sufficient. In a world upended by outsourcing, deluged with data, and choked with choices, the abilities that matter most are now closer in spirit to the specialties of the right hemisphere–artistry, empathy, seeing the big picture, and pursuing the transcendent.

The right-brain does not retreat into categories; it goes wherever its interest, or the truth, may lead. This is good for us spiritually, for it protects us from fundamentalism, which is when spirituality becomes frozen in fear and set in a close-minded, self-embedded, constricted, and brittle integrity.

To question is to have faith in the sanctity of truth.

–52–

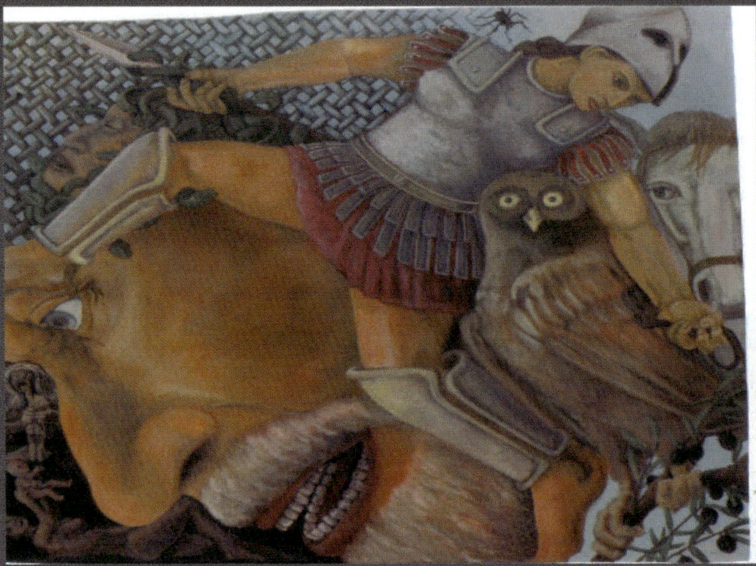

"The Birth of Athena" by David Curtis

In a complex world, mastery of metaphor—a whole-minded ability that some cognitive scientists have called "imaginative rationality"—has become ever more valuable. Each morning, when we rise from our slumber and flick on the lights, we know we'll spend much of the day paddling through a torrent of data and information. Certain kinds of software can sort these bits and offer glimpses into patterns. But only the human mind can think metaphorically and see relationships that computers could never detect.

Daniel Pink

The notion of scientifically managing the educational endeavor is ailing. The socialistic operating metaphor guiding American schooling has never been aligned with our core democratic values. Our teachers and students have known, in their hearts, that something was amiss, even if they couldn't fully realize or articulate it. The systemic costs are accumulating and escalating. Resentment and resistance, in both our teachers and students, are increasing. Formulas of manipulation are reaping a growing atmosphere of mistrust and disconnection. The social mental health of many of our schools and classrooms has diminished to the level that worthwhile learning is a rarity and even safety cannot be assumed. The paradigm of programmed instruction has generated a progressive disorder that is reaching systemic collapse.

Schooling cannot continue under these conditions. Worse ramifications will emerge if we don't change them. It is our responsibility to understand and establish the conditions in our schools (and in our homes and communities) that generate both learning and maturation. Leonard Shlain, in *Art and Physics: Parallel Visions in Space, Time and Light,* writes:

> To help the ailing Zeus [suffering from a throbbing headache], Hermes brought another god, who placed a wedge on Zeus' brow and, with a sharp blow of a hammer, cleaved his forehead. From out of this central fissure sprang the goddess Athena, full-grown and dressed in armor, without infancy, childhood, or any rite of passage to adulthood.
>
> That Athena was the goddess of wisdom meant she was the goddess of learning from trial and error and combining past knowledge with intuition to predict future outcomes. Wisdom is synonymous with good judgment. It is based on experience that integrates information from both the right and left hemispheres [of the human brain].
>
> . . . According to Greek myth, wisdom, in the form of Athena, came into the world because of the mythological hemispheric lateralization of the single most potent god. And who among all the gods and goddesses did Hermes summon to wield the wedge and hammer that split Zeus' brow? None other than Prometheus, the god of forethought, the only god capable of such radical neurosurgery. . . . The god whose name means forethought midwifed the birth of wisdom.

The potent god of science is now being cleaved into two hemispheres of concern and capability. Newtonian physics is making room for quantum physics. Neither supersedes nor negates the other; together, they constitute our best pathway toward wisdom and capability. This postmodern Prometheus will not create another Frankenstein for it will not forget about the magic of life, the synergy of the whole. It will help us gain organic cohesion in our educational perspectives and practices by melding the capabilities of new science and its imagination and concern for dynamic complexity with classical science and its focus and concern for the practical and measurable. Learning Redefined invites the organic nightingale into our schools and classrooms.

Education, at the confluence of all human endeavors, is, in its best spirit, a Promethean task. Our profession has become too closely identified with the characteristics of Apollo, a serious, humorless warrior who had stolen the gift of prophecy from Pan. But Apollo has turned out to be a false prophet, for despite all the testing and assertions of achievement, increasing numbers of our students either drop out or fail to learn essential capabilities. Apollo has his strengths, but we cannot depend on him to the exclusion of the other gods.

Knowledge synergized by meaning constructs understanding and leads us toward wisdom. It is time we turned toward making sense of what we are teaching and learning. When we fixate on facts and neglect inspiration, we are allowing the coldness of Apollo to crowd out the fire of Prometheus, which, after all, was given to him by Athena. When we suppress initiative in a flood of training, we are allowing Prometheus to be bound to the rocks. We must not forget that it was Prometheus who set us free from the machinations of the gods, who gave us imagination and free-will, who gave us the spirit that carries forth the democratic experiment. We need both Apollo and Athena. The ways of Apollo have generated too many systemic poisons and must be balanced with the wisdom of Athena. Education must become the hammer and wedge of Prometheus, setting Athena free and alleviating the throbbing headache of Zeus.

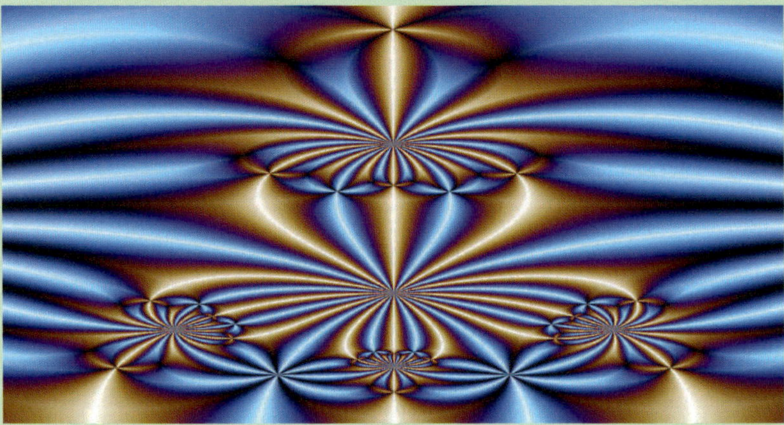

"Fountain" by Kerry Mitchell

The plasticity of the brain, and thus the mind, is greater in children and the young than in the older. But an essential characteristic of people we deem wise is a greater plasticity in their operating metaphors. In the gathering of their experience, they have learned that there is always "more than one way to skin a cat." They have felt the patterns change, the ground shift beneath their feet: forced by the pressures of life to change their images, their visions about life and themselves. They have seen certainties come and go, within cultures and within themselves—but manage to maintain curiosity, courage, and kinetic stability. The psychologist/philosopher James Hillman, in his book *The Force of Character and the Lasting Life*, discusses the work of Sherwin B. Nuland: "For every decade after age fifty, the brain loses 2 percent of its weight. . . . Yet parallel with this rapid deterioration of substructures, something else is going on: The higher intellectual areas of the cerebral cortex have a significantly lower degree of cell disappearance. . . . It may even be that the fewer neurons increase their activity. . . . Recent research suggests that certain cortical neurons seem actually to become *more abundant* [my italics] after maturity. . . . the filamentous branchings (dendrites) of many neurons continue to grow in healthy old people. . . . Neuroscientists may actually have discovered the source of the wisdom which we like to think we can accumulate with advancing age."

Closure

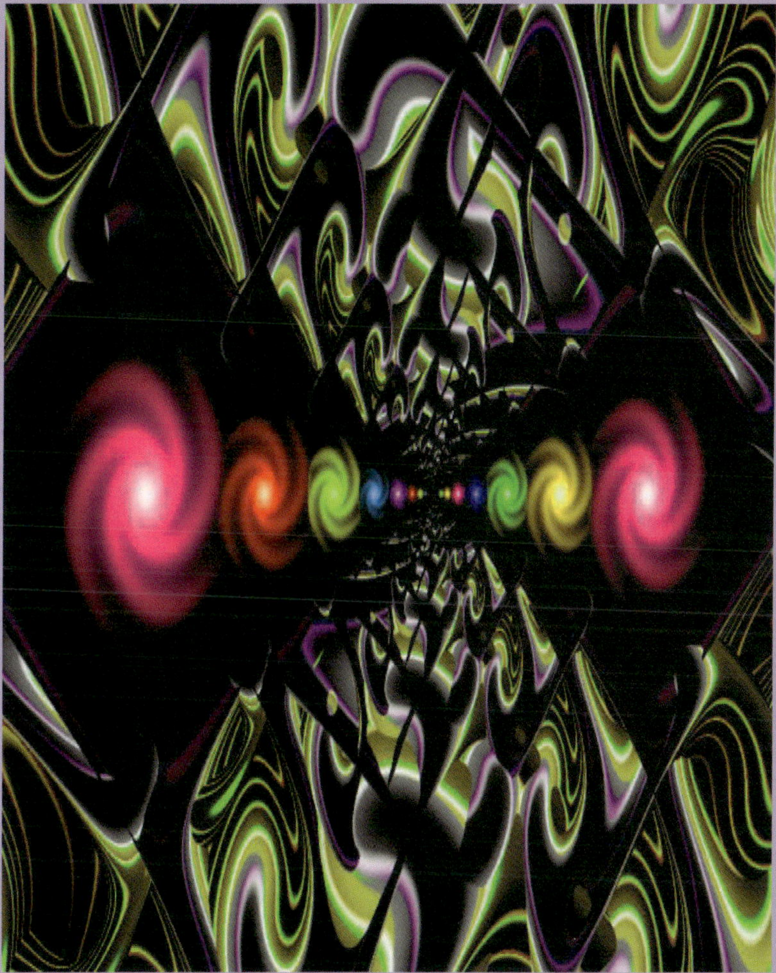

"Order from Chaos" by Ann Coffey

The left and right brain agree that order is necessary. But the left brain accepts the order as given while the right brain searches for new order. Thus a little chaos is also necessary. The left likes training while the right prefers initiative. Both are required, but, as the poet Paul Valery warned us: **There are only two things to fear: order—and disorder**.

Hopefully, these vignettes contribute to the ongoing conversation regarding the nature of learning past and learning future. What will be our new definition of learning?

–53–

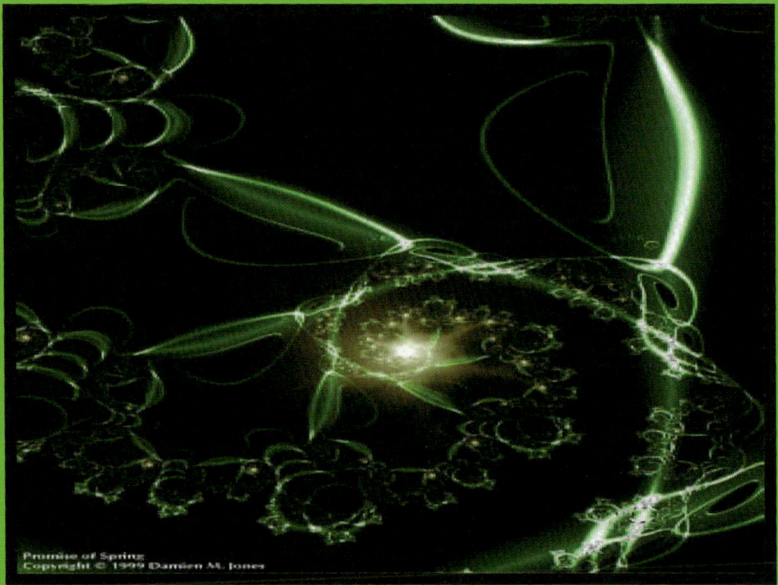

"Promise of Spring" by Damien M. Jones

God bless the grass that grows through the cement.

Malvina Reynolds

What Can We Do?

The cement is how we school our children: through incessant lecture, top-down driven curriculum, and the ubiquitous, standardized tests—all based on top-down, bureaucratic, centralized management—generally referred to as **Socialism**. The **Grass** is the teachers, administrators, citizens, and students who perceive not only the waste of time but the damage to our potential as a nation caused by the current system.

We can be the grass that grows through the cement. We have the responsibility, as citizens of a democracy, to grow through the procedures and policies dictated by a socialistic education system. We, as teachers, administrators, concerned community members, and students can start with the power of the question: **Do we not, as American citizens, have the right to question?**

Students, hopefully with the support of teachers, family, and community, should understand that they not only have the right, they have the responsibility to question. If educators complain that students do not know how to question, then students should demand to be taught to question with perspective and purpose. If the education managers complain that questions disrupt curriculum and testing, then they should be challenged to answer why they value curriculum and testing more than the concerned questions of its citizens. We should not allow anyone or anything to squelch the power of questioning, for it is the most powerful tool for the learning mind—and it is essential to democracy.

This is what we can do: WE CAN QUESTION and insist that our questions are answered. The curriculum and the tests are important—but questions are much more important—especially about the curriculum and tests. Questions express and inform interest, imagination, initiative, and responsibility. The democratic student insists on schooling responsive to her questions—so that he can establish ownership of who she is and will be. Everyone needs to learn how to read, write, problem-solve, and think, but questioning is the best way of learning any of those. The unquestioning student is a passive learner—who cannot shoulder the responsibility of democratic citizenship.

> Questions, and the conversations resulting from them, are essential to the democratic process, and the best way to learn anything. Each question is a chip away at the cement of the socialistic system of curriculum-control and standardized testing. Each question is an expression of initiative, imagination, interest, and, most importantly, ownership and responsibility.

Malvina Reynold's blessing should become the rallying motto for the challenge to bring initiative back into our schools. With initiative comes questions and conversations; both prevent hardening of the educational process. Questions not only free the imagination, they generate effectiveness and ownership, for the individual free to question is also free to innovate and, most importantly, choose responsibility and allegiance. Despite all of the accumulated, socialistic concrete, George B. Leonard, as he expressed in his book, *Education and Ecstasy,* believes there is hope for our schools:

> And yet, life and joy cannot be subdued, The blade of grass shatters the concrete. The spring flowers bloom in Hiroshima. An Einstein emerges from the European academies. Those who would reduce, control, quell must lose in the end. The ecstatic forces of life, growth, and change are too numerous, too various, too tumultuous.

New economic realities (always at the core of historic changes) demand more initiative, and thus creativity and real learning. Also, the growing ressentiment in our students and teachers indicates a free-floating resentment, that, if given direction, could dismantle the socialistic structure of our schooling suddenly and dramatically. But for right now, we can muster forth the guerilla power of questions against the cement of centralized control. Alfie Kohn, in *The Schools our Children Deserve*, writes:

> Deborah Meier and her colleagues . . . have anchored their teaching in what they call five "habits of mind." They contend that the study of virtually any topic in any discipline will benefit from raising questions about *evidence* ("How do we know what we know?"), *point of view* ("Whose perspective does this represent?"), *connections* ("How is this related to that?"), *supposition* ("How might things have been otherwise?"), and *relevance* ("Why is this important?"). The last of these, nominated by Meier as the one that matters most, recalls the response "Who cares?" It is a stimulus for adults to think about what matters enough to teach and an organizing principle for thinking (with students) about how to teach it.

Armed with these questions, students, along with teachers and administrators, can disrupt the metaphors, methods, and materials presently governing the process. Every question asked, every conversation that unfolds, is movement toward the redefinition of learning.

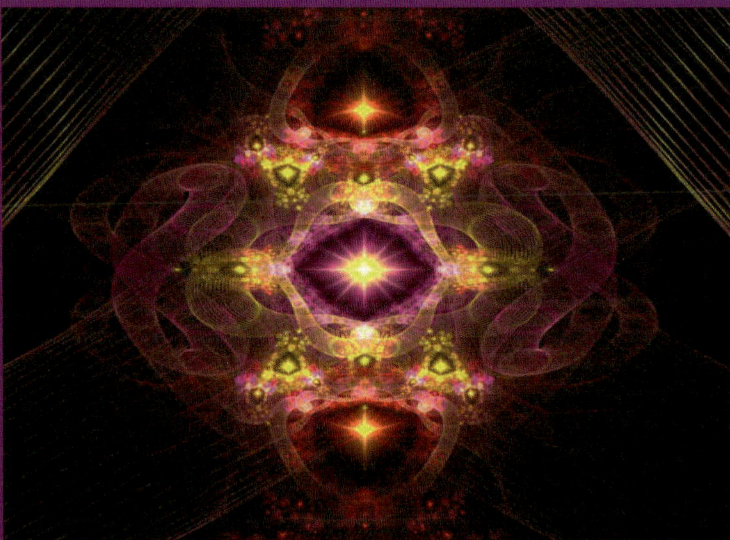

"Hope" by Colourinside

Human existence, because it came into being through asking questions, is at the root of change in the world. There is a radical element to existence, which is the radical act of asking questions. At root human existence involves surprise, questioning, and risk. And because of all this, it involves actions and change. Bureaucratization, however, means adaptation with a minimum of risk, with no surprises, without asking questions. And so we have a pedagogy of answers, which is a pedagogy of adaptation, not a pedagogy of creativity.

Paulo Freire—*Learning to Question: A Pedagogy of Liberation*

In *Catching Up or Leading the Way,* Yong Zhao writes: "Since 1997, Singapore . . . . has engaged in a major curriculum reform initiative. Titled *Thinking Schools, Learning Nation,* this initiative aims to develop all students into active learners with critical thinking skills and to develop a creative and critical thinking culture within schools. Its key strategies include the following:

- Explicitly teach critical and creative thinking skills.
- Reduce subject content.
- Revise assessment modes.
- Place greater emphasis on processes instead of on outcomes when appraising schools."

Zhao talks about how South Korea, China, and Japan are developing the conditions conducive to grass growing through the cement. These nations, and a few others, strive to redefine learning, teaching, and schooling—while we cram more content and tests.

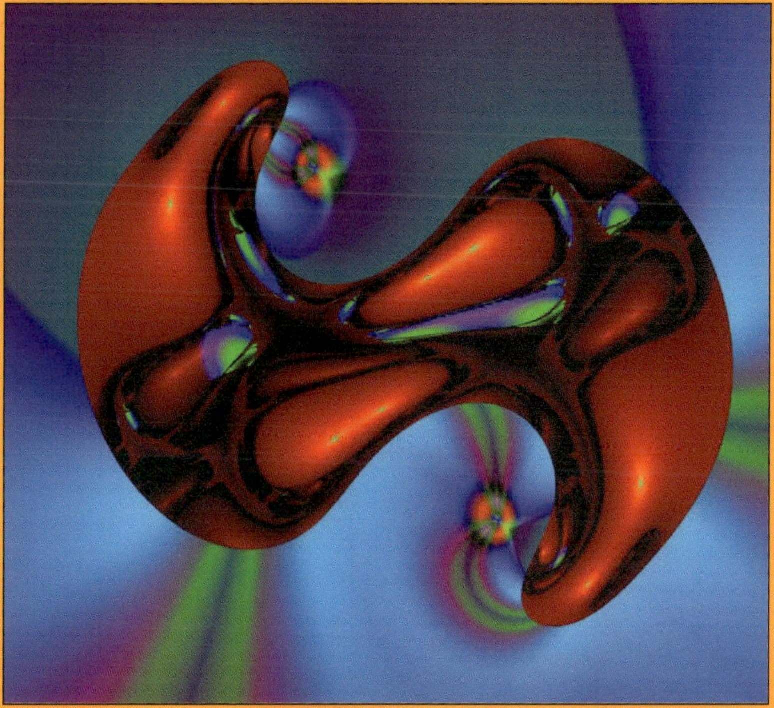

"Chrysalid" by Cameron O'Phee

A Cautionary Thought—The necessary growth need not happen in this country. Learning does not have to be redefined in American education. The grass can grow somewhere else—where conditions are more hospitable to the democratic ideals necessary for its cultivation.

–54–

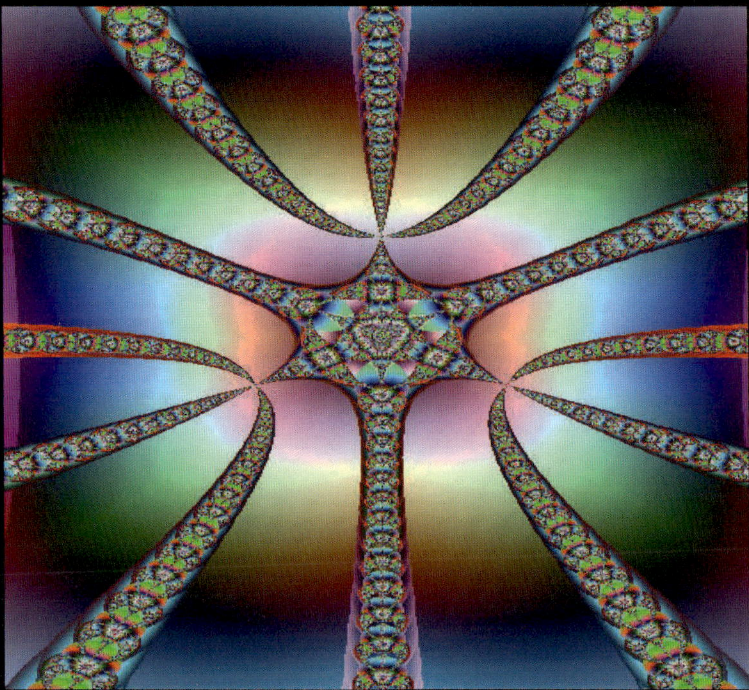

"Touch" by Ken Keller

The most powerful agent of growth and transformation is something much more basic than any technique: a change of heart.

John Welwood

Whenever students arrive at a classroom, make their way to their seats, and compose themselves sufficiently—or not—for the lesson, a question either arises or has already been answered: What is the agenda of the teacher? They know, or think they know, the answer. It may be to cram them with more stuff for the tests, to protect their own behinds, to control student behavior, to somehow do away with the days until they get to summer break or retirement. Or the agenda may be to inspire the students with the teacher's love of the subject, to excite them to think, to become engaged, to ask questions, to explore the nature of their potential. Students know when teachers are there for them—or when they have another agenda.

Agenda is the foundation of any meeting, formal or informal. We forget that at our peril. The question of agenda is a philosophical one. We ask, "What is on his or her mind?" and "What are they trying to accomplish?" and "What is really going on here?" Such questions are answered by our understanding of what is in their hearts. Trust is reliance on another's integrity, and who can trust the agendas of people with their hearts in the wrong place? And without trust, credibility does not exist—so the meeting is either a waste of time and energy or, worse, further incitement of resentment, resistance, and mistrust.

A frequent arrow thrown at the heart of philosophy is that "it bakes no bread." This is short-sighted perception, fed by a lack of systemic wisdom. Ultimately, all bread is baked by philosophy—on a daily basis, in every cultural nook and cranny. As the economist Lord Keynes pointed out earlier, underneath whatever dominant theory governs our present economic behavior lie the value-decisions of dead economists—their philosophies. The question of agenda is the search for the operating metaphor guiding the heart of the speaker or teacher, and the question then arises whether it fits in with the agenda of the participant. Philosophy underlies every interaction, either supporting or suppressing its purposes and potential. Philosophy—since it is the inherited (or lack thereof) personal and cultural wisdom—bakes all bread. Philosophy establishes and defines the practicalities of everyday life.

The premise of this book is that many of our problems ultimately derive from philosophy, the agendas set by the operating metaphors guiding learning, teaching, and schooling. We need to reset the agenda, in ourselves as individuals and within the culture of the profession. We need to change our hearts—as well as the heart of the system that currently perceives the endeavor of schooling as a top-down management exercise geared toward standardized assessment. At this point in time, anything other than the education of our hearts is a waste of time and energy, a Sisyphean endeavor, a systemic stupidity. We don't need more stuff about techniques or curricula, we need a fundamental change of heart, of understanding, values, and intentions.

There is no need to get better at what we shouldn't be doing. As the famous marksman Davy Crockett said,

"Be sure you are right, then go ahead."

We, as individual practitioners, too often let the proverbial "they" control the agendas and dynamics of classrooms and schools through standardized tests and set curriculum. In our hearts, we know that the socialistic top down mandarins should not have so much control, but it has become such an entrenched status quo that it is hard to imagine otherwise. So we allow ourselves to become lost in the practicalities set by the agendas of others. So we get better and better at doing what we really don't want to do—that are not aligned with either our perspectives or our values, with our philosophies.

Here is the secret to changing American education:

In a democracy, we the citizens set the agendas.

It is <u>our</u> philosophies, <u>our</u> operating metaphors, that should determine the methods and materials—not those of top down bureaucrats in the state or national capitals. As David Mathews of the Kettering Institute reminds us: "We citizens are not customers of government—we own the store." It is time we started acting like proprietors instead of customers limited to the metaphors, methods, and materials provided by centralized command and control centers.

Teachers are, by the nature of their profession, pragmatists. They must find or create the most effective ways of being successful at a very complicated endeavor. There is nothing wrong with pragmatism. It is, after all, an American-bred philosophy. However, the current educational system depends upon teachers who are pragmatic within the boxes provided by the current philosophy. Thomas M. Skrtic, in *Behind Special Education: A Critical Analysis of Professional Culture and School Organization*, provides this insight:

> Ultimately, however, whether the current crisis leads to positive growth and renewal depends upon the manner in which we make pragmatic choices and take pragmatic actions relative to our current situation. The manner in which we make these decisions can take one of two general forms: *naive pragmatism* or *critical pragmatism.*
>
> Naive pragmatism values functional efficiency—pure utility or expediency. It is premised on unreflective acceptance of the explicit and implicit assumptions that lie behind our practices and discourses. According to Cherryholmes (1988), naive pragmatism is "socially reproductive, instrumentally and functionally reproducing accepted meanings and conventional organizations, institutions, and ways of doing things for good or ill" (p.151). Conversely, critical pragmatism approaches decision making in a way that treats such assumptions themselves as problematic; it "results when a sense of crisis is brought to our choices" (Cherryholmes, 1988, p.151), when it is accepted that our assumptions themselves require evaluation and reappraisal.

Teachers are treated as mere curriculum technicians who are not expected to question either their tasks or instructions. The significant is defined for them. Often, teachers collude with such diminishment, because they lack the political literacy to realize they don't have to accept their debasement. But not always—as one experienced practitioner complained:

> I get so tired of administrators treating us teachers like rat terriers. People used to throw rat terriers into pits full of rats and see how long it took for them to kill them all. Then the specially bred dogs were immediately thrown into other pits of rats to repeat the process all over again. The first rat terrier to finish the marathon of rat pits was the winner. Well, that's how I feel with all these changes they keep throwing at us. No sooner do we learn the ins and outs of the latest craze in teaching than they throw another one at us. They keep us from becoming better teachers by consuming our time and energy with all their rat pits. I am a consistently successful teacher. But what works for me doesn't always work for

> someone else. We each have to find our own ways of being effective. And I have managed to do that. I should therefore be treated like a professional. Who are they to define my work for me?

The woman quoted above has, through dedication and initiative, developed her heart and her intellect, not just her techniques, as a teacher—and her interest in medieval life provides a dramatic analogy. She understands her endeavor; she defines the significant. She has reflected on her practice; she is an experienced teacher. She possesses a critical pragmatism regarding the task of teaching. She chafes at being treated like a rat terrier instead of a professional. She resents a system that digs pits, fills them with rats, and then compels her to be trained on how to deal with them. The ultimate impracticality, after all, is when people lack the autonomy to set their own agendas. Disrespect for teachers is a logical result of a Taylorist mindset about the educational process.

Skrtic writes:

> Managing and governing schools as if they were machine bureaucracies misconceptualizes teaching as simple work that can be rationalized and formalized. This reduces professional discretion, which, in turn, lessens the degree to which teachers can personalize instruction to meet the particular needs of their students. Complex work cannot be formalized through rules.
>
> . . . The goal of critical pragmatism is not certainty; it does not seek objective knowledge or monological truth. Rather, the goal of critical pragmatism is *education*, or *self-formation*; it is a pedagogical process of remaking ourselves as we think, act, write, read, and talk more about ourselves and our practices and discourses (Gadamer, 1975). As such, critical pragmatism is premised on the notion of continually searching for "a new and more interesting way of expressing ourselves, and thus of coping with the world. . . ." (Rorty, 1979, p. 359).

True professionals develop a critical pragmatism regarding their endeavor. They never become so busy improving effectiveness that they lose sight of what they actually do, thus allowing their values to be suppressed by a culture of compliance to Tayloristic beliefs about management and control. Our best practitioners know what works in teaching, and they find ways of developing their personal effectiveness despite an ethos of socialistic control. Teaching is not a science; it is an art that can be informed, but not managed, by science. The task is to become good consumers of research, to use it with a critical instead of naïve pragmatism.

> In a democracy, producing thoughtful, informed citizens is the real point of schooling, and the real basics are what the next generation will need to continue what Lincoln thought of as a great democratic experiment.
>
> Joseph Featherstone

–55–

The Next Step—Self-Reliance

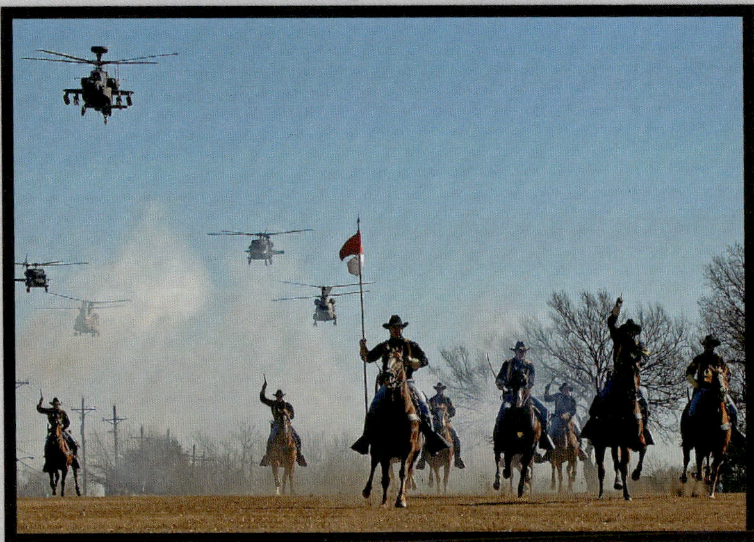

U.S. Army photo by Pfc. Phillip Turner

John Wayne, leading the cavalry, is not coming. He never will. Get over it. Leaving the responsibility in the hands of the bureaucrats is un-American. Placing the responsibility in the hands of outside experts is also un-American. Waiting for some kind of John Wayne (or magic bullet) to ride out of the woods to save us is, in its very spirit, un-American. It is up to us, whether as individuals, communities, districts, schools, or classrooms, to understand our situations and forge a way through our problems toward our potential. We can look to others for advice but not direction, for help but not salvation; we must take responsibility for our individual endeavors. We must work our way to the simplicities for ourselves, for only we can fully perceive and recognize the dynamic complexities that presently confuse us. It is up to us to muster the necessary self-reliance. Then we can generate neurogenic classrooms and schools and reinvigorate the spirit of democracy in our nation.

It's all about clarity. Those who can't grow their own <u>will pay the costs</u> of getting it from somewhere else.

So what can schools and teachers do? First of all, they must stop walking down the same primrose path that has resulted in the present "rosy" picture. They must stop paying the costs of getting their clarity from somewhere else and grow their own.

Things <u>not</u> needed:

—New and improved curriculum packages. Enough already; they cost too much money and disrespect teachers as well as generate sameness; choose or construct your own.
—Experts to lead you out of the woods. You don't, or shouldn't, need them.
—Ever more strident and stringent mandates from on high. Begin the resistance necessary to reclaim your schools for democracy; establish your own vision of and voice about schooling; define your own path.

What <u>is</u> needed:

—Conversation, in order to construct the clarities.
—A sense of community, in order to implement them.
—Most of all, courage, for without it, nothing else follows.

Neither the voices of communities nor teachers are heard in a culture dominated by a Taylorist mindset. The endeavor can be scientifically managed, insist the bureaucratic managers, consistently disregarding either the desires or the judgment of communities and teachers. They have gained such control that neither communities nor teachers feel like they own their schools. David Mathews, in *Reclaiming Public Education by Reclaiming Our Democracy*, writes:

> In 1996, the Kettering Foundation published *Is There a Public for Public Schools?* It reported on a decade of studies that all pointed to one alarming conclusion: many Americans doubted the public schools were really their schools. They weren't just critical of the instruction; they didn't think there was much they could do about any of their concerns. They couldn't change the schools, and the schools appeared to be incapable of reforming themselves.
>
> . . . Teachers complain that they are captives of externally imposed reforms, with little or no voice. . . .Reforms were handed down from on high, one teacher said; typically she and her colleagues were only "empowered" to implement what others had decreed. . . . The [Kettering] foundation has found the absence of a sense of agency widespread in other groups of educators, as well as members of school boards.

Taking ownership of our schools will require teachers to become active and communities to coalesce in a focus on taking back their schools. Our teachers, however, have been trained by the system to be passive curriculum implementation specialists. And, as Mathews pointed out, our communities don't feel like they own the situation. Schooling seems firmly in the hand of the socialistic bureaucrats who constantly push research-proven and data-driven education, which fits into their allegiance to the Taylorist ideal of "scientific" management. Can our teachers and communities grow beyond the fatalism that compels the belief that they cannot fix the problem?

Teachers have been trained to be passive and communities are distracted. Everyone is so busy and the system seems so huge, pervasive, and set. What can possibly be done to take back the schools from the nameless powers that control the metaphors that control the methods of instruction and assessment? Can teachers and communities learn that their schooling is controlled by a socialistic operating metaphor? Can we realize that is why we suffer from the same old schools, regardless of the diversity of community or faculty? Can we understand that much of our discipline, drop-out, burn-out, and ineffectiveness issues can be traced to the systemic toxins of the Taylorist process?

Perhaps we got lazy and allowed outside forces to impose their clarities upon us. Or perhaps we were hoodwinked by the Taylorist mindset claiming their prediction and control machinations as scientifically based. The supposed clarities of Taylorism never really worked in this, in its very essence, democratic country—it is time we grew our own.

Our only hope is that the democratic spirit is not beyond revitalization. But that is a reasonable hope. Scratch an American hard, and you will find the desire for self-rule intense and alive. But here is the rub, where we are reminded of H.G. Well's warning that history is the race between education and catastrophe: Can teachers and communities be awakened to how they have slowly, systemically lost control of their schools to a socialistic mindset? Can the flame of democracy be rekindled enough in our teachers and communities to take control of our schools?

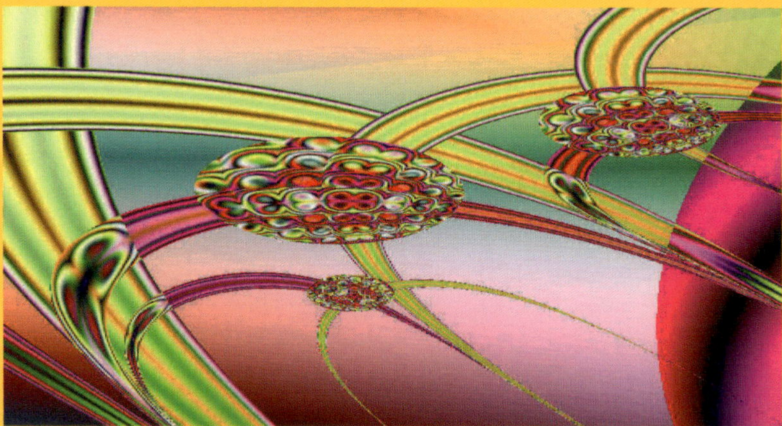

"Super Balls" by Ken Keller

An American isn't after a free ride, if he can help it. He wants to sail his own boat, which means getting a grip on the strings attached.

Roy Blount, Jr.

Cautionary Considerations

Let's face it: teachers have been born and raised in the belly of the beast. They have been acculturated for generations to believe that gavaging is teaching and that standardized assessment is effective at measuring worthwhile learning. They have been so systematically and systemically disrespected by the system that they think current conditions are just the way it is. They have been successful at jumping through the hoops; after all, they have become teachers within the system. Americans are by nature anti-intellectual and teachers even more so. Some have chosen the profession as a second choice because they couldn't achieve their initial ambition; others just like their summers off; timidity is their habitual temperament. Teachers have also undergone reform after reform; they are justifiably cynical about the possibility of worthwhile, long-lasting, effective change. BUT there has been a lot of guerilla activity over the years. Many teachers have gone behind their closed doors and sniped at the system as best they could. They have seen the damage done to the souls, hearts, and intellects of so many students by a top-down, socialistic system. They have felt the constant, degrading disrespect. They have seen their judgments consistently discounted and their initiative constantly suppressed. They may be in the belly of the beast but they are not yet digested by it. They still have enough integrity to see the damage that it does, to find ways of irritating the system, to muster aggravations against its walls.

"We teachers can resist the Standardisto imperative that would turn us into train conductors, programmed to keep our students operating on an ideal schedule devised by a complicity of politicians and bureaucrats."

Susan Ohanian

The hope is that teachers and other educators will understand that real reform is impossible without revision—a fundamental reconstruction of how learning, and thus teaching and schooling, is defined. The troublesome, and exciting, part of that equation is that the revisioning can only come from them; it must be the practitioners themselves who create the metaphors, methods, and materials that define learning, teaching, and schooling. After all, a philosophy that is not self-constructed is a hand-me-down and the American spirit does not like hand-outs. Ressentiment has been building in teachers, students, administrators, and community members against the present educational system for many decades now. In addition, the exploding field of neuroscience is accumulating scientific evidence that is pulling the sand from underneath the socialistic metaphors, methods, and materials that currently dominate educational practice.

In other words, conditions are ripe for a revolution.

The Secret Engine of the Democratic Spirit

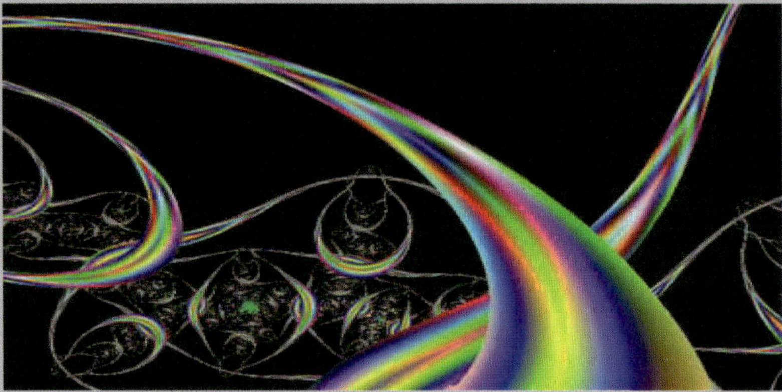

"Transports" by Beth Windozer

While supervising a student teacher at a school in San Diego, I waited for her arrival in the main office. The principal arrived, apparently from a meeting with the superintendent. Several teachers were waiting for him, and an intense discussion ensued, one that I could not hear. The impromptu meeting broke up, and I could tell that the teachers were not happy. One of them called out in frustration to the back of the principal as he entered his office: **Don't they get it? When it's ours—We will make it work!** The teachers did not want to be either customers or clients or cogs of the governing system. They wanted to own the store—but they were thwarted by a socialistic, bureaucratic mindset. They wanted to grow their own clarities, the very essence of the democratic spirit. Mary Parker Follet defines democracy as self-creating coherence—not one handed down or imposed by others. There is a special competence in ownership that experts and bureaucrats don't realize. This is why the spirit of democracy is superior to other forms of government. Democracy is messy and chaotic but, in the final analysis, the most effective approach, especially when situations are dynamic and complex. Socialism is addicted to order, even at the cost of effectiveness or common sense. Democracy understands that a little disorder is necessary in order to gain the power and just plain fairness of ownership. Socialism places its faith in a monoculture governed by bureaucrats. Democracy places its faith in a community of divergent viewpoints with the cooperation and co-intelligence to better deal with its predicaments and opportunities.

One thing is certain: Whatever happens to public education will certainly affect America's ongoing experiment in self-rule. That is the reason the public schools are ultimately accountable to democracy, not just to parents or taxpayers.

David Mathews

–56–

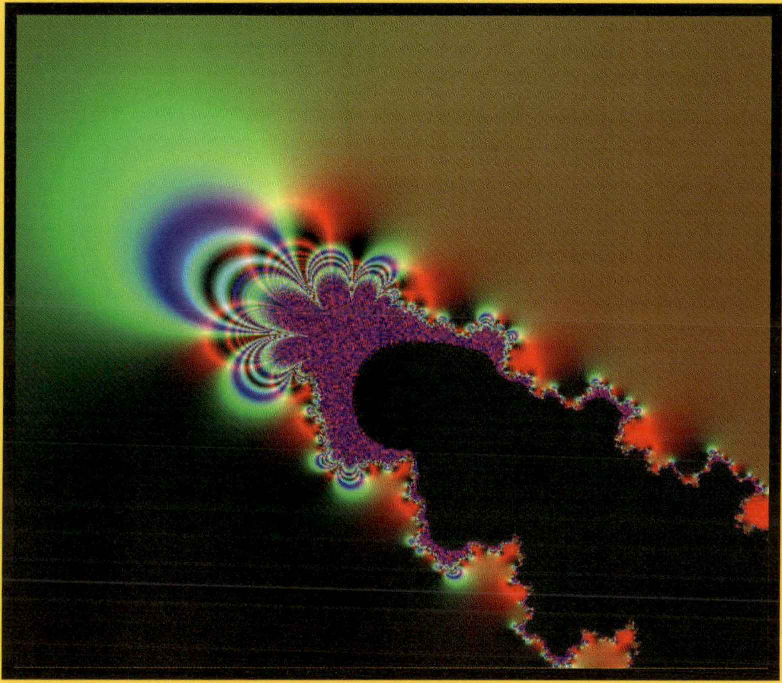

"Flight into the Future" by Eugenia Senkevich

Perhaps it's time to toss the very word "management" onto the linguistic ash heap alongside "icebox" and "horseless carriage." This era doesn't call for better management. It calls for a renaissance of self-direction.

Daniel H. Pink

It's the AUTONOMY, stupid.

The metaphorical, perhaps even literal, dendritic thread that interconnects this hodgepodge mosaic of essay vignettes, quotes, and stories is faith in the ideas and principles of democracy. As the human story progresses from striving to merely survive to a reasonable economic and political security, the human spirit advances toward the need for autonomy. Autonomy is the universal urge to be causal agents of our own life while acting in harmony with our integrated self. Autonomy is the drive to increasingly author ourselves. This doesn't mean we want to be independent of others; it means to be less enmeshed and embedded, thus able to both choose and contribute more of our ourselves if we so choose.

We want to be individuals rather than simply products of our cultures and circumstances. We want to be self-directed, though not self-enclosed.

The right brain characteristics of imagination, interest, and initiative are essential to autonomy. The intricacies of the interactive dynamics are beyond any one of us—but thousands of neuroscientists are beginning to put their oars into the ocean of ignorance of how the mind works. One important unfolding picture is the following:

> The spirit of democracy is no longer just desirable, it is becoming necessary, for without its vital and substantial presence, we cannot learn well enough and creatively enough to deal with our problems and seize our opportunities. Self-directed learners may one day not be the ideal, but the required. Self-directed contribution in the business world is now becoming increasingly recognized as desirable. The old management assumptions about control through extrinsic rewards and punishment don't work in such terrain; new ways of leading, and teaching, are becoming necessary.

The Red Queen World demands more democracy, more individual autonomy. It turns out that democracy, the philosophy that best supports individual initiative and responsibility, is more in tune with our natural minds. Daniel H. Pink, in *Drive: The Surprising Truth About What Motivates Us,* writes:

> . . . Our basic nature is to be curious and self-directed. And I say that not because I'm a dewy-eyed idealist, but because I have been around young children and because my wife and I have three children of our own. Have you ever seen a six-month-old or a one-year-old who's *not* curious and self-directed? I haven't. That's how we are out of the box. If, at age fourteen or forty-three, we're passive and inert, that's not because it's our nature. It's because something flipped our default setting.
>
> That something could well be management—not merely how bosses treat us at work, but also how the broader ethos has leeched into schools, families, and many other aspects of our lives. Perhaps management isn't *responding* to our supposedly natural state of passive inertia. Perhaps management is one of the forces that's switching our default setting and *producing* that state. . . . But today economic accomplishment, not to mention personal fulfillment, more often swings on a different hinge. It depends not on keeping our nature submerged but on allowing it to surface. It requires resisting the temptation to control people—and instead doing everything we can to reawaken their deep-seated sense of autonomy.

The drive to be autonomous runs counter to the management ethos that controls most business and educational theories. Workers, and students, the current perspective believes, must be subjected to carrots and sticks to get them to either work or learn. Extrinsic motivation machinations, in other words, are necessary.

But the drive for autonomy is fueled by intrinsic motivation; it comes from within the mind, a strange Alice-in-Wonderland kind of place where general rules don't always apply. In fact, extrinsic motivation schemes tend to suppress intrinsic motivation, decreasing the very things we most desire, such as self-motivated, self-directed learners. Pay students to learn math, for example, and the result is a systemic, long-term loss of interest in math. As Pink points out, "This is one of the most robust findings in social science—and also one of the most ignored." The power of intrinsic motivation is ignored, for it threatens the present educational perspective, since it calls into question its coverage-fixation and test-addiction.

A revolution in our understanding about motivation has been brewing since the publication of Edward Deci's *Intrinsic Motivation* in 1971. Deci and a former graduate student, Richard Ryan, have developed Self-Determination Theory, which consists of three psychological needs: competence, autonomy, and relatedness. Autonomy is the cardinal need, for through it we develop our special and unique competence. It is also essential to relatedness, for we want to produce something that contributes to others—that has purpose.

David Osborne and Ted Gaebler, in their book, *Reinventing Government: How the Entrepreneurial Spirit is Transforming the Public Sector,* write:

> John Chubb and Terry Moe, authors of a Brookings Institution book called *Politics, Markets, and America's Schools,* studied data on 500 high schools around the nation to discover what factors most influenced student performance. The greatest influence was, of course, the aptitude the student brought to school—something determined largely by family background. But the second most important influence was the school itself. Yet the traditional factors we often emphasize—teacher salaries, per pupil expenditures, class size, graduation requirements—had no impact on school performance. Instead, the keys were parental control, the clarity of the school's mission, strong leadership, and the degree of freedom and respect offered the teachers (in our terms, community ownership, a mission-driven [not rules-driven] organization, and decentralized authority). To develop these attributes, Chubb and Moe found, schools needed autonomy from external control—from administrators, unions, and school boards. "The more freedom that the school was granted to chart its own course," they discovered, "the more likely it was to become effectively organized".
>
> "The real issue in school reform, then, is: how do you provide autonomy and still hold schools accountable? After all, you can't just turn over the keys of the school to the teachers and principals and be sure that they're going to be held accountable. . . . The only empirically and logically compelling way in which autonomy and accountability can be maintained is to move to a different system of accountability. You need a system that holds schools accountable not from the top down, but through the market process, through the competitive process. You need a system that holds schools accountable by giving them

autonomy—and by observing how well the schools succeed in winning the support of parents and students."

Competition is our road to effectiveness. David Miller and Saul Estrin write, in their article, "Market Socialism, a Policy for Socialists," about the survival of the helpful—rather than the survival of the bureaucratically entrenched or politically powerful. Those administrators and teachers who can help accomplish the mission of delivering worthwhile education will become apparent when given autonomy. The deadwood will also become apparent.

With autonomy, people find a way to grow through the cement—which encourages the growth of more autonomy.

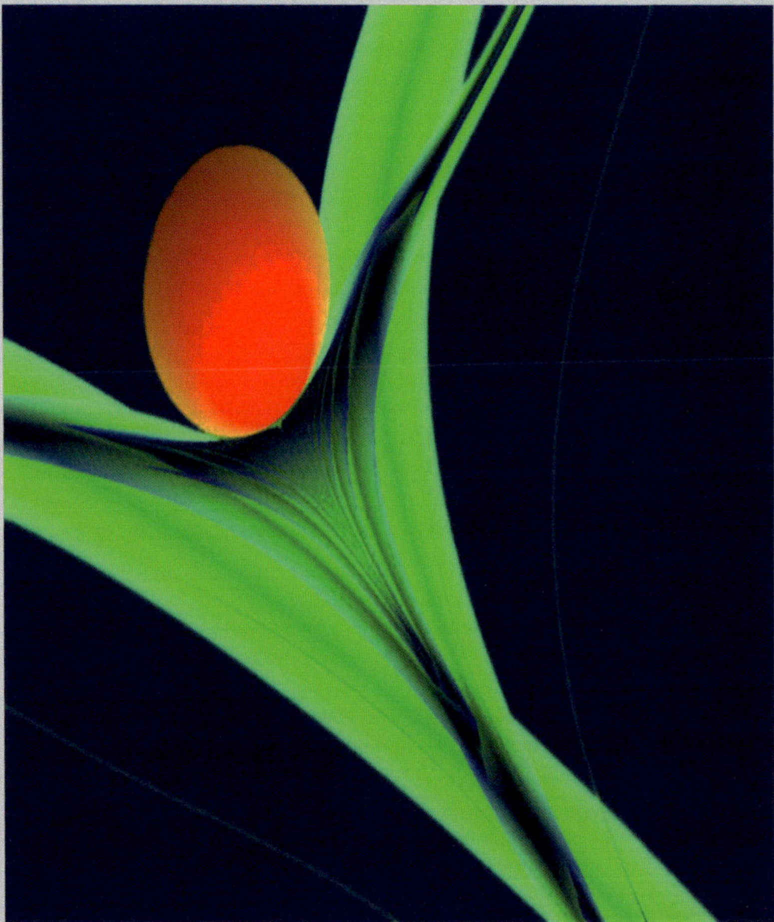

"Rising Sun Flower" by Marie Luise Schmidt

We have it in our power to begin the world over again.

Thomas Paine

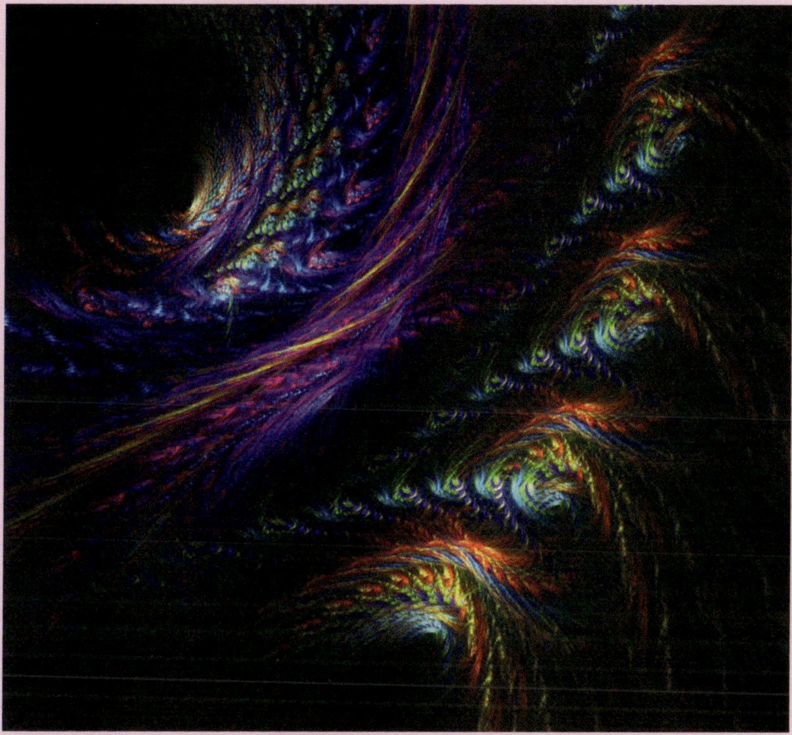

"Renaissance" by Lauren Zorn

The word government is from a Greek word, which means "to steer." The job of government is to steer, not row the boat. Delivering services is rowing, and government is not very good at rowing.

E. S. Savas

Strong people hate to be micromanaged; only the weak acquiesce to, or worse, take refuge in it. When government tries to take over the rowing, it goes beyond its purpose. The rules that cascade down from on-high usually translate to rowing the boat, and interfere with any effective delivery plan. This causes the strong to either resist or leave the situation. The result is a weakened system as it gradually pushes away the strong who demand autonomy, leaving an increasing percentage of those who can accommodate to the lack of it. Strong people also resist rowing the boat in a direction they don't respect. And a key principle of democracy is that citizens have a say in the direction steered. In our hearts, we know that addiction to the easily measured in educational assessment has steered us away from what is good for students or for our potential as a democracy. The principle of self-direction is in our democratic bones. We deny that truth only when we feel too weak or confused to demand the necessary autonomy.

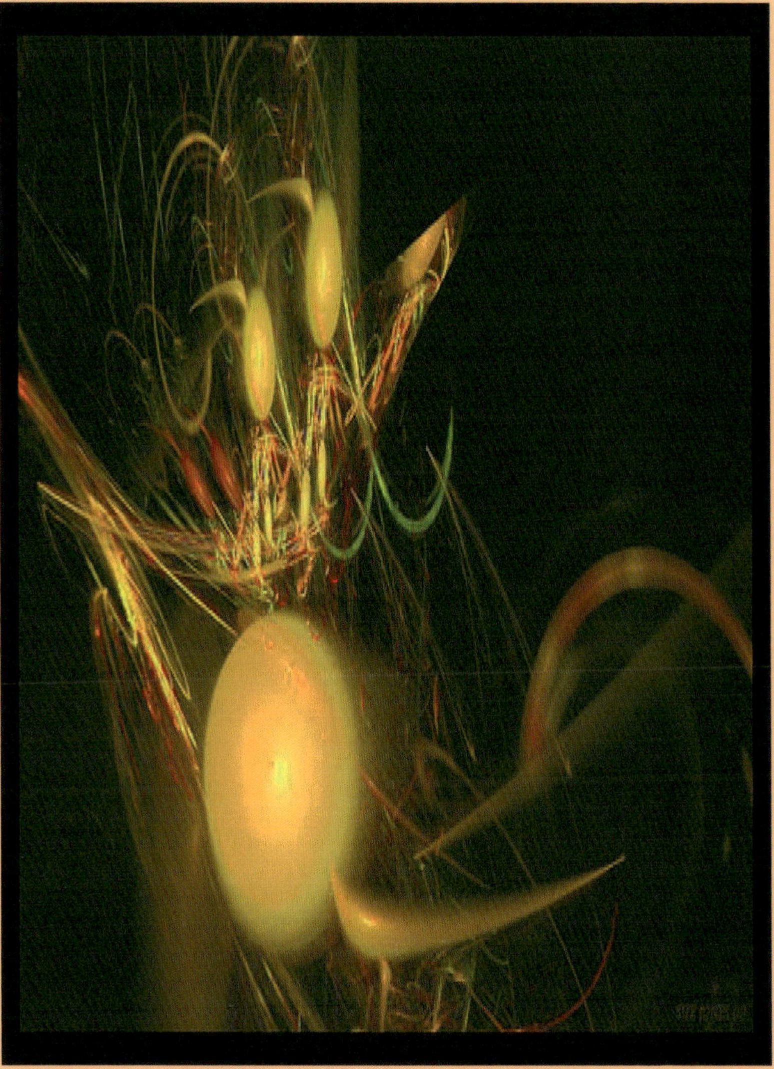

"Intrepid Travelers" from Sue Tortoise's photostream

We're born to be players, not pawns. We're meant to be autonomous individuals, not individual automatons.

Daniel H. Pink

What luck for rulers that men do not think.

Adolph Hitler

CONSIDER—The Responsibility of the Grass

The image of GRASS ROOTS is integral to the redefinition of learning. Originally a mining term, it indicated gold so easy to find that all you had to do was search the grass roots. Within a few decades the term grew into an analogy—grass roots meant getting down to "brass tacks" and looking at the "underlying principles or basic facts of a matter." [Charles Earle Funk] At the grass roots is where understanding interactive dynamics is at its best, where effective response is most likely. When politicians claim grass roots support, they assert both a better realization of the things that matter and connection to the real power of a democracy. "Grass roots" is a particularly democratic image, for it indicates changing conditions at the sources of power and effectiveness, individuals and local communities. This is where the redefinition of learning must begin and grow.

Grass roots has 3 meanings: 1. the essential foundation or source. 2. the common people at a local level (instead of the centers of political activity.)
3. something totally new, not adapted to an existing facility or operation; built from the ground up.

Peter Block, in *Community: The Structure of Belonging,* articulates the need for citizens to act autonomously and responsibly in order to take control of their communities: "John McKnight found that most sustainable improvements in community occur when citizens discover their own power to act. . . . It is when citizens stop waiting for professionals or elected leadership to do something and decide they can reclaim what they have delegated to others that things really happen." Engagement comes from empowerment. Remember: "If it's ours—we'll make it work." Two powerful positives result from a grass roots movement: increased effectiveness and sense of community. Autonomy is integral to democracy; the notion of self-direction is embedded in our cultural and personal definition. The Tayloristic mindset, using ersatz science as its cudgel, took control of educational metaphors, methods, and materials. But the conditions are right for a new Zeitgeist, a democratic one, supported by neuroscience, where the grass grows through the socialistic cement and takes control.

Our problems are not unsolvable, our obstacles not insurmountable, but they require a faith in democracy, a steady and insistent belief that we, as individuals and communities, can solve them ourselves. We don't need more top-down directives to answer our educational challenges. We certainly don't need more standardized goals. We don't even need more money. What we do need is less management from centralized power centers and their outside experts—and more self-direction and self-definition. We need a groundswell of autonomy and responsibility from the grass roots to grow through the cement of systemic stupidities. We need more democracy.

–57–

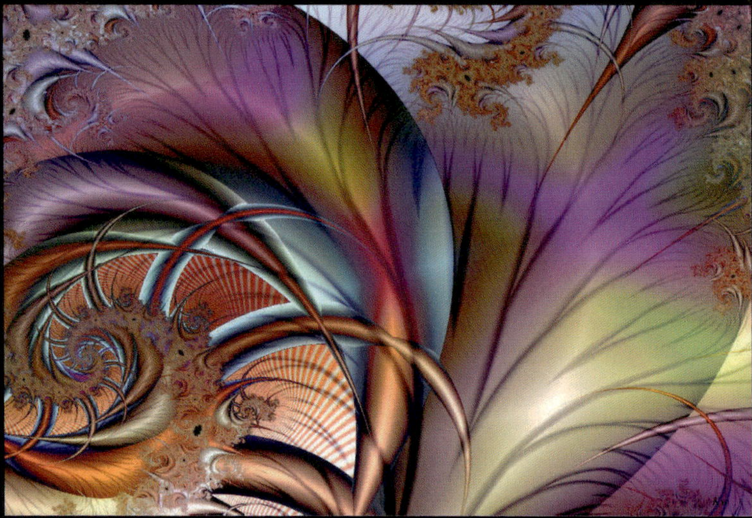

"Sayonara" by Ken Worden

In the mid-1980s, the Union of Soviet Socialist Republics had existed for nearly three-quarters of a century, and it stood as a seemingly permanent fixture on the world stage . . . . In 1987, one would have had to scour the journals of history and political science to find even a tentative suggestion that the U.S.S.R. might collapse within half a century, let alone in the coming decade. Then, to everyone's amazement, the unthinkable became a reality—in just a few years.

Mark Buchanan

The grass is growing that will eventually break through the cement. The conditions (in particular: scientism and expertism) that have supported the socialistic operating metaphors guiding present educational practice in America are dissolving. Personal initiative and responsibility can be suppressed only so long before they reassert themselves—as the Soviet hierarchy found out. Individual assertion comprises the grass that grows through the cement.

The word "assert" carries an important image for us to consider:

> Assert comes from the Latin *asserere*—"to join to oneself." Assertion is an expression of identity: "This is who I am, where I stand, and what matters to me."

Assertion is essential to a sense of community—the place where we contribute and thus belong. This is especially true for a democratic community, one imbued with the principles of individual uniqueness and responsibility. We withdraw, when and to the degree we can, our sense of belonging from the places that do not respect our capacity for contribution. Logically, emotionally, and spiritually, we prefer to belong to communities that cherish our contributions. Suppressed assertion fuels both ressentiment and disengagement in both teachers and students. After all, our very identities are at stake. The present definition of schooling therefore generates an increasing percentage of teacher burn-out and student drop-out.*

Teachers burn-out when they cannot apply their initiative to their dynamically complex endeavor; that they are not allowed to assert themselves, to join their individuality to their work. Students drop-out when their individual imagination, interests, and initiative are crowded out of the learning environment by set curriculum and ubiquitous, all-powerful tests. When individuals are not allowed to join the endeavors, of either teaching or learning, to themselves, why should we be surprised at the increasing burn-out and drop-out rate? We need community, especially one that respects and cherishes our individual desires, assertions, and contributions—our autonomy.

Teachers, taught by the system to be curriculum implementation specialists, are trained out of their assertiveness by the overwhelming weight and systemic perniciousness of a top-down, bureaucratic and socialistic process. Students, taught to be passive recipients of learning by schooling, will not question. The right to question, to assert one's perspective and concerns in pursuit of the truth is a fundamental democratic principle. The grass will grow through the socialistic cement as our teachers and students assert their right to question the process and therefore the products of schooling. The issues of drop-out and burn-out will then dissipate.

Teachers, students, and communities need to do their part to help us grow through the cement. The fundamental educational task is to serve as the liver for the social body and cleanse it of such poisons as ignorance, prejudice, apathy, incapability, and weakness. But that task is harder than ever in today's Red Queen World. A faith in democracy demands that we trust the judgment and initiative of individuals—rather than a top-down socialistic process—to best accomplish that task. Assertiveness, after all, is integral to a sense of community, especially one imbued with the spirit of democracy. Our present educational system is not a permanent fixture; we could dismantle it quickly if we chose.

*Both burn-out and drop-out are on a continuum. The teacher is burning-out who decreases contribution of imagination, interest, and initiative because the systemic conditions are toxic to them. The Educational Council of Taipei City [Taiwan] coined the term "drop-out-at-heart" to indicate someone who was physically present but not engaged in classroom learning, says Li-juing Wu in *The International Journal on School Disaffection* (2004). A hot concern in the educational world at the moment is engagement. Perhaps we need to look at the conditions that generate the general feeling of disaffection that can grow into burn-out and drop-out at heart or in fact. Concern for engagement is a good thing, because democratic, not socialistic, processes are the best at generating engagement, the application of personal assertiveness through individual imagination, interest, and initiative—through respect for personal autonomy.

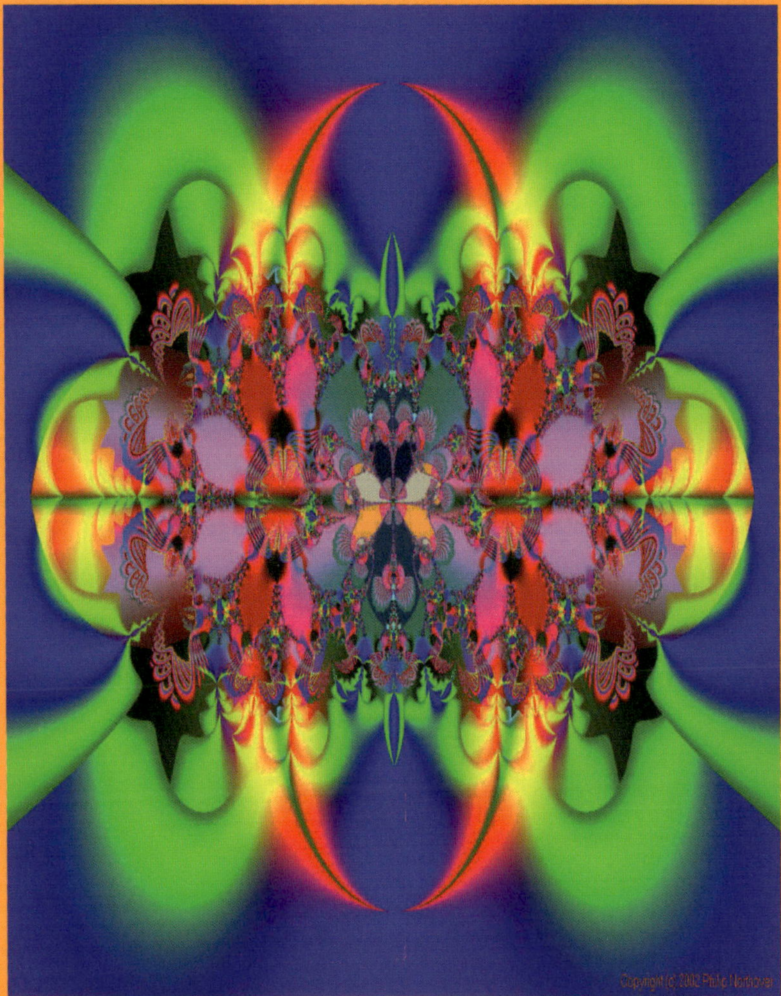

"Newton's Cradle" by Philip Northover

"May God us keep from single vision and Newton's sleep."

Over 150 years ago, the poet William Blake saw the danger of scientism and expertism to our cultural health and vitality. What he meant by "Newton's sleep" is the loss of our autonomy and assertiveness through the worship of scientific managers, who, through centralized top-down procedures, would supplant our individual judgment and initiative. The Newtonian image promised a world of prediction and control—of this-then-that. Blake's poetic soul harbored the truth of Quantum reality, and he feared the seductiveness of the Newtonian operating metaphor to those who desired simplistic clarities.

Democratic Assertiveness

"The ability of our citizens to inquire has profound implications for whether we can fulfill the promise of our democracy."

Andrea Batista Schlesinger

The democratic spirit demands self-reliance. It also demands diversity and inclusion which requires understanding and wisdom. This is why the educational process is so entwined with the spirit of democracy. It takes an educated citizenry to maintain a democratic process. The persistence, quality, and clarity of our questions are essential to our health and vitality. Can we ask assertive questions that seek to find systemic wisdom instead of laying blame? After all, our problems are systemic—not personal. We can trust that most of us want to learn, grow, and contribute.

Teacher Assertiveness

We can begin the dismantling of our same old and ineffective schools by changing the educational culture to where teacher assertiveness is encouraged and supported. In a recent classroom scuffle over cell phone use in my classroom, an incoming freshman student dared to use foul language (muttered) in her reaction to my threat (not an empty one) to confiscate it. My angry response to her attitude was one of ironic exasperation: "What do you think I am, a public school teacher? I am a college professor. I don't have to put up with this kind of crap. I can color you gone in a New York minute."

My response was neither mature nor effective nor good teaching. But the key thing here was her assumption that she could get away with her behavior, and that I found it necessary to point out that I was not a public school teacher. What have we done in this society when public school teachers feel virtually powerless to educate for polite and civil behavior—to establish prices of admission to their classrooms? That is a systemic stupidity. If teachers fail to educate for polite and civil behavior, who will? School systems constantly buy into complicated discipline packages and bring in outside experts to train teachers to get on the same page. Such programs wash through our school systems on a regular basis. Teachers have also been prevented from generating learning environments by mandated curriculum and policies—and students are justifiably resistive to classrooms that gavage them.

The answer to increasingly uncivil behavior—as well as Same Old Schools and classrooms toxic to learning—is teacher assertiveness. Allow teachers, while providing the necessary support structures, to become captains of their own ships, to establish prices of admission to their classrooms. There will be problems, such as unreasonable teachers and irritated students, but they will be democratic problems instead of bureaucratic ones.

Student Assertiveness

"External pressure designed to produce learning or intelligence violates the fundamental rule:

A healthy brain stimulates itself by active interaction with what it finds challenging and interesting in its environment."

Jane M. Healy, Ph.D

Students should assert their right to have TEACHERS—not representatives of the system governed by the CYA operating metaphor, not curriculum implementation specialists—but TEACHERS. Students should ask, "Okay, teach, you got this price of admission thing going on, why should I want to pay it? You got anything neurogenic happening in there?" They should assert their right to have learning environments, where their imagination, interest, and initiative are respected—not curriculum implementation centers, where they are constantly gavaged, forced to do make believe work, and compelled to temporarily memorize meaningless stuff for the pernicious tests, which only takes care of the system, not them. They should demand their democratic right to have a voice regarding the conditions within which they live, to be allowed to state their case, to follow their imagination, interests, and initiative, to have opportunities for conversation and reflection—to learn intrinsically. Most importantly, students should demand a culture of schooling that respects their right to inquire, one where their questions are addressed respectfully and fully.

Community Assertiveness

Where are our communities in this struggle? Do they not see the harm being done to their children? Do they not perceive the continuous decline of civil behavior? Are they not aware of how much teachers are both overloaded and discounted? Have they so bought into the socialistic operating metaphor that they assume the state and federal governments should be in control? Certain principles, such as diversity and equality of opportunity, should be universally maintained. However, what about individuality and uniqueness? Should every school and classroom be defined by the same old policies and curriculum? The socialistic operating metaphor wants to standardize the methods and the results. But is that what we really want? Can you standardize a democratic entity? Doesn't a faith in democracy demand the emergence of individual uniqueness? Charter schools and home-schooling sometimes provide models of democratic, or at least less socialistically controlled, schooling. They contain the seeds of our renewal, and some of our public schools are beginning to learn from them. Communities need to reclaim their schools and make them more individualistic and democratic.

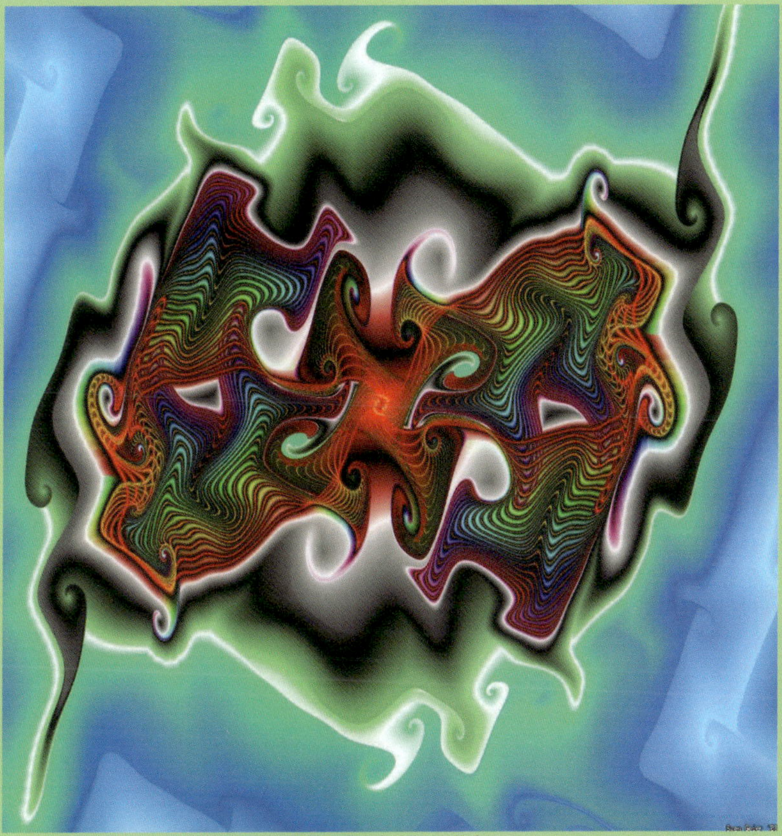

"Butterfly" by Sven Geier

. . . We will transform our schools and colleges and universities to meet the demands of a new age. . . . Now, there are some who question the scale of our ambitions, who suggest that our system cannot tolerate too many big plans. Their memories are short, for they have forgotten what this country has already done, what free men and women can achieve when imagination is joined to common purpose, and necessity to courage. What the cynics fail to understand is that the ground has shifted beneath them, that the stale political arguments that have consumed us for so long no longer apply. . . . What is required of us now is a new era of responsibility—a recognition on the part of every American that we have duties to ourselves, our nation and the world; duties that we do not grudgingly accept, but rather seize gladly, firm in the knowledge that there is nothing so satisfying to the spirit, so defining of our character than giving our all to a difficult task.

President Barack Obama

–58–

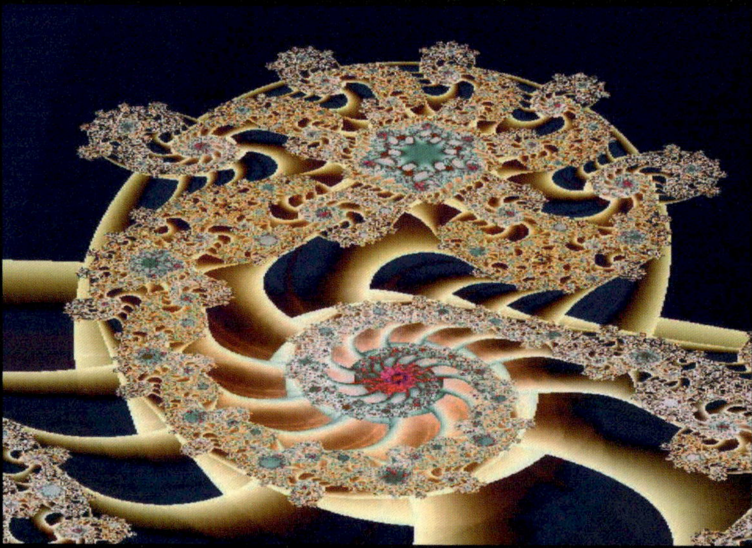

"Breaking the Egg" by Ken Keller

The classroom, with all its limitations, remains a location of possibility. In that field of possibility we have the opportunity to labor for freedom, to demand of ourselves and our comrades, an openness of mind and heart that allow us to face reality even as we collectively imagine ways to move beyond boundaries, to transgress. This is education as the practice of freedom.

bell hooks

Some value decisions have to be made. Do we value individual initiative and personal responsibility? If so, then we will have to place more trust in our teachers and allow them to design and forge learning communities in their classrooms. If so, then we will have to not only allow but support and encourage the constructivist nature of learning. Students and teachers, allowed to practice democracy in our schooling, will not only learn better, actively and constructively—but also how to become a democratic citizenry.

> The classroom is the crucible of possibility. Do we continue poisoning that crucible with socialistic notions of prediction and control? Do we instead value democratic principles enough to allow them to operate within our schooling?

We need to challenge how three people in particular think about the pedagogical process. Those individuals are President Obama, First Lady Michelle Obama, and Arne Duncan, Secretary of Education. The image that could guide that transformation is not far from the White House. The President and First Lady only need to follow their children to school. There, they will learn some important lessons about educating for freedom.

David Marshak asks an insightful question in the title of his article "If a Post-modern,* Whole Child School is the Choice for Malia and Sasha Obama, Why Not for Everyone?" The Obama children attend the Sidwell Friends School in the District of Columbia. It is expensive, almost thirty grand a year, but as Marshak points out, the real issue is not money but values, and, ultimately, the school's definition of learning.

Marshak is particularly upset by the operating metaphor guiding the actions of our Secretary of Education: "Arne Duncan wants to intensify the industrial, modernist character of American public schools. He wants a longer school day, a longer school week, and a longer school year. And he wants national subject standards, which will inevitably lead to one national test. And Duncan wants to institute merit pay, which is a euphemism for paying teachers to produce higher test scores." Marshak writes:

"Sidwell rejects the modernist, industrial paradigm of schooling that makes school like an assembly line engaged in mass production, that claims that all children should learn the same stuff at the same time. Sidwell also rejects the modernist claim that children's individuality and inner knowing are irrelevant to education. Sidwell embraces a post-modern paradigm of schooling defined by the following elements:"

—Sidwell is a pre-kindergarten through 12th grade school, with 1097 students. This is about 84 children in each grade, a small enough number so that no child is lost in the crowd.

—Sidwell offers "a *rich and rigorous interdisciplinary* curriculum designed to stimulate creative inquiry, intellectual achievement and independent thinking in a world increasingly without borders." It does not limit its curriculum to the antiquated 19th century subjects, as does every set of state curriculum standards—or the new national standards that Arne Duncan is pitching.

—Sidwell encourages its students "*...to give expression to their artistic abilities.*" It does not cut the arts out of the curriculum to focus only on math and reading as so many schools have done in our testing-obsessed era but understands that the arts needs to be an integral element in every child's education.

—Sidwell's Friends School is a community that values *"the power of individual and collective reflection..."* Sidwell encourages reflection and inner knowing, neither of which are acknowledged in any state's academic standards.

—Sidwell explicitly acknowledges *multiple forms of accessing knowledge and truth:* "through scientific investigation, through creative expression, through conversation…through service within the school community and beyond." All state standards are far more simple minded.

—Sidwell recognizes that schooling is both about individual learning and about young people learning how to work well with others. "*Work on individual skills and knowledge is balanced with group learning*, in which each person's unique insights contributes to a collective understanding.

—Sidwell is a school that focuses on ***personalization of learning*** and on ***educating the whole person.*** "Above all, we seek to be a school that nurtures a genuine love of learning and teaches students 'to let their lives speak.'"

Not all of the elements listed by Marshak are included here, but the image of the Sidwell Friends School is clear. It is not a place fixated on gavaging students. It understands the synergistic importance of the right brain. It treasures reflection and conversation. It encourages the arts. It teaches to the child's unique potential—not to the test.

The search for a picture of "the way the world really is" is an enterprise that transcends the narrow interests of the theoretical physicists. For better or for worse, humans have tended to pattern their domestic, social, and political arrangements according to the dominant vision of physical reality. Inevitably the cosmic view trickles down to the most mundane details of everyday life.

Nick Herbert
Quantum Reality

*The much abused but still useful term **postmodern** returns us to the images of the Newtonian and Quantum worlds. The modern era can be thought of as one guided by clockwork, cause-to-effect, linear connections, while the postmodern era is characterized by chaos points, unpredictable synergies, and non-linear realities. The operating metaphor guiding the modernistic mindset is Newtonian. The operating metaphor guiding the postmodern mindset is Quantum. Truth and wisdom reside within the interaction between the two perspectives.

In their hearts, the President and First Lady know that the modernist model of schooling, of gavage and regurgitation, is neither effective nor good for children. Perhaps they feel that a postmodern perspective works only for children of privilege, of children with supportive parents, who have learned intrinsic motivation from home. Perhaps they are elitest. Or perhaps they have lost their democratic faith, the belief that the strength and vitality of a democracy resides in educating an increasingly high percentage of the individuals that comprise community.

I believe the problem resides in none of these suppositions. I believe the problem is that the Obamas, like so many others, have been blinded by the rays of yesterday's light. They have been enculturated into the assumption that the modernist structure is the way schooling has to be. (Though not for their children.) The President and First Lady, as bright and well-meaning as they are, still harbor the operating metaphor of top-down command and control schooling. We can hope that they will stop nourishing that socialistic mindset, that they will entertain a new perspective, one modeled by the very school they have chosen to send their children to attend.

> Here is a chaos point of possibility: the disconnect between the schooling the Obamas push upon public school students and the one provided their own children. Two results are possible: their credibility can be questioned and their arguments for bureaucratic control of schooling discounted, or they can reflect upon the error of their ways and rethink their definition of learning—as applied to children other than their own. We can hope for resonance in their hearts and minds to the butterflies of possibility.

The Frankenstein will eventually be dismantled; most likely because of pressures from the bottom up, but the revolution can be helped immensely when those at the top realize how their behavior is disconnected from changing conditions—or even their own expressed values. Just as Gorbachev helped dismantle the stupidity of the soviet system, Obama could help dismantle the socialism of our educational system.

The Obamas want to bring their children up to be good democratic citizens. They want capable and responsible children, who can question, who can think for themselves, who can imagine and initiate, who are intrinsic, life-long learners. Perhaps they will come to understand that such capability and responsibility needs to be spread throughout the citizenry, that that is what it means to believe in democracy. Perhaps they will also see how the top-down educational bureaucracy addicted to the easily measured and therefore readily controlled is socialism—and against the very soul of a democracy.

We labor for freedom, as teachers and as students, and as parents and politicians, when we pressure for initiative in the process. Bringing initiative, along with imagination and inquiry, back into the pedagogical equation will move us back toward our democratic principles. We labor for freedom in the field of possibility as we become aware of the socialistic designs of the current educational process and replace them with metaphors, methods, and materials more in line with our democratic values.

> To educate for freedom, then, we have to challenge and change the way everyone thinks about pedagogical process. This is especially true for students. Before we try to engage them in a dialectical discussion of ideas that is mutual, we have to teach about process.
>
> bell hooks
>
> *Teaching to Transgress: Education as the Practice of Freedom*

–59–

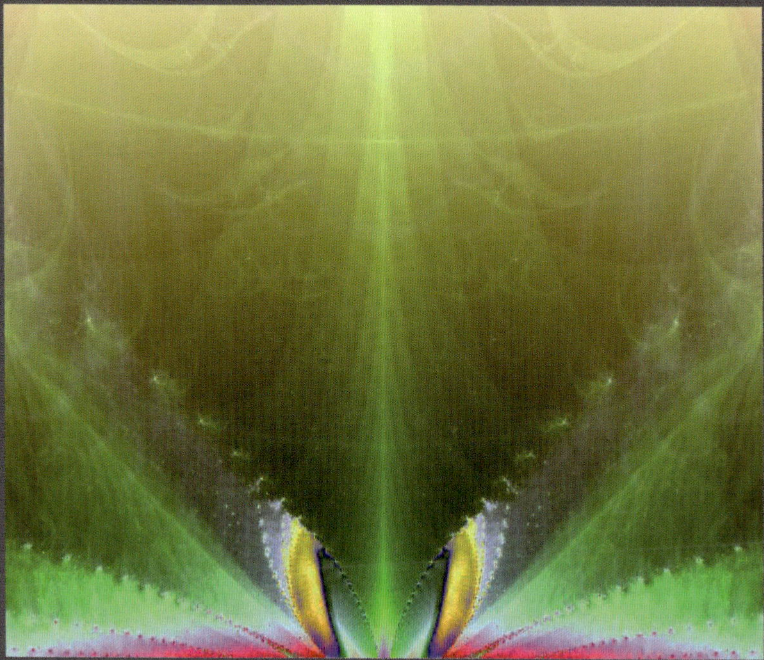

"Enlightened Butterfly" by J. Gebelein

The fatal metaphor of progress, which means leaving things behind, has utterly obscured the real idea of growth, which means leaving things inside us.

G. K. Chesterton

In order to grow, we must let go of the operating metaphors, the guiding images, that presently limit our wisdom and our potential for maturation. We must leave the old definition of learning inside us in order to progress enough to deal with the challenges and opportunities of the postmodern world. Learning redefined will in turn redefine teaching and eventually schooling.

Jacqueline Grennon Brooks and Martin G. Brooks, in their book, *The Case for Constructivist Classrooms: in Search of Understanding,* write:

> What images are evoked in most people's minds upon hearing the word "school?" Raising one's hand before answering questions, listening to teachers and taking notes, taking tests, lugging textooks from class to class, writing book reports, standing in straight lines, seeking permission to visit the restroom. These are the very images, practices,

> and expectations upon which schooling has been structured since the first common schools were erected well over a century ago. They are images of control, not of learning.
>
> A new set of images, reflective of new practices, is needed—images that portray the student as thinker, a creator, and a constructor. Schools can become settings in which students are encouraged to develop hypotheses, to test out their own and others' ideas, to make connections among "content" areas, to explore issues and problems of personal relevance (either existing or emerging), to work cooperatively with peers and adults in the pursuit of understanding, and to form the disposition to be life-long learners. The old images of school do not speak directly to the central issue of school reform—ways to evoke student learning through their search for understanding.

The new definition of learning will have a much increased focus on thinking, creating, and constructing. The new definition of teaching will respond accordingly, as teachers become facilitators of the new image of learning. They will become less like trainers and more like people who inspire and inform initiative within their students.

"We have seen the enemy and the enemy is us," as the cartoon character Pogo once said. Part of the problem is the increasing dynamic complexity of the world, but we can't change that. What we can change are the operating metaphors within us that keep us from growing. The Trojan Horse within us is intentional ignorance, which results in intentional blindness and weakness. It is a psychological truism that we can only see what we either know we can deal with or believe we can grow the necessary strength. When the challenge either is, or believed to be, too much for us, we escape into some form of denial.

The Future of Schooling

We need to return to the ancient image of school, from which the word is derived, a place where leisure time is given to learning, where students have the space to think, converse, and work on projects. Correct-answer schooling can only hurry, and hurry harder, in the World of the Red Queen. Education for understanding is better preparation for an increasingly right-brain world, where many of the jobs haven't even been invented yet. As we learn about teaching and learning from neuroscience, coverage-fixated factors such as expensive workbooks, worksheets, and make-do homework will disappear—replaced by conversation, reflection, and projects. The image of schools as gavage factories, (or injection molding plants) will fade away—replaced by learrning environments focused on conditions and resources. Passive and bulimic learning will subside—replaced by active, symphogenetic factors such as imagination, interest, and initiative. Intrinsic, instead of extrinsic, motivation will become (the always elusive) Holy Grail. But the fundamental difference will be the Demise of Sisyphus.

A Vocabulary of Freedom

What do words do? Diane Ackerman, in her beautiful synergy of poetry and neuroscience, *The Alchemy of Mind,* writes: "Words can act like tongs to drag a squirming thought into view, or like a set of lenses to help focus our thoughts. Words can cap gushing emotions, and trawl for memories. They can highlight and frame things when we need perspective, and they're excellent handles when we need to grip a slippery notion. As social beasts, we trade words with others, negotiate meanings, use words as currency. Words form the backbone of what we think."

Words, the important ones, are messy, sometimes in denotation but always in connotation. They both enlighten and confuse. Words are trouble—but they are also the magic of us, for, as we construct interpretations and thus dissonances and resonances, words constitute our individual variety and social flexibility. We live in a world of words; they comprise the substance of our thoughts and the foundation of our actions. They can be toxic, and they can be nourishing. And the important words are living things; they squirm with change and growth, birth and death. The denotations of words are attempts at solidification, and do not have the powerful but often idiosyncratic impact of their connotations. When two people say they love each other but their minds harbor two completely different images of the concept, there can be hell to pay.

When students say they wish to learn, do they mean the development of their intellects or the begrudging acceptance of the required hoops? Is there curiosity or merely compliance in their assertion? Is their learning intrinsically or extrinsically motivated? Does their definition of learning have anything to do with growth, of mind, of heart, of soul? Or is it wrapped around the acquisition of certifications, of tickets punched in order to move on down the line? When people call themselves teachers, do they mean lecturer, indoctrinator, or gavager? When people talk of schooling, do they envision a socialistic, Tayloristic process, or do they instead envision a democratic process, where individuals learn how to empower themselves? What are the images behind the words?

After all, Dixon is correct:

> **The human mind is not, as philosophers would have you think, a debating hall, but a picture gallery.**

Images such as chaos points/The Butterfly Effect, neurogenesis, gavage, passive and bulimic learning, sciolistic versus symphogenetic learning, ressentiment, The Red Queen World, operating metaphors, organic conditions versus mechanistic machinations, the right and left brains, kinetic stability, Same Old Schools, teachers as rat terriers, and democratic compared to socialistic schooling will, hopefully, find a thoughtful resonance—or even a thoughtful dissonance—in the minds of readers.

Words can be the bars that enslave us—or the chisels that break through the mindsets that hold us back. The educational world does not need any more programs of reform; it needs **Conversations of Revision**—that, by "turning" the images this way and that, critically examine the words that currently define learning, teaching, and schooling—that presently shape and sometimes limit our potential.

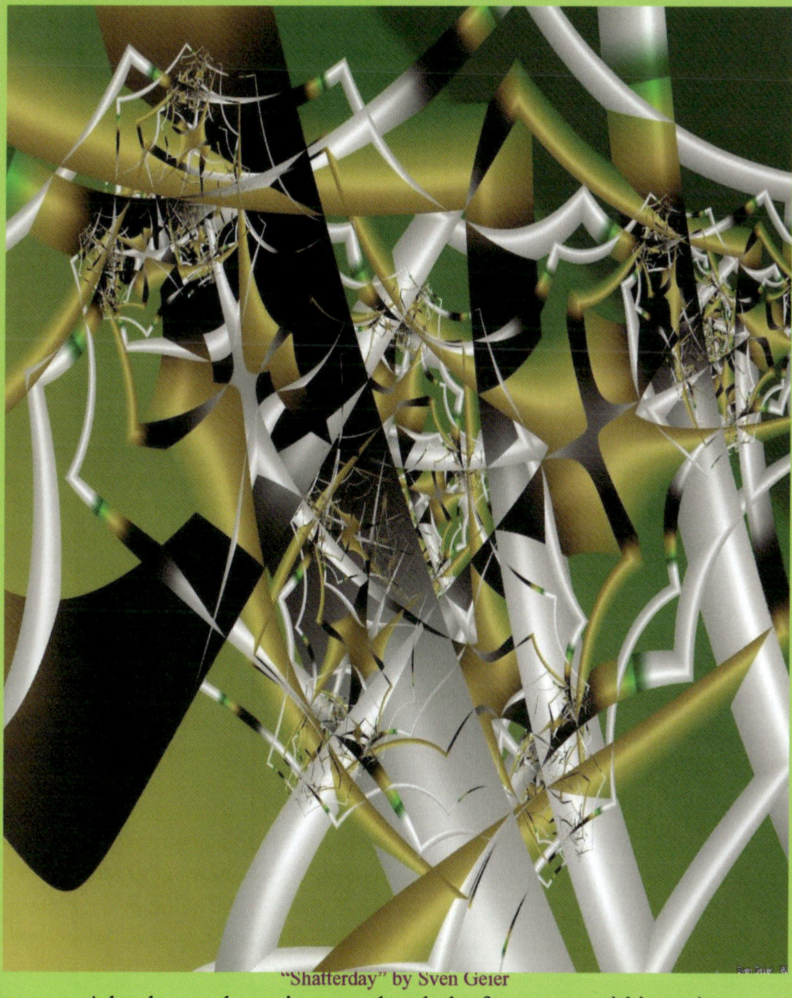

"Shatterday" by Sven Geier

A book must be an ice ax to break the frozen sea within us.*

Franz Kafka

*Or, at least, an attempt

–60–

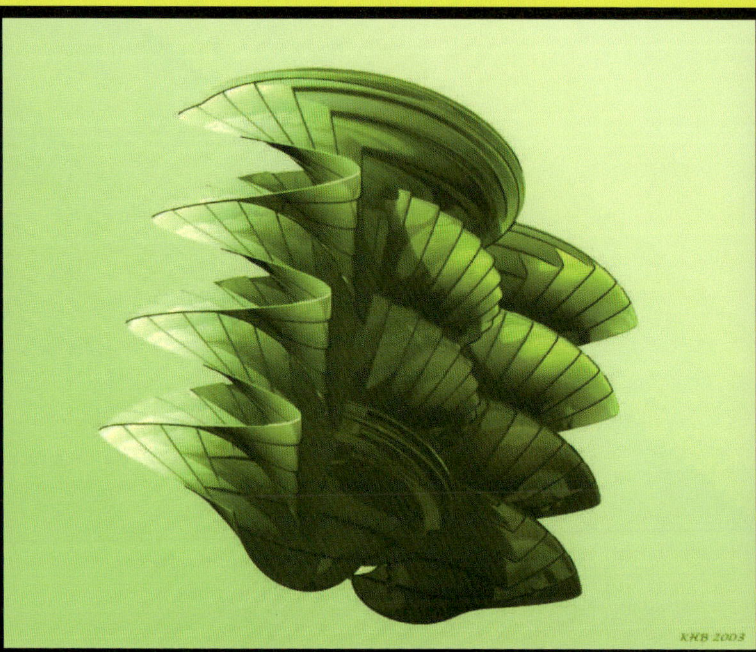

"Blooming Shell" by Panny Brawley

The world we have made as a result of the level of the thinking we have done thus far creates problems that we cannot solve at the same level of consciousness at which we have created them. . . . We shall require a substantially new level of thinking and learning if humankind is to survive.

Einstein

Our definition of learning is an integral component of our consciousness—and thus our awareness and capability. It governs how we go about the human specialty of learning. The present definition, the passive acquisition of easily measured knowledge bits, has caused many of our problems. Unless we redefine learning, we will not redefine our teaching and our schooling. We will therefore remain on our present path. We will stay within our present consciousness.

The question is whether that is acceptable. It should not be, if for no other reason than the socialistic metaphors guiding the delivery plans fail to align with our democratic values. The present definition of learning suppresses interest, intelligence, imagination, initiative, individuality, and, ultimately, our integrity. In its failure to encourage and inform our democratic faith, it degrades both our capability and responsibility as citizens.

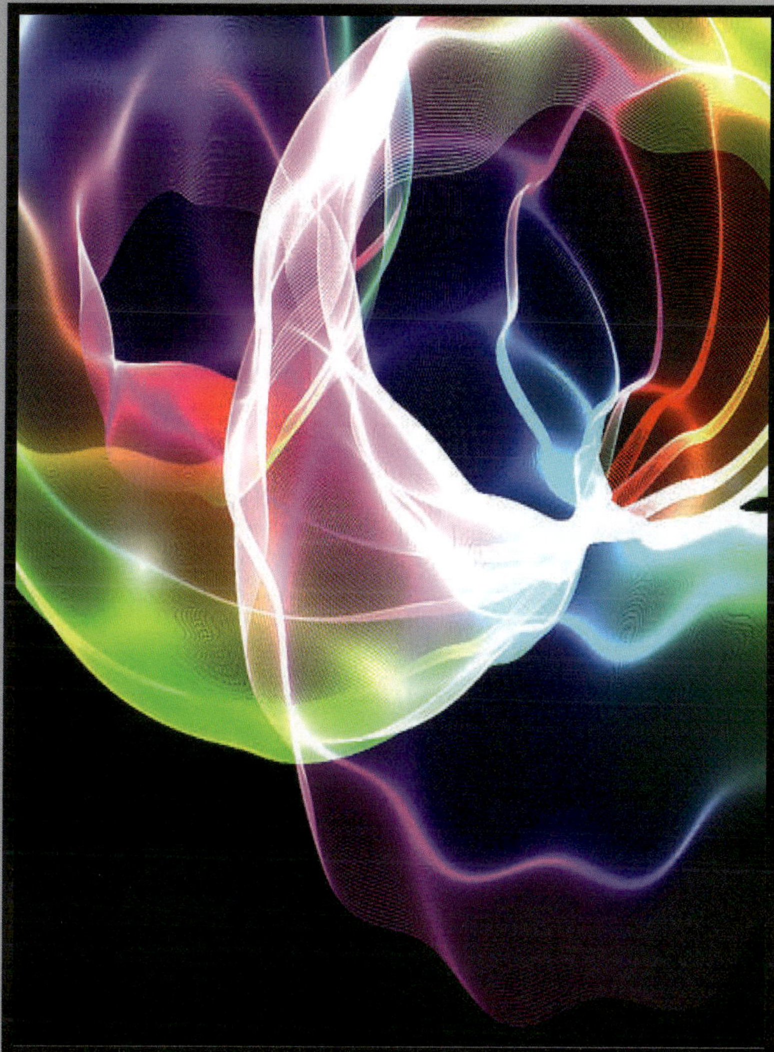

"The Birth of a Rainbow" from realeoni's photostream

Can we change our consciousness to where we can recognize and solve our problems? Can we change the images—the operating metaphors—that guide our behavior? Can we develop the kinetic stability necessary for these chaotic times? Can we incorporate the insights and understandings of neuroscience in order to establish and implement the organic image of learning in our schooling? Can we redefine learning, and thus teaching and schooling, and, in so doing, redefine ourselves?

Our future waits, impatiently, for our answer.

Learning is not compulsory—Neither is Survival.

Edward Deming

"Atropos" (cuts the thread of destiny) by Janet Parke

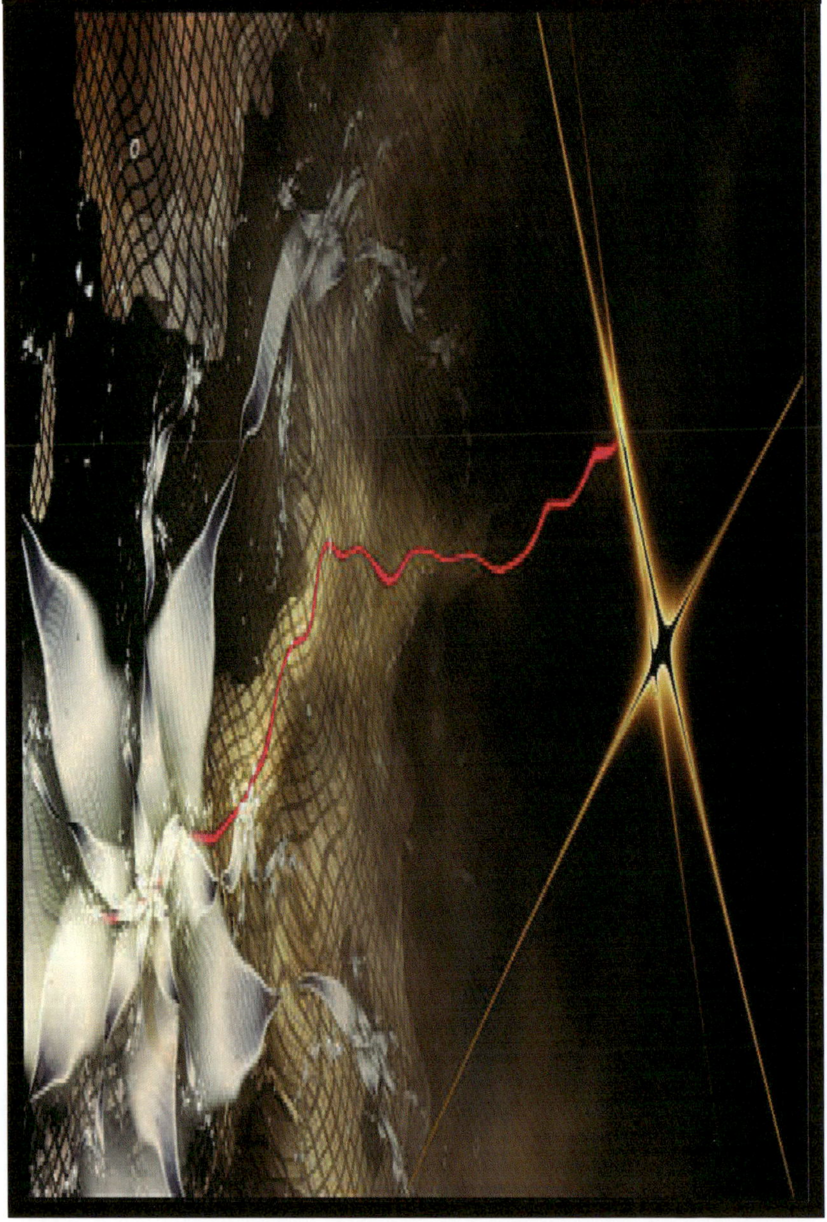

Acknowledgements

> In the matter of indebtedness of idea and motive I find that there are so many to whom I owe so much that I have the feeling of being only a nexus of the momentum of others' thoughts and despair of claiming anything herein to be original. I am like a coral animal who stands ready to take something from every passing tidal current, and I feel not only grateful but almost guilty for turning the wisdom, money, love, and time of others into so much rock, or, as the case may be, carbon dioxide.
>
> Paul Shepard

How do you acknowledge the contribution of everyone to the development of a book that has taken inspiration, guidance, and support from so many different sources? My mind grows dizzy from trying to track down everyone to whom I owe thanks. Shepard's thoughts neatly cut through that Gordian knot. When another's words are better than one can possibly create, it is best to use theirs.

Some individuals do stand out as particularly helpful, but many are lost in the confusion of ebbing and flowing tides. Thanks, first of all, to Serendipity (a goddess, in my definition), who has brought so many unexpected threads into my weaving, so many nutrients in the ever-changing passing tidal currents. Like a coral critter, I am more of an opportunist than a scholar, and opportunists are always striving to make treasures out of messes, and Serendipity loves to help make the messy connections that fuel excitement and growth.

A serendipitous conversation with a colleague informed me that the author bell hooks was at Berea College in Kentucky, only seventy-five miles down the road. Since her book, *Teaching to Transgress: Education as the Practice of Freedom*, was instrumental in my thinking, I sent her a copy of the unfolding manuscript. Wanting to meet her, I checked out the college website and found, to my delight, that she was speaking the following week. I showed up at the appropriate time at the proper venue, to find something entirely different going on. A woman came over to help out this obviously confused man. It turned out that I was a year too late; the website and I had miscommunicated. Frustrated, I walked downtown to look for a birthday card for my sister.

While shopping, my cell phone rang and bell hooks wanted to know when I was next going to be in Berea. Informing her that I happened to be in Berea at that very moment, bell and Serendipity invited me to come over to her house, only a few blocks away, and talk about the book, becoming the first of our many wonderful conversations. Sadly, we had to cut that initial conversation short, for bell had a friend coming over to work on a project. Her friend arrived, two hours later, calling out as she entered the back door, "Bell, this guy showed up to hear the talk you gave last year." It was the woman who had helped me out of my earlier confusion at the college. She did a double take when she saw me sitting with bell in the living room: "How did you get here?" The answer was, of course,

Serendipity. Bell has, in her writing and in personal conversations, inspired and informed me in a thousand ways.

Brenda Richardson, an innovative professor at Berea College, then contributed her inspiration to the momentum. In addition to her intellectual and aesthetic contributions, Brenda connected me with Bob Cornett. Bob is the kind of citizen every democracy needs, full of gumption, a responsible individual to the bone, with a wide-ranging imagination and intellect, dedicated to the spirit of initiative and responsibility, and committed to building community. He saw how the book fit in with his grass-roots democracy work and has been financially, intellectually, and spiritually very helpful.

Tashery Shannon brought her scholarship and creative writing ability to bear on helping me clean up some of the messiness and intellectual weakness in my writing. (She did not completely succeed, of course; some of my weaknesses are genetic while others are too dear to be seen clearly, much less dealt with—some of the flies in my eyes are pets.) Sheila Anderson realized that I lacked the necessary organization and detective skills and offered to help me track down the fractal artists and request permission for using their work. Without her assistance, I may have gone berserk. Conversations with Joe Blackbourn over the years have always stimulated the right side of my brain.

The generosity of the fractal artists has been amazing. Three deserve particular mention: Sven Geier, Ken Keller, and Judy Hart. I urge everyone to explore the fractal art world. The best way to do that is to google **fractal art contests** and dive in. A Michigan organization of home-schoolers gave early resonance and encouragement. Working with them on designing a learning environment called The Hatchery has been both fun and stimulating. Cindy Fadel deserves particular mention. Mindy Nathan has also helped enormously.

Others that deserve mention are Richard Farrell, Dave Garnet, Keith Crabtree, Ella and Claude Hensley, John Gould, Judy Paxton, Nancy Lyn McWhorter, James and Mary Pennell, Pat Greer, Mark and Diane Garrison, Liz Taylor, Sonya Boyd, Joyce Reid, Ed Councill, and Pat Bacon. The crew at Office Depot has helped tremendously—especially Justin Harper. Betsi Darden-Jones, who exemplifies Adrienne Rich's definition of friendship as refining the truths you can tell one another, offered constant support, helpful insights, and the occasional chiding. Don Jeffers took time out from beating me up on the tennis courts to offer unexpected and very generous support for my writing efforts.

These individuals and numerous others lost to poor memory and disorganization deserve credit for helping me produce anything of substance—the rock, so to speak. The carbon dioxide is my own.

Dennis R. Rader
Frankfort, Kentucky
April, 2010

About the Author

Dr. Rader is an experienced teacher at all levels. He has also worked as an educational therapist, an assistant editor for a series of textbooks with Alvin Toffler, author of *Future Shock*, and the emotional intelligence coach for a university football team. He is an experienced speaker and storyteller. His most recent work is as a consultant for the design of a learning center, The Hatchery, for a large organization of home-schoolers in Michigan, supported by the Kellogg Foundation. He wrote the first doctoral dissertation on personal integrity in the United States. From a non-academic, low-income background in east Tennessee, he was never expected to attend college much less achieve a higher degree. As writer, teacher, and speaker he is dedicated to helping people build bridges across the personal and cultural barriers that stifle potential. The combination of his Appalachian heritage, "rising above his raisin's," and interest in the relationship between the educational process and the development of personal integrity led him to co-found , with Bob Cornett, The Gumption Community, a gathering of people dedicated to the task of revitalizing the concept of gumption in our language and the perception of "gumption traps." America used to be a community alive with the unspoken motto: GUMPTION GROWN HERE. It can be again, revitalized by a resurgence of individual initiative and responsibility—the very foundation of the democratic spirit.

More about The Gumption Community can be found by visiting its website at www.TheGumptionCommunity.com. More about Dr. Rader's work can be found at www.Learning-Redefined.com. The best way to reach him is through Hogsonice@yahoo.com

Building Democracy Press

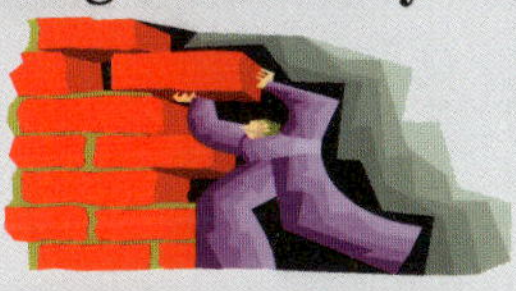

The consortium of individuals supporting Building Democracy Press results from the concern that we are losing the imagination, initiative, and integrity necessary to maintain and nourish the democratic spirit. *Learning Redefined* is part of that community of effort. The consortium is comprised of individuals from various backgrounds in Kentucky, Michigan, Tennessee, and Mississippi. Building Democracy Press is an arm of The Gumption Community. It is looking for those who wish to contribute—in any way—to a resurgence of the democratic spirit.

Democracy has to be born anew in each generation—and education is its midwife.

John Dewey

LaVergne, TN USA
12 August 2010
192976LV00001B